Veronica's Diary IV

Angels Among Us

1994–1996

Veronica Esagui, DC

PAPYRUS
PRESS, LLC

Oregon, USA

Library of Congress Control Number: 2014953763
ISBN 9780982648445

First Edition
Veronica Esagui, DC

Illustrations: Derrick Freeland
Book Cover/Graphic Designer: Jean Sheldon

PAPYRUS
PRESS, LLC

21860 Willamette Drive, West Linn, OR 97068

To order additional copies of this book
www.veronicaesagui.net

Printed in the United States of America

To my teacher, R.H. Sheldon,

and the women that have been
a significant part of my life's journey
in the last thirty-five years,

Vicki Duke, Jean Sheldon, Nancy McDonald,
Genene Valleau, Karen Sorbel, Linda Becker,
Amalie J. Hill, Alice Lynn, Julie Wickman,
Erica Haugen, Fay Zealand, Terri Flannigan,
Barbara Schiavonne and Dr. Clari Faerman

Author's notes

The people and the stories portrayed in this book are all true as to my recollection but I have changed the names of some individuals to protect their privacy.

By disregarding our inner wisdom,
we can become our worst enemies.

—Veronica Esagui, DC

Contents

Illustrations

Photos

~ Chapter One ~

The Trip to New Jersey

Spring of 1994

What an experience, traveling by train from Atlanta, Georgia to Newark, New Jersey!

The conductor had assured me that once the train began moving, the air conditioner would kick on, but that never happened. A hot, moist blanket of air swallowed my small compartment, and left me barely able to breathe. I stripped off my clothes and lay on the bottom bunk as still as a corpse.

For an hour I refused to move, taking slow shallow breaths. Passengers stood in the hallway, outside my compartment. They complained about the heat, their voices as thick and sticky as the air. Obviously, that whole section of the train I stayed in had some kind of electrical malfunction.

I eased off the bunk bed and slipped on my green silk pajama top. Without my bottoms, it would give me the grand look of someone who was suffering from heat exhaustion. I opened the door and stepped into the hallway. A cloud of hot steamy air assaulted my lungs. When the conductor saw me, he yelled that I was not decently dressed and should get back into my cabin.

I pulled out my natural talent for Portuguese melodrama. "I'm two months pregnant! I can't breathe in my cabin, and I'm scared that I'll have a miscarriage if I spend the night in there. I need to move into a cabin, with air conditioning. Can you help me?" I pleaded at the conductor.

My façade of despair was worthy of an academy award.

The conductor's face softened and he said if I got dressed he would find me a cool place for the night. I returned to my cabin and slipped into my jeans and T-shirt and followed him under the assumption that he was taking me to another private compartment. I was very disappointed when he pointed to three seats in the back of the train, with a heavyset woman sitting in the window seat. "Sorry, but this is the best that I can do for you. This part of the train is cooler and you should be fine. Have a good night." He walked away.

The woman slept with her head resting on a rolled up sweater against the glass window. I could lie across two seats. There weren't any sounds coming from the passengers except for the woman by the window, snoring up a storm. The soft amber lighting throughout the car was conducive to sleeping and I laid down in a tight fetal position, making sure that my feet didn't stick out into the aisle. The sharp edges in-between both seats were digging into my ribs but if I were going to get any rest my sleeping arrangements would have to do. I closed my eyes and concentrated on the soothing hum of the wheels rolling on the tracks while being rocked by the train's swaying motion. I had just dozed off when I woke up to the sudden jilting sound of screeching brakes as the train came to a stop. Soon afterwards I heard the bustle and hustle of passengers leaving the train and others getting on board. I used that opportunity to get up, stretch and switch sides, hoping that someone wouldn't bump into my head now resting on the aisle seat. Then the inevitable happened. An older man, holding a train ticket, tapped on my shoulder, and asked me courteously to get up and give him the aisle seat.

Mr. Rogers was on his way to New Jersey, to visit his son and daughter-in-law. He was a 68 years old widow, who worked for forty-five years as a barber and was looking forward to retirement. He was glad to sit next to me because I reminded him of Doris, his first wife. She was also the quiet type, but a wonderful woman who had bared him five wonderful children. Being a barber for so many years it was ironic that he had lost most of his hair, not that he would have gone to one of those new modern, so-called hair stylists. The art of cutting a man's hair was a thing of the past just like the old horse and buggy days, he added. I was trapped between a snoring ogre and Mr. Rogers's constant yakking. I closed my eyes, crossed my arms, and put my head back as if I was ready to sleep. But he didn't get the hint.

I held out to one o'clock, and then excused myself to go to the bathroom. I went directly to my cabin to quietly die in there. Laying my face close to the window, I felt fortunate for the little air I could get and thanked God for my situation. I could have been in a train with hundreds of others on the way to a concentration camp. I cried thinking about those who had died from suffocation. Finally, the cool night air made its way into my cabin, and I fell asleep.

My ex-husband, Al, my daughter-in-law, Diane, and her baby, Jacob—my first grandson—who I had never met, were waiting at the Newark train station. My son, Steve, couldn't be there, he had to stay at his music store, which—according to Diane, his wife—was doing quite well. It didn't surprise me. Steve has a natural talent for dealing with customers.

While we were walking to the car, Al tried to hold my hand, as if we were still married. I understand how he feels given that we were married close to thirty years, but we have been divorced for two years now. I took my hand away.

"We're no longer married." I said.

"Ronnie, you are still my sweetheart."

"Please don't call me Ronnie. My name is Veronica."

"To me, you'll always be my Ronnie." He lovingly perked up his lips and blew me two kisses.

Diane handed Jacob to me. I was holding him in my arms for the very first time and I didn't let go of him until we got into the car. Jacob was only six months old but I could see a close family resemblance to Ralph, Steve's brother. Jacob kept smiling at me and it is my opinion as a grandmother that he is the most beautiful baby I have ever seen. I was looking forward to baby-sit for him as much as possible.

Al drove us directly to his apartment, saying he had made lunch for us.

His driving had not changed. If anything, it had gotten worse. Besides zigzagging between two lanes, and tailgating, he was still not using the directions lights.

When we got divorced two years ago I told Al that he could keep the apartment and all the contents since I was the one that asked for a divorce. The stale air inside the apartment reminded me that he was still keeping the shades down and the windows closed all year round. The small lamp over the dining room table wasn't enough to light up the room and the annexed living room space. I felt like I had stepped into a dungeon.

He had prepared a feast of cold cuts, potato and macaroni salad, pickles and all the extra condiments needed to make sandwiches. A large sushi platter stood in the center of the table. I was very touched by his efforts. He's the father of both my sons, and I can never say that he ever did anything to hurt me; if anything, he always gave me the freedom to do whatever I wanted. Some people might classify me as greedy. After nearly thirty years of marriage I still wanted more. Yes, I enjoy affection and acts of kindness, which, Al always provided, but our marriage lacked the mental and physical stimuli, I consider a vital part of any relationship.

One thing about Al that used to bug me—and does to this day—is that he says exactly what's on his mind without regard for anyone's feelings. I was in the kitchen putting the dishes in the dishwasher and Diane sat in the living room entertaining Jacob.

"Ronnie, you'll be sorry if you stay with Steve and Diane. She can't cook, and they never have any food at home. Stay here. You can sleep in my bed and I'll sleep on the sofa." Al tends to talk loud even when he whispers and I was worried that she could hear him.

"Thanks. But I already promised to stay with them." I was doing my best not to hurt his feelings and I was glad when he finally gave up trying to persuade me. If I had to stay with Al, I would surely have taken the next train back to Georgia.

He showed us around his apartment. He had redecorated it with new furnishings but had kept the old wall-to-wall bar now filled with dozens of ceramic Asian figurines. Then we entered the bedroom. A large framed picture of me when I was fifteen years old hung over his bed. I told him that we needed to talk, alone, and he said he would pick me up for lunch the next day.

When Diane and I were about to leave with Jacob I noticed a framed poster of a flying eagle hung above the sofa.

"That's new," I said.

"It reminds me of you, always reaching higher. It has inspired me greatly. I've joined the Air Force as a volunteer and have gotten into detective work and bounty hunting. It's something I always wanted to do. Before you leave, let me show you my latest collection of uniforms."

He proudly showed us his coat closet full of uniforms. Then he turned on three spotlights aimed at the living room wall, which until then had been obscured. A dozen plaques and awards glistened in the light advertising his work as an Air Force volunteer. I was happy to see that he was doing something he enjoyed. During our marriage he had no hobbies or interests of any kind.

It was wonderful to see Steve again. Except for a little weight around the waist he had not changed much. He was still flamboyant and full of energy. He ran towards me and did his usual welcome greeting. He lifted me up in the air, and spun me around. Then he tried a new karate move on me, but when he lifted his leg in my direction, I grabbed his foot and didn't let go. He was impressed with my quick response. "Mom, you still got what it takes."

After Diane put Jacob to sleep in his crib, we sat for dinner. Diane prepared Steve's favorite, broiled chicken and a Caesar salad and then we sat in the living room talking. He hoped to be as good a father as I had been a mother to him. I told him he already was.

Diane worked full time. Every morning she left at five and didn't come home until five in the afternoon. I don't know how she managed that and still took care of Jacob, and Steve who was very demanding about his needs. No wonder she had no time to cook.

The next day, Al came by and took me to his favorite German restaurant. A few years before, I had found a cockroach in their asparagus soup. This time, I played it safe. I ordered a salad and half a sandwich.

He laughed. "You keep that going. You'll turn into a rabbit."

He was still making the same comments he had when we were married, and I took his remark as an encouragement to discuss our divorce. He wasn't listening. He waved his hands in the air. "Yeah, yeah, don't worry. I know we're divorced, but I still love you."

"Al, please listen. You have no monetary obligations towards me anymore. I'm doing well on my own." He was well aware that I had a full scholarship and extra money coming in from financial aid. "I keep telling you not to send me money." I pull an envelope out of my purse and hand it to him across the table. "This belongs to you."

"No, it's yours. I don't want it." He pushed the envelope back to me.

"Al, it's *your* money. You are not rich. You work for a living. I asked for the divorce, not you. This money belongs to you." I pushed the envelope back to him.

The envelope went back and forth until I said, "Okay, if you don't want it, I'll leave it as a tip."

"All right. All right! How about, if you keep it and I'll promise not to send anymore?"

"Deal." I shook his hand.

Steve took me to see his new music store in Howell. It was right across from the one that Al and I used to own, before we went bankrupt. He kept the name of our store, Howell Music Center, for two reasons. Mr. Crocker, the owner of the music store in Freehold, where I used to teach guitar, banjo, and bass prior to opening the music store with Al had told me that whenever you open a business, the name of the town is a very powerful tool towards its success. I had passed that tidbit of information to Steve. The other reason was that the name, Howell Music Center was well established in the community and that was a plus for keeping the old customers.

Considering that the store was a quarter of the size we used to have, I was flabbergasted with what Steve had done. He had built three rooms in the back for private teaching and a luncheonette with a small counter up front, where the younger crowd could buy drinks and food. He had installed wall to all mirrors behind the baby grands with a crystal chandelier hanging from the center of the ceiling and organized two rows of acoustic and electric guitars, banjos, and bass guitars along the walls, producing an outstanding display of string instruments. He had layered several wood platforms and stocked them with full drum sets, cellos and upright basses. The music store reminded me of Aladdin's treasure cave, the way everything glittered while wrapping its arms around me.

What Steve lacked in a business degree he made up with his creative insight. I watched him as he took care of customers. No one left without buying an instrument and or signing up for music lessons with one of his teaching staff.

Diane was a petite perky young woman with a natural spunk for life, except for when she came home at the end of the day. She would collapse in the living room couch with her arms lying to the sides and her legs open and stretched out.

She wore her blonde hair shorter on one side, and I believed that the reason it looked good on her was because she had beautiful features. She smiled all the time and even when she didn't say anything her eyes did. Jacob was a lot like her in that aspect.

I took Diane to work one morning so that I could have her car for the day, and a much needed heart-to-heart talk.

"I want to apologize for having been so reserved when you and Steve were dating. He used to date so many women that I preferred not to get involved."

"I know, Mom. He used to be a playboy, when I met him." She responded along with a few light giggles.

"Calling me Mom is very sweet of you when you already have a mom. I've always wanted to have a daughter, so thank you."

Her eyes smiled back at me.

"I could not have asked for anyone better than you to come into Steve's life. And now that you are Jacob's mother, I can say without holding my feelings back that I love you."

She giggled once again and said, "I love you too! And I'm glad that you were able to visit us."

Before she got out of the car I told her that if for any reason anything went wrong between her and Steve, she could move in with me. I wanted her to know that she had a friend for life.

I couldn't take a trip to New Jersey and not visit my two best friends Tracey and Francis. Tracy was my fun friend. She always enjoyed telling a dirty joke and she was my partner for most of the years I owned The Simy Dinner Theater, in Howell. We sat at her kitchen table having her famous spaghetti with homemade meatballs and tomato sauce. Once again, she told me I was wrong for leaving Al.

"He's a real sweetheart, and any woman lucky enough to have him as a husband should be kissing the ground he walks on."

She was entitled to her own opinion but I wondered if she weren't being a bit too personal about her feelings towards him.

In the evening I met with Francis at the diner across from the Kobe Japanese Restaurant. I made sure that I went to the restaurant before meeting with her and said hello to Mr. and Mrs. Ounuma, the restaurant owners. We reminisced about the Simy Dinner Theater I had founded ten years ago in their upstairs conference room. The theater was still going, but the current productions were attracting a different kind of clientele.

"They are cheap people, they only come for play and don't want to buy dinner," complained Mr. Ounuma.

"We miss you. Stay for dinner with us?" Mrs. Ounuma asked.

I promised them to come back the next day since I was meeting Francis, that evening.

Francis and I had met seven years prior when she came to the Howell Music Center to buy strings for her daughter's violin. We became friends, and later, we worked together as members of the Howell Cultural Arts Committee. Francis was the kind of friend that I could trust, with my most intimate secrets. Francis and her husband had bought a house in Newark, for the sole purpose of providing a place where children with AIDS could live and get the care they deserved.

I told her about my new life as a student at Life Chiropractic College and how happy I was that someday I would be like her, useful to others.

The very sad part of my trip was seeing my old friend Rosanna. I called to let her know I was in town. When she picked me up for lunch, what I saw was not my old friend Rosanna, but an odd, strange version of what she used to be. Jacob was playing on the living room floor, and when he saw her, he started to cry. They say children in their innocence can tell when someone has gone mad, and now I believed it.

On the way to a seafood restaurant in Belmar, no matter what I said to Rosanna there was little or no response. I took it that at her age she wanted to pay better attention to her driving. At the restaurant, she snatched the menu from my hands and insisted on ordering lobsters for both of us.

"Please tell the cook not to remove the tomalley from inside my lobster." She told the waiter, and then yelled, "Stop staring at me! Just tell the cook and he'll know what I mean."

"The green stuff, hum? Are you sure? That's the… the…. the lobster digestive system." He said, with a disgusted look on his face.

"You may call it crap, if you like, but that's what I want."

"And you, miss, do you also want your tomalley?" The waiter asked me with a distinct attitude in his voice.

"Yes, I do." I turned to Rosanna. "You can have it."

"You don't have to do me any favors, but I'll take it."

When I asked her how she was doing, her answer was, "What do you care?"

I told her one of my funniest experiences at college. Her reaction was barely a contorted smile followed by a deep sigh. We finished our main course in silence.

Then she ordered our favorite dessert, chocolate mousse. I told her that I wouldn't eat it until she told me what bothered her.

"You know very well what you've done to me." She answered.

I pushed the dessert plate away. She finished eating hers in silence.

"No reason to let it go to waste." She grabbed my dessert.

I would have liked to get up and leave, but depended on her to drive me home. I remained quiet, glancing at her every so often.

"You missed out on the dessert." She wiped her mouth with her napkin.

I pointed to my left side of the face where she had missed a chocolate smudge.

"I'll never forgive you for not meeting me in Florida, like you promised me."

"Rosanna, I had just gotten a divorce from Al. Those two weeks that I had as a school break were the only time available to find out if my new relationship was going to work out. I would have understood if you had been in my situation. I would have been happy for you."

"You abandoned me when you made "him" your priority in life." She began putting her lipstick on.

"When I told you on the phone that I couldn't meet you in Florida you said you understood. I believed you."

"When you abandoned me I was deeply hurt, but I didn't want you to know it."

"Here you go again using the same word. You make it sound like I deserted you. I'm still your friend. I will always be your friend through thick and thin. You know that."

"No matter what you say, nothing is going to make me trust you again." She stood.

"I'm sorry that I hurt you in any way. That was not my intention and I feel really bad."

She grabbed my credit card from the check holder and tossed it back at me. "Keep your money. I don't need your help."

Rosanna had turned into a mean, angry person. She drove me home. Before I got out of the car I tried to hug her, but she stiffened up and pushed me away, saying despondently, "It's not necessary."

"Why did you invite me for lunch, if you hate me so much?"

"I want you to know how much you're missing without my friendship."

Oh my goodness, she had gone nuts! She had gone over the edge, but I couldn't bring myself to tell her, even though we had made a promise a few years back that we would warn each other if one of us were to lose our mind. I held my tears, till I was inside the apartment. My stomach tightened into spasms. I ran to the bathroom and vomited everything I'd eaten.

Diane worked in the blood lab at the old Fitkins Hospital, but her dream was to become a medical doctor. I took her shopping at the mall and bought us identical wristwatches with a picture of Bugs Bunny holding a carrot and the words, "What's up, Doc?"

I felt that the wristwatches were a very appropriate gift for us to share, given that someday I would be a chiropractor and she would be a medical doctor.

I devoted the last two days to Jacob. He loved it when I lay with my back on the floor, put him over my knees and lifted him up in the air. I have never seen such a happy baby, and so easy to please. Steve was right, about Jacob being thankful when he got his diapers changed. His smiles were broader. I regretted that by being in school so far away, I was missing an important part of my life, the joy of being a grandmother.

~ *Chapter Two* ~

Back to School

March 29

The train trip back to Georgia went well, except for the inside latch on my cabin door being broken and anyone could have walked in during the night. The air conditioner worked and the railroad company apologized for my miserable trip up to New Jersey. As a token of goodwill, they were going to send me a complimentary round-trip ticket to use any time within a year.

Leila, my classmate and friend, picked me up at the Atlanta train station and took me to a Korean restaurant for lunch in Smyrna, where we live. For the incredible price of $2.95, we each received a plate of fresh thinly sliced meat to cook ourselves over a small broiler in the center of our table. The meal also included rice and an exotic array of six mini dishes with very hot-and-spicy pickled Korean delicacies. Leila had discovered this restaurant the previous quarter and had been eating there about three times a week because it was cheaper than bringing lunch to school or buying food in the cafeteria. Besides, she loved the food and believed it was fresh and very nutritious.

When I got into my apartment, the phone rang. It was Robert, a chiropractic student one quarter behind me. I had met him just before I left for New Jersey, when he had borrowed my notes. He wanted to know if I would go with him to the movies that afternoon. My heart was beating faster. I told him I looked forward to seeing him again, but had to be home no later than seven. I was waiting for a call from Stewart, my soon-to-be roommate, from New York. I had promised to pick him up that evening at the Atlanta Airport.

At two in the afternoon, Robert knocked at the front door of my apartment. We hugged each other as is customary between students, and once again I had to force myself to let him go.

We went to see *The Fugitive,* and he held my hand. That was a good sign. To me, it meant Robert was normal. My last boyfriend, Dexter, would never hold my hand or show any type of affection outside the bedroom. I hated Dexter for not being complete. I hated Michael for not fighting for me and Al too for loving me but being incapable of making me happy.

After the movie, Robert and I returned to my apartment, where I learned that Robert had been an aspiring musician before he started chiropractic college. He played one of his original compositions on my electric keyboard, and I showed off by playing *Romance Antigua* on my classical guitar and then the Beverly Hillbillies theme song on my five-string banjo. When we ran out of music to play, we sat on the Asian couch and looked at each other in silence.

Robert was a young black man, with the most beautiful green eyes I had ever seen. I didn't feel the need to tell him that I was fifteen years older than he was. He already had told me before I left to New Jersey that he was divorced and had two children. That made him old enough for me. We had nothing to talk about, and our only form of communication was lust for each other. We hugged, caressed and kissed each other. He moaned in my ear and I responded by taking his breath into my lungs to utter the sound of my own hunger. The fire in his eyes promised me a tale of infinite pleasure. I wanted to remain in his arms at whatever price it might cost me. I had to go along with the next step—or, as they say in dating, to second and third base—if I was going to remain in his arms for the rest of day. I hungered for the intimacy, the nurturing of being close—something Dexter could not provide. I was ready when he carried me like a bride over the threshold to my bedroom. He set me on my bed as though I had a stamp on my forehead, "Handle with care."

He studied me while he slowly removed his jacket and laid it in the back of the chair and then just as slow he took his tie off. He reminded me of a male version of a stripper, when he unbuttoned his white starched shirt and smiled at me before taking it off. I smiled back in anticipation and proceeded to take my t-shirt by pulling it over my head and then tossing it towards the chair. We were both taken aback when it landed on the silk maroon flowers and tipped over its crystal vase, which miraculously remained on the tabletop. We smiled. I combed my fingers through my hair. He took off his shoes and socks. I kicked off my sandals and let them fall on the floor. He peeled off his pants and underwear. I wiggled out of my tight jeans and pulled my bra and panties. He stood naked before me. Chocolate came to my mind, dark, smooth, luscious chocolate.

The light seeped through the bedroom window shade and spread a golden glow across his toned dark body, with every swollen muscle appropriately displayed. He looked like Michelangelo's David, only glimmering black.

Robert turned the bedroom light on. I reached for the bed sheet to cover myself. His mellow voice like that of a finely tuned sax protruded my senses. "I want to look at you when we make love." He pulled the bed sheet away.

During the next hour, we had sex three times. So much for the myth that a man needs half-hour to re-charge. What bothered me was that he thanked me after each time he penetrated me. I felt like a saloon girl entertaining a polite cowboy at some whorehouse on the prairie.

He was content for his personal reasons, and so was I. The best part being in his arms that way. Tears filled my eyes, and

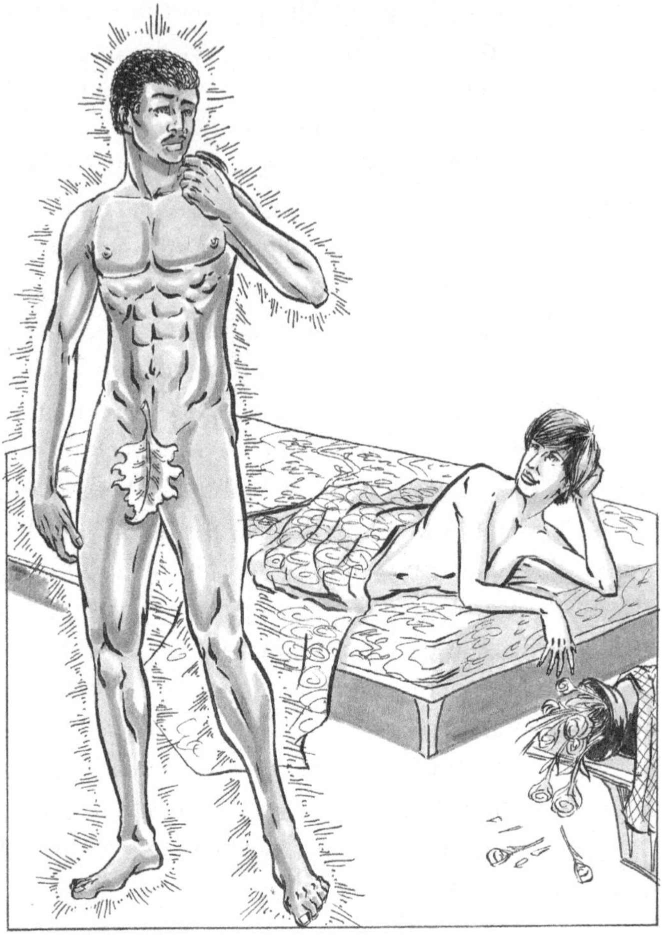

The Masterpiece

I finally understood what someone had told me many years before, that she had sex in order to be held.

Robert asked me why I was crying. “You make me happy,” I said.

We remained that way for a while longer, not letting go of the joy of our interlocked bodies.

It was eight o’clock in the evening. Stewart would be calling me soon to pick him up from the airport.

Before Robert left, he gave me his African wrist bracelet. "This is a token of my love. I hope you'll wear it." He whispered in my ear, "I love you."

I slipped the bracelet onto my wrist but felt overwhelmed by his declaration of love.

"It's a nice bracelet. Thank you." I was not sure of what else to say.

When he left, I took the bracelet off and put it away in my jewelry box. I didn't even know his last name. We had sex that was all. It had nothing to do with love.

Maybe I was wrong for feeling this way, but I felt ashamed for not waiting a few more dates before jumping into bed. Just because he was a student like me didn't make him anything less of a stranger. I couldn't believe I once again had unprotected sex.

AIDS, Veronica. Wake up! This was not a joking matter. I must have been out of my mind! But so what? I caught AIDS, big deal. It was too late now and it did me no good to cry over spilled milk. *But I love life. So, what's the matter with me? Am I suicidal?*

I missed Michael. He was the first man I ever loved and even though many years had gone by since we said goodbye, whenever I felt sad or lonely, thinking of him comforted me. I knew these were crazy thoughts but sometimes I believed I couldn't survive my life without him. *No, I will not allow dark negative thoughts to take over my life.*

There was a storm warning in effect. I called the airport. Stewart's plane was going to be late.

I lay on my bed and waited for the phone to ring.

Stewart showed up at the apartment at one in the morning with a large backpack and a sleeping bag. I didn't expect him to be so young; but he had a clean shaved look and his clothes spoke of coming from a well-to-do family. His belongings were being delivered at the end of the week.

I gave him the key to our apartment and he gave me one month's rent.

"Feel free to decorate your room and bathroom as you like it." I told him.

"Yow, your accent sounds familiar," he said with a New York accent.

"It should. I lived in New Jersey for almost thirty years." I couldn't help yawning.

"Na, there's something else in there."

"Oh yeah, I forgot. I was born in Portugal. I was eighteen when I came to America in 1962, but I never lost the accent."

"You can't be that old."

"Right, and I'll look even younger after I get some sleep. Goodnight."

We both laughed and I went back to my bedroom and closed the door.

The staff at Life Chiropractic College did a great job at passing the word out to new students that were looking for rooms to rent.

April 7

Classes started last week at full steam. I have been busy settling into the school curriculum and have not had a chance to do much writing. We seem to have better teachers this quarter or at least the subjects are a lot more enticing. Time will tell. My favorite is the Toggle Adjusting Technique class I have so impatiently been waiting for.

I passed my first quarter class notes to Stewart. Meanwhile, Robert and I are planning our second date, at his apartment, for the coming Saturday night.

April 8

Ralph called. His trip to Oregon turned out to be a traumatic and expensive experience. He did well from Georgia to New Jersey but from New Jersey to Oregon, he had to replace the transmission on his new Plymouth Duster three times. The dealer had told him the car was fine to pull the small storage trailer with all his belongings. He arrived at Western States Chiropractic College on the first morning of classes. He left his car and trailer with his belongings in the school parking lot and attended his first class.

Sometimes I felt like I should have gone with him as he asked. He's my son and my best friend, but I had a free scholarship, and I liked it here in Smyrna. I felt comfortable in this school environment. I knew what to expect. Besides, Oregon didn't sound appealing to me. I had heard that it rained every day.

I caught a cold on Friday, and by Saturday morning felt pretty miserable. I called Robert to tell him. He said he wasn't worried about catching my cold. He believed in the chiropractic philosophy that with regular chiropractic adjustments his immune system was infallible. I let the subject drop. In this school there were too many fanatical teachers and students who believed that spinal adjustments guarded against all illnesses.

I lay in bed thinking about Robert and decided to conduct an experiment. I put on my tightest blue jeans and my Boy Scout uniform shirt, which had been a prop for one of the plays I produced years earlier. As a final touch, I added a belt with a large buckle. It represented my chastity belt. The belt wouldn't come off unless I believed without a doubt that we had something more meaningful than sex between us.

When I got to Robert's apartment, he enveloped me in his arms and began kissing me on the neck like a suckling vampire. He said a woman in uniform turned him on, and he tried to open my shirt. I pulled myself away from him.

"Sorry, but I really don't feel good." A whiff of his cucumber salad scented cologne caused me to sneeze repeatedly. I blew my nose. My eyes filled with tears as I coughed green phlegm into a Kleenex tissue I took out of my pocket. How could anyone be turned on by this?

"Would you like to see my music room?" He grabbed my hand and led me into a small room that was bare except for a full size keyboard on a stand, a bench, a standing lamp next to it and a few piles of music books on the floor. He asked me to sit on the bench with him while he played and sang one of his original tunes. His voice was sweet, mellow like honey dripping, but the speed of the tune and the repeated words of, *here you come, baby,* over and over again, was too much for me to endure. I felt like I was going to keel over. The thought that he might want to do that for hours scared me. I was too sick to withstand the ordeal.

A friend in New Jersey once told me, that when artists ask for your opinion and you don't want to offend them, just say, "It's very interesting."

That advice came in handy when Robert upon finishing, turned and kissed me very sweetly on the lips. "Nice, hum? Did you like it?"

"It's very interesting." I assumed he meant the song.

"Everyone that has heard me play this tune has told me the same. Would you like to hear another?" He put his arm around my shoulder and gave me a squeeze.

"Is it as good as this one?" I asked, my voice cracking up.

"Absolutely. Just listen."

"Baby, baby, baby, baby, baby, baby," he crooned the words out emphasizing the *b's*. Just as I rolled my eyes up to the ceiling asking for some divine intervention he changed the lyrics to repeating the word *now* while emphasizing the *ow's*. Same tune different words? I couldn't tell the difference. My head was too heavy to hold up on its own and I dropped it on his shoulder.

"What do you think? Really good, hum?" He asked after hammering down the last chord.

I was on automatic pilot. "It's very interesting." I emphasized the *V,* while seating up straight like a good German soldier.

He put his arms around my waist and nibbled at my ear. Then he reached for my belt buckle.

I pushed him firmly away. "How about we talk? I'd like to know more about you." I stood.

He said nothing for a moment, only stared, and then grabbed my hand. "Would you like to see my wardrobe?"

"Sure," I said. Hardly my idea of getting to know someone.

He led me to his bedroom and opened the wall-to-wall closet. I had a feeling of déjà vu,—Al showing me his closet full of uniforms.

His suits took half of the left side of the closet, and on the right hung a variety of long colorful robes called djellabas, I'd seen Muslim men wear in North Africa.

"Wow, Robert, you could open a couple of clothing stores—one here and one in Morocco!"

"I enjoy spending money on clothes." It didn't surprise me.

"Which side do you prefer? The suits or the djellabas?"

"They are gorgeous!" I pointed to the right side of the closet.

"Which is your favorite?" He began pulling out one robe at a time. He held a robe in front of himself, took a pause, and waited for me to wave my hand to put it away. I felt like I was back in Tangier, Morocco looking at carpets. I picked the creamy yellow one with the dark brown embroidery.

"That's my favorite too," he said.

We hugged. We touched. We kissed. He maneuvered me inch-by-inch towards his bed.

"Let me make love to you. It will help you with your cold." His voice sounded deeper, warmer, and sexier than ever.

I had no doubt it would help me. I'm a strong believer that sex can heal just about any sickness out there, but I wasn't there to be treated.

"I want to talk. I don't even know your last name or where were you born. What are the names of your children?"

He shot out the names of his children, then lamented about his marriage. He wrapped up the questionnaire by saying, "Would you like to watch TV?" He didn't care if I wanted to watch television. He led me back to the living room, turned on the TV, and eased me into the couch, where we sat holding hands. A few minutes later, he draped his arm over my shoulders—the biggest mistake he could have made. I again thought of Al.

Al's old favorite cops/robbers TV series was on. Robert hummed along with the theme song after he turned it up. Al never hummed along, but like Robert, he always listened to TV at full blast. I began coughing. I was sure that I had a fever.

"You should go to the school's clinic tomorrow and get your spine adjusted. Your cold will be gone, just like that." He snapped his fingers.

I rubbed my sinus steadily. His cucumber cologne was getting the best of me. Al used to wash himself on a daily basis with cologne. Just one of the many reasons I had asked for a divorce.

The phone rang. He lowered the sound, stood, and slipped into the kitchen. I could tell he was talking to a female on the other end. The perfect time to get out of there had arrived.

I waved goodbye and said, "I'll see you in school."

I was not going to settle for any man just so that I could get hugs. The man of my dreams would offer me his complete love and devotion—like Al did—and he would be honest, creative and idealistic—like Michael used to be—and he would have

Dexter's intellect, and Robert's sexual endowments. And I wanted a man who was intelligent, adventurous, sensitive, and willing to travel and dare the impossible. Now my wish list was complete.

Robert called me in the middle of the week. I told him that I had a new boyfriend and we couldn't see each other anymore. He believed me.

Ralph found a two-bedroom apartment and a roommate to pay half the rent. He definitely wasn't sorry he transferred to Western States College. He loved the teachers and the curriculum. There was only one small but important detail missing; no chiropractic philosophy was being taught. The school was so dedicated to the sciences that he could swear he was in medical school. He still didn't like my college but he was thankful that he spent his first two quarters attending it with me. He relied on what he had learned here to think now in chiropractic terms over there.

Chiropractic philosophy was supposed to co-exist with the science and art of chiropractic but at this college we were mostly immersed in philosophy. In chiropractic philosophy class we were told over and over again that Universal Intelligence was what brought organization to all matter, and maintained its existence. All living things had inborn, or *Innate Intelligence,* which adapted universal forces and matter for use in the body. Every living thing had ALL the Innate Intelligence it required to maintain its life and optimal health. Health was the expression of the Innate Intelligence through Innate Matter, via Innate Energy. When there was interference with the transmission of Innate Energy, the result was a decrease in the expression of Innate Intelligence, which chiropractors called dis-ease, not to be confused with disease.

To many people all of this could sound like some form of nonsense or religion, but to chiropractors and the patients that had experienced the healing power of chiropractic, it was all elementary.

Leila and I were having lunch at the cafeteria in school. "Veronica, you have the perfect ex. You told him that you didn't want any money and he still sends it to you. I tried using the same psychology on mine because he's either late with his checks or tries to gyp me out of my alimony, but it failed miserably."

"I still don't want Al's money, and I even told him that when I was in New Jersey."

"That's right. Because you don't want it, he wants you to have it."

Leila was a psychotherapist before coming to chiropractic college and tended to examine everything too in depth.

"Leila, your ex is paying for your tuition and all your living expenses, of course he was happy to hear that you no longer wanted his financial help. Al just sends me whatever he wants and isn't under any obligation. That's the difference." I was laughing.

She went back to calling her ex to remind him of his financial duties. They have no children; I don't see why he has to pay her just because she was his wife. What a rip off for the poor guy.

Sara was one of my classmates in radiology, someone I'd known since second quarter. She came over to my apartment quite often, and during study breaks we talked about life. Mostly we talked about the opposite sex. I told her about my experiences with men and how disappointed I was with dating.

"I don't need men," Sara said. "When I feel lonely I give myself a hug and I'm fine."

She stood, crossed both her arms over her chest, and turned her back on me. Then she said in a serious voice, "See? See my hands on my back? I'm hugging myself. It works really well and I don't have to put up with any jerks."

I laughed heartily.

"My last boyfriend was from the middle east," Sara said. "Middle Eastern men love women with nice round bellies like mine. He used to say that a woman with a flat belly was like having sex with a scarecrow." She pushed out her stomach proudly.

She can be a riot sometimes. Leila and Sara are my best friends.

Motion Palpation was an important diagnostic technique that students of chiropractic had to master if they were going to be successful at locating joint dysfunction within the spinal column and extremities. Once achieved, that segment of the spine was addressed with the proper chiropractic adjustment to increase mobility to the joint. Too forceful a palpation could cause reactive muscle spasms, a very painful experience. Harold, a student in my palpation class last quarter—appropriately called Harold the Hateful, by most students including myself, was known for his negative attitude, racist comments, and most of all his lack of thoughtfulness when palpating. I stayed away from him like the plague.

Friday night he showed up at my front door.

"What do you want?" I wasn't going to invite him in.

"I want to apologize if I hurt you during motion palpation class."

"It wasn't just me that complained."

"I know. Nobody wants to partner with me in class. That's why I'm here. I need you to teach me how to do it."

"Ask the teacher to show you."

"I did. She's too busy. You are the only one that can help me. Please."

I had him sit on a chair and cross his arms across his chest. I stood behind him as we've been taught in class and I put my left arm around his upper torso to help me control the bilateral flexion and rotation of his torso. With my right hand, I moved my thumb and index finger along his spine, one vertebra at a time while flexing and rotating his thoracic region.

"Harold, as you know the purpose of motion palpation is to evaluate the dynamic movement of the joints and assess any dysfunctions, without causing any discomfort to the patient."

"Unless I go deep into the spine with my fingers I won't be able to find the bones that form that particular articulation." He stood, frustrated.

"Have you ever played a musical instrument?"

"I tried the guitar. It didn't work for me."

Yeah. I bet he broke the strings.

"Okay, I'm going to let you palpate my neck, but if you hurt me, even a little, we're done. Try closing your eyes and let your innate intelligence guide you."

He laid his left hand over my head like a ton of bricks and proceeded to clasp his fingers of the right hand like a wrench on a water pipe. He wasn't human.

"Stop," I screamed. "Would you like to know how that feels?"

I didn't give him a chance to answer. I climbed on top of the other chair and bent forward enough to put my left elbow on top of his head, using my shoulder to press down, grabbed the back of his neck with my right hand and squeezed as hard as I could.

It was the first time I saw Harold laugh. He was laughing but he was also holding the top of his head. I had made my point.

Even though I don't drink tea, I appreciated that he took me out for tea. It was his way of saying thank you. He would be returning Tuesday evening.

On Tuesday, I blindfolded him and told him to use the sensory feeling we all have in our fingertips to palpate my spine. He was able to name each vertebra without hurting me. I appreciated his offer to take me out for ice cream, but as before, he didn't use stop signs and was speeding. I was sure that his tiny sports car was a death trap. I clenched my teeth in anticipation and gripped tightly to my seat. While driving he displayed a nervous blinking of his eyes and twitching of his features while his head moved rapidly from side to side. He reminded me of a squirrel holding on to his precious nuts while running up a tree. He cursed when he had to stop for a light and he cursed when it started to rain.

"Have you noticed the Jews at school have their own clique?" he asked.

"No. I haven't"

"Yeah. And they don't invite anyone to their parties unless they're Jewish."

"Really?" Why would anyone want to invite *him* to a party?

"They own the banks. That's where they keep their money. Unless you're a Jew, they won't share any with you."

"How greedy of them." Would he have asked me to teach him Motion Palpation, if he knew I was Jewish?

"Yeah, I'm just sick of them. They're always ready to help each other in time of need. That's what they are known best for."

"Isn't it good that they help each other? If everybody did the same, there wouldn't be people out there begging." I was breathing deep and slow, trying to remain cool.

"Not me. When I graduate from this damn college and start making money, I'm not sharing my hard-earned money with any beggars. Let them work for it."

I had been married to Al long enough to know that nothing I say would change Harold's thinking. Like Sara kept telling me, I had to stop trying to save every Tom, Dick, and Harry that showed up at my door.

I was walking at the flea market Saturday morning when I noticed a vendor selling used guns. After my experience last quarter with pepper spray, where I was walking in a parking lot and that was all I had to defend myself, against a suspicious looking character, it might be a good idea to have something more effective. What if the cop that came to my rescue had not been there?

The gun dealer told me I didn't need a license and I could pay him cash for the gun of my choice. He would include a box of bullets.

"I'd like to be able to defend myself in a dangerous situation, but I don't have the first idea of how to use a gun."

"It's no big deal, just point and shoot." He handed me a small handgun, which he said would be perfect to carry inside my coat pocket.

The gun fit the palm of my outstretched hand. The forbidden fruit of crime felt light, cold and motionless. I was surprised to see how rusty it looked, but he said, "What do you expect? It's seen a lot of action."

I kept my hand flat, appropriately supported by my other hand, afraid that any movement of my fingers might trigger it to go off into the crowd.

He wrapped the gun and the box of bullets in newspaper and put them into a plastic bag.

I paid him $145, believing I had gotten a real bargain.

On the way home, I stopped at a shooting gallery not too far from where I live and signed up for shooting lessons. The man behind the counter said my gun was old and far from safe. Its parts were corroded and he couldn't guarantee that it would shoot properly. He advised me to take it back and exchange it for something better.

I took my gun back to the flea market and for $50 more exchanged it for a better one. When I took my new and improved gun to the shooting range, Gregg, the salesman, advised me not to use it because it wasn't much safer than the previous one. He wouldn't be surprised if it backfired in my face. He recommended that I return the gun and get my money back. I could hear the faintly sound of gunshots coming from inside the shooting range. I was experiencing an Adrenaline rush. For a nominal fee, Gregg said that I could practice with one of his guns in the shooting range and I wasn't under any obligation.

"I've never shot a gun in my life."

"I'm going in with you. You'll need "muffs" for your ears and "eyes" to protect you from hot spent casings that eject from semi-automatics." I followed him wondering if I wasn't biting more than I could chew.

The range reminded me of a dark, narrow bowling alley and had a cold surreal feeling. The pins were the bullseye targets and the bowling ball was my gun. He showed me body stance, how to grip the gun; trigger control, and use of the sight. It was a lot of things to remember, and a lot of work to shoot a bullet. Even with the supporting hand stabilizing the gun, and my feet firmly on the ground I felt the hard backward impact on my body with each shot. I could see a man with strong hands having no problem shooting for hours but I was done after attempting ten times to hit the target. My hands were shaking, and the right shoulder felt like it was going to fall out of the socket. Gregg said that I had a lot of potential and with practice, I would get better at it.

I left the shooting range feeling like a female Clint Eastwood.

"You've got to be pulling my leg. I don't take guns back. There was nothing wrong with either gun I sold you. I was already nice enough to exchange the first one," said the gun dealer as he left to take care of someone else.

"I was told at the shooting range that both guns you sold me were not safe to use."

"You heard me. There's nothing I can do for you. Now, get lost."

I drove to the police station and asked to speak with their chief of police. I needed his advice as to what to do next and showed him the gun.

The chief took me under his wing and told me to go back to the flea market and tell the "good-for-nothing son-of-a-gun" he'd come have a chat with him if he didn't return my money. "You go get yourself a gun from a reputable place and leave it underneath your car seat. If someone comes up to your window and you feel threatened, just grab your loaded gun and shoot him between the eyes."

I stared at him in shock and pulled myself back into the chair.

He then told me his wife never left their house without her *special* shoulder bag, which looked like any normal over-the-shoulder purse, but there was a slit for her gun. She kept it loaded and ready to fire. They sell those purses at several gun shops. The chief also encouraged me to take lessons on how to handle a gun safely and how to shoot so that I wouldn't miss my target.

"Keep your gun under your pillow when you go to sleep. If someone breaks into your bedroom, no one in Georgia will blame you for shooting the bastard."

I headed to the flea market.

When I relayed the police chief's message to the gun dealer, he handed me my money. These people in the south are tough.

I returned to the gun range shop. Gregg showed me several guns and provided statistics on each one. I understood little of what he was saying.

"What does that mean, automatic?"

"Why waste time cocking the gun? That's what automatic means."

"I spoke to my ex a few days ago and he told me to get a Smith & Wesson. Do they come in automatic?"

"You bet they do. Here is a .38 automatic that carries five bullets and it's ready to fire.

"Pretty." I said running the tips of my fingers over its polished, inviting metal surface.

I signed up for a gun education class provided at no charge by the police department and I registered my gun.

Even though I'm through with Dexter, I still enjoy talking to him, as a friend. He usually calls on weekends.

"The teachers at this college are outstanding." He bragged again when he called this morning.

"I believe you, but I don't want to move to California."

"Why not?"

"Earthquakes..."

"The media exaggerates everything. They are just little tremors, nothing to worry about.

"I see. But I'm going to school for free. I would have to be nuts to waste my scholarship."

"Veronica, your one year scholarship will be finished the end of next quarter. Besides, I have great news to share with you. I've spoken with a well renowned psychologist in San Francisco who said she could help me overcome some of my issues. If I promise you to seek care, will you give me a second chance?"

"I need to think about that." I told him.

I wasn't very excited about the idea. Our relationship was far from good when we dated, and I don't want to repeat the same mistake.

My friends Sara and Russell have been talking about going to Portugal with me, during our next school break. Russell's wife called me to confirm the plans. We are getting together on Sunday to discuss all the fine details. I already phoned my parents and they are looking forward to seeing me and meeting my school friends.

I've been spreading the word, that my birthday is May 7. When I was younger, I was too shy to let everyone know. Now that I'm half a century old I feel like I should celebrate it with as many friends as I can.

I studied all morning and then Cida, my Brazilian friend and classmate, took me out for lunch. A few hours later, Sara came by my apartment with a bunch of fresh tomatoes that she grows in plastic garbage cans. Harold showed up and insisted on treating me to his favorite tea place even though I don't drink tea. After he brought me back, I walked to the park, ate dinner, and caught up on homework. I was already in my pajamas when the phone rang. It was Leila.

"Veronica, what are you doing for your birthday?" She always puts a stronger pitch in the *ro* of my name. She was from Argentina and her first language was Spanish which is what most likely made it easy for her to roll out the letter R.

"I'm going to bed."

"What are you talking about? It's only ten. I'm taking you out on the town and I don't want to hear any excuses. Just be ready."

One hour later, I was dozing on the couch when I was awakened by the doorbell.

"Leila, you are amazing," I said, hugging her and feeling suddenly, energized.

We drove to Atlanta, and were soon seated on high stools outside a bar, surrounded by a large crowd, most people a lot younger than either of us. Leila is 45 years old, five years younger than me. Speakers blasted out the festive sounds of Caribbean music. Lights glittered from one end of the street to the next. A hot clammy breeze swept past us, leaving a faint blend of sweat, perfume and tobacco clinging to our clothes. We both drank a fancy pineapple juice drink from a coconut shell, filled with chunks of fresh pineapple and sliced strawberries.

At half-past midnight, we stepped into a dancehall. We barely had a chance to sit down when we were approached by two Latino men. An hour later, we crossed the street to another club. At two-thirty, we agreed it was time to head home.

While Leila drove, I taught her my favorite song, and we were singing it loud. *Oh what a beautiful evening, everything's going my way.*

When we stopped for a traffic light, two men in an open-top sports car pulled up next to us. They heard us singing and they began singing along with us. We sang back and forth without moving, despite the green light, singing the same tune over and over again. Then a car pulled up behind us and the driver blew the horn. We waved goodbye and drove off. Our joyful mood remained until Leila dropped me off at my apartment.

"Veronica, swear that you won't tell anyone at school what we did tonight."

"We didn't do anything wrong."

"I don't want anyone at school to know that we were dancing with Mexicans. I feel kind of embarrassed about that."

"That's silly. Tonight was the most fun I've ever had on my birthday. But okay. I won't tell anyone we know."

The ratio of women to men in my gun safety class was six to one, and we learned a lot of good advice from our teachers, the local sheriff and his deputy.

If someone breaks into my apartment, I should hide in my bedroom with the door closed. I should sit in the furthest corner of the room and point the gun at the door. When the robber opens the door, I should aim the gun at his heart and keep shooting until he goes down. If I hit him but he runs outside, I must go after him and shoot him, then grab his body and pull him back into the house. Otherwise, if he lives, he could sue me for hurting him. Most robbers who break into homes are on heavy-duty drugs. A single bullet isn't going to kill them; if anything, it will annoy them.

The instructors also advised that we use brass-jacketed, hollow-point bullets because once they enter the criminal's body; he has no chance of living. I diligently exchanged my bullets.

"If any of you feel sorry for the intruder and can't defend yourselves," the deputy said, "he will most likely kill you. So it's your choice if you live or die."

The instructors also showed us how to use a pillow to our advantage. If we're not sure whether the robber has left the house, we should open the bedroom door and toss out the pillow. If the robber goes to grab it, he becomes an easy mark.

I barely saw Stewart, my roommate. During the week, he left at five to go to the gym, and then spent his days in classes. He hung out with his own group of friends in the evening and on weekends.

Stewart never brought anyone home, but he did ask if it was all right to have his girlfriend, visiting from New York, stay with him during the next school break. Of course, I said it was fine.

Stewart was into bodybuilding and had a special diet of tuna and rice. He also cooked a lot of pasta dishes, like lasagna. The beauty about him was that when he finished cooking, he left the kitchen spotless. He was polite, quiet, and very clean. Ralph said I'd hit gold with my perfect roommate.

I decided not to carry my gun or put it under my car seat. I put it under my mattress but pointing away from my head. I was no longer sure that I wanted it.

I showed the gun to Harold and he showed an interest in buying it from me. I would have to think about that.

Leila called.

"Veronica, I need you to be my psychotherapist."

"I don't know anything about it."

"It's no big deal I can teach."

"You think too highly of me. You need to see a professional."

"Honey, my ex-husband doesn't give me enough alimony to cover psychotherapy sessions. I need your help."

"Okay, what do I have to do?"

"I'll tell you when I get to your place."

She came over that afternoon. She set a box of tissues next to her and used them to wipe her tears as she told me all the things that bothered her. I had to do only one thing—keep quiet and listen. It wasn't easy for me to keep quiet when the answers to her problems were within her reach. It would have been so easy to guide her, but she didn't want help; she wanted to vent. Like Dexter, she was addicted to being a victim and liked to dwell on her own misery.

I wish some of the teachers were more serious about their job. I get frustrated listening about their hobbies, their philosophies, or whatever they think is more important than teaching. No wonder Ralph was so much happier at Western States College, even if they don't offer any chiropractic philosophy courses. One particular new teacher, Mr. Random is infatuated with the TV show, *The X-Files.* All he does is talk about conspiracy theories, which could seriously affect obsessed minds, such as Harold. Mr. Random is not as radical as Harold, but he spends most of our time trying to convince us to mistrust the government. His stories annoy me to no end—especially when taking the place of lectures.

Considering how hard I studied, I still didn't test as well as I wished for and couldn't bring my grade point average above a 3.5. I had lived in America most of my life, but I had to accept that English would always be my second language.

Illegal copies of exam tests for finals and mid-term were always available, as they cruised from one student to another, but I couldn't make myself remember answers word-for-word like a parrot. If I didn't understand the questions, memorizing the answers were a waste of my time because when testing time comes, I couldn't recall the answers. I'm a hands-on learner, and I had always been that way. I have to understand the material from the inside out to get a firm grip on the subject. There were no cheating exam copies available for national and state boards. I couldn't kid myself, if I didn't study hard and understand each subject to the fullest, I would fail the board tests, and never be a chiropractor. I couldn't even conceive such personal failure.

I began listening more attentively to Dexter's description of the chiropractic college in California. According to him, the classes were small and the teachers cared enough to stay after class to answer questions. I knew that I would thrive in such environment but, moving to California at that time, sounded like a huge endeavor.

May 20

Every year I buy myself a present for my birthday. A little late now but today I found what I wanted. For the amazing price of $300, I bought a used, portable adjusting table, including the carrying bag, and a small head-drop piece called Toggle that is made specifically for manual upper cervical adjustments. I intend to practice the Toggle technique on Joe, my stuffed dummy. I've gotten my money back tenfold since I bought Joe. About a year ago, I took Joe to Florida as a passenger dummy. Carjacking was wild down there, but I felt safe with Joe. With his football cap, a pair of snazzy sunglasses to bring out his healthy features, and his well-built upper torso, no one would believe that Joe wasn't real. The bottom half of his body was missing but he made the perfect volunteer for practicing chiropractic neck adjustments. Students flocked to my apartment to practice on Joe.

Every day I practice on my Toggle piece five important exercises. The wrist stretch increases the ability to stabilize my hands into extension. The wrist traction helps with flexibility. The thumb web exercise for better thrust. The arch exercise helps to establish a good, solid arched hand so that only the fingers and the pisiform, a small knobbly, pea-shaped wrist bone, is in contact with the vertebra to be moved.

Leila and I made a pact— if we go in different directions after we graduate and don't see each other for, let's say, another fifty years, our best way to recognize each other will be to say, "Pisiform!" and do a high five.

My favorite of all the exercises is the Toggle flick, but until we get proficient at using both hands during this move we are allowed to Toggle only raw eggs. There are no seats in Toggle class, only a Toggle adjusting table with a headpiece that needs to be cocked in order to drop along with the egg. The table stands in the center of the room, covered by black, thick plastic that extends to the four walls. If the headpiece doesn't drop because we forgot to cock it, we are guaranteed to get egged out. We stand in a circle, holding three eggs each. No one smiles. When someone successfully toggles their egg without breaking, we clap politely. It's a nerve wrecking experience to see how many eggs we get splashed with. The day I can be swift enough to make a hand trust on a raw egg and move the head piece without breaking the egg, is the day that I'm ready to Toggle someone's neck with confidence.

The school requires that all students have a clinician and get adjusted at least once a week at the school's clinic. I allow my clinician to perform only Toggle on me. This technique helped me recover when a herniated disc on my lower back prevented me from walking three years ago. I was still married to Al and living in New Jersey.

From studying Toggle this quarter, I've realized why my first experience with a chiropractic adjustment had been so painful; Dr. Peruzzi, the chiropractor I went to, forgot to cock the headpiece on the table, and it didn't drop when he Toggle my upper neck. No wonder it was extremely painful and it felt as if my brain flew out of my skull, like in one of those crazy cartoon scenes. If my head had been a raw egg, I wouldn't have lived to talk about it. Still, I feel that Toggle is the most gentle and safest technique, when performed properly.

June 5

After finals next week, I will be traveling to Portugal with Sara, Russell, his wife, Joyce, and Ruth, their three-year-old girl.

I've made arrangements for all of us to stay at a pensão in Lisbon which is very close to where my parents live. The day after we arrive, my traveling companions will rent a car and head north to the city of Coimbra for a week. I will remain in Lisbon, with my parents.

~ Chapter Three ~

Mama's Sacrifice

July 13

It was ten at night when the plane hovered over the city of Lisbon, the capital of Portugal. Below us the familiar city lights glimmered like a red carpet for its homeward daughter. I was home, even if it was only for ten days.

Because of the language barrier, everyone depended on me to make a smooth transition out of the airport and into a taxi. Russell and Joyce took turns carrying Ruth, three large suitcases, a hefty baby carriage and two over the shoulder bags with baby accessories and toys. Sara dragged along a large suitcase and I carried an old military duffel bag with gifts for my parents, and Luisa, their caregiver. My real luggage was a backpack. I like to travel light and with my hands free.

My old bargaining Portuguese talents came on handy when the taxi driver complained about the excessive amount of baggage and wanted to charge us extra.

Ruth who had slept throughout the eight-hour flight was ready to be entertained. Sara whispered that the kid was nothing but a brat and was driving her crazy. Sara was no longer looking forward to traveling with them.

"For an American, you speak pretty good Portuguese," said the taxi driver.

"I *am* Portuguese."

"Which island?"

"I was born here, in Lisbon." I wasn't going to tip him much after that last insult.

Joyce stared out the window. "I'm surprised the city is so alive this late at night. Where's everyone out there going?"

she said. Everyone agreed even Ruth was pounding excitedly with both hands at the glass.

"A lot of these people had their usual late dinner at home and now they are enjoying an evening walk." I said. "On a nice warm night like tonight everybody goes out. The ones you see walking are most likely meeting with friends at a coffee shop or just going out for a good time. The Portuguese love the night life."

The driver glanced over his shoulder. "Lisbon's night life is considered to be one of the best in Europe," he said in English. "The bars don't close until two in the morning and the discos are open until six, or even later. A city that never sleeps." He glanced back once more. "By the way, can one of you stop that kid from hitting the window? It's very annoying."

"So you speak English?" said Russell.

"When I want to." He laughed.

Portuguese humor is one of a kind, and only the Portuguese find it funny.

A pensão is not as luxurious as a hotel but it's a lot more affordable and because of that, travelers like us, on student budgets tended to use them. Pensão Areeiro was situated at Praça Francisco Sa Carneiro, a public square near a subway entrance and bus stop. Both transportation methods were ideal to access the airport and any place in the city.

Russell pointed to the pensão's rusted metal elevator. "Is this thing safe?" he said. "I didn't know they still made elevators like this."

"They don't," I said. "It's probably about seventy-five years old. Just don't catch your fingers between the railings when you close the door." I laughed and entered the elevator followed by Sara and Joyce who were carrying their luggage but not laughing as much as me.

"I'm going to take the steps." Russell said, and picked up Ruth. She kicked and yelled that she wanted to take the elevator with her mother.

The next morning my traveling companions left for Coimbra. I had encouraged them to stop at Eiriceira, a small, picturesque fishing village that was dear to my heart.

I headed to my parents' home, a brisk twenty-minute walk. They lived across the Avenue Dom Afonso Henriques, named after the first king of Portugal. At the end of the avenue stood the Fonte Luminosa, a twentieth-century water fountain with three waterfalls bathing the bigger-than-life statues of naked men on horses and beautiful naked nymphs. At least that's the way I remembered it, from when my two brothers and I had dangled our feet over the pool and were sprayed with chlorinated water brought to us by a gentle breeze. It was there that I had learned to dream of adventure in faraway lands. Now I was an adult, feeling more like an American than ever, a foreigner to the surroundings that no longer held the magic it possessed when I was a child. The fountain was dry and under major repairs.

Just to please Mama, I deliberately wore a tight, sexy short red dress and red high heel shoes. I had even put on red lipstick for the first time in my life.

Wearing red on that day was for me the biggest sacrifice a daughter could make for her mother. I would rather have worn black or earth tones like burnt orange, brown mustard or a harvest-gold shirt with my usual blue jeans. When Mama saw me, she was thrilled.

"Veronica, I know you got dressed like that—just to make me happy." Tears walled up in her eyes. "You look so beautiful, and believe me when I say that red is your color."

Mama—according to my calculations was around eighty-seven. The reason I wasn't sure of her age was her refusal to share that information with anyone, including me. I was surprised that she no longer used make-up. It was as if she had lost her zest for life.

Papa at ninety-one years old had the energy of a twenty-year-old. He still went out every day and came home only for his meals. He possessed a quixotic attitude and was focused on only one thing: find Alice, his former "employee," and bring her to justice. Maids in Portugal were now addressed as employees. After lunch, we sat in the living room and he elaborated.

"Alice murdered your brother José, and if it wasn't for Luisa, an employee at the time, your mother and I would also be dead. Luisa saw Alice putting drugs into our food and told me about it when Mama was taken to the hospital with severe stomach pain."

"Papa, why didn't you call me? All I knew was that you sold everything, including your home. It didn't make sense to me."

"It was a critical time. I had two weeks to dispose of everything and get out. You were too far away to help. I called your brother Max-Leão, twice, but there was no answer. Well, you know him. He leaves the country and doesn't tell your mother or me where he is. We hardly see him anyway."

"Why didn't you go to the police, for help?"

"Luisa and I were scared for our lives. If we called the cops, Alice's boyfriend could have come after us. He was being hunted by the police as a criminal. I only had one option, give Alice a two-week paid furlough, and sell everything before she came back. The idea was for her not to be able to find us. Luisa was kind enough to offer us a room to rent in her apartment."

Mama didn't respond, but her eyes spoke a thousand words.

I could only imagine what Mama had felt at the time. She came out of the hospital and found all her belongings gone, and had to live in Luisa's house for the rest of her life.

After lunch, Papa left for his nap, Mama and I remained in the room and she showed me a letter that he had written to Luisa. In it, he offered to marry Luisa as soon as she got a divorce—and then when Papa died she could collect his pension. Since he was still married to Mama, it was beyond me how he could do that. Mama excused him by saying that Papa was developing slight dementia and she just wanted me to see what she was going through with him.

"I don't know how much money Luisa's husband makes as a chauffeur, but your father gives her all his pension money and most of the money his cousins in England send us every month to help out with *our* living expenses. With the money he made from selling our possessions, he paid for remodeling Luisa's apartment and bought her a new television, stereo, furniture and home appliances." She grew quiet when Luisa came in the room and sat with us.

No doubt, whatever money Papa had made from selling everything was long gone. Luisa had my father by his heart and Mama knew it.

"In case you are wondering, your parents have the room where my son and daughter used to sleep." Luisa said. "It was only right that your father buy this couch, which opens into a bed at night. This is where my son Raul sleeps. In order for me to have your parents living here my family had to make a lot of concessions. Our ten-year-old daughter Tania sleeps in my room with my husband and me. It's definitely tight living in this small apartment and sometimes I even wonder why I took them in."

Either, she was a good kind person or she needed the money.

Luisa's apartment was on the second floor, and because Mama was too weak to use the steps, she never went out. The only time she left the apartment was because of her health issues, such as her heart problems. Then, she would be taken down the steps on a stretcher and driven by ambulance to the hospital.

"Your father is sleeping. I'll show you our bedroom later. Let's sit on the kitchen veranda." Mama held onto my arm. Their small kitchen apartment sat two people at a round kitchenette table. Two French doors opened to a three-by-five foot terrace overlooking a dead-end street. Mama told me that when she needed fresh air and solitude, she would sit out there; her little piece of heaven.

"Isn't Luisa nice?" Mama said. "When she found out you were coming, she put my rocking chair in here and arranged those geraniums. Isn't she nice?" She raised her voice for Luisa to hear in the kitchen.

I could feel the tension in the air, as if Mama was trying to tell me just the opposite. I told Mama how happy I was being single again, and how much I was looking forward to the day I would start practicing with Ralph. She had many questions about my life in America, about my divorce, my sons and my grandson Jacob. I was delighted to see her laugh and enjoying herself.

Luisa came to the veranda and said, "I know you're having fun talking but it's five 'clock and I need to start preparing dinner."

"Yes, thank you for reminding me," Mama said joyfully. "I will be overseeing the preparation of *caldeirada,* one of my favorite meals. The secret to making a perfect *caldeirada,* (fish stew) is the way each ingredient is cut and laid in the cooking pot." Mama sat on a kitchen chair next to the stove and asked me to stand next to her.

Mama said, "Tania, there's eight of us for dinner that includes your father, your brother and his girl, we'll need the largest cooking pot you can find."

Tania took a large pot from under the kitchen sink and showed it to Mama.

"Perfect" she said. "Put it on top of the stove, but don't turn it on yet. Your job is to peel and slice twelve potatoes one inch thick. Luisa we will need six garlic cloves chopped and three onions, thinly sliced, ring shape. Let's keep all the ingredients separate, until we have everything ready. Luisa, did you get fresh cod fish?"

"Yes, mam, I also bought sword and haddock like you asked me to."

I picked up a knife and started peeling the potatoes.

"Next, we need to peel three tomatoes and chop them up."

"I'll do that," said Luisa.

"Can I cut the green peppers?" Tania asked.

"The peppers don't get cut with a knife. They must be broken in large pieces, by hand. I'll do that."

Papa came in after his afternoon walk. "No man allowed in here, scoot," said Luisa.

"Oh I see, we men can go to war but we aren't allowed in the kitchen, hum?"

"That's why it's so peaceful here." I answered him.

We laughed.

Mama stood with a bottle of olive oil in her hand. She poured about two tablespoons into the cooking pot and said, " First layer starts with potatoes, a bit of garlic, next onions, then fish, followed by tomatoes, bay leaf salt, pepper, paprika, pepper, nice chunky peppers, back to potatoes, garlic, onions and so on"

"Don't be shy with the white wine." Mama said to Luisa. "Pour about half. Very good, now bring me two cups of the hot water. Pour it in. That should do it. Now we let it cook slowly for about an hour and fifteen minutes."

Everybody was tired after all the cooking and cleaning up the kitchen. We sat in the living room with Papa, watching the news on television. Tania asked me, "What do you have in that big bag in the hallway?"

"Oh my goodness I forgot all about it. Gifts for everyone!" I announced.

I felt like Santa, taking the presents off my duffel bag. Tania was delighted with the doll and stuffed dog and Luisa ran to her room to try on two dresses. Mama looked beautiful in all her new tops and I used some of the make-up I had brought along for her, to do her face. She loved the softness of the new slippers. Two ties and a box of handkerchiefs went to Papa and a tie for Luisa's husband. Everybody was happy. I was glad when Luisa's son and his girlfriend didn't show up, because I had not brought anything for them.

The delicious smell from the fish stew was beckoning us to get seated at the dining room table. *Caldeirada* was not my favorite Portuguese dish, but knowing that Mama loved it, was good enough for me. The flavor was smooth, not spicy and I was glad when I found cod fish in my plate versus the other fish. It was a perfect meal for a cold winter day. I used to hate bread when I was a kid and now I was appreciating its crispy texture when soaked into the juices. I noticed that the right lens on Mama's reading glasses had a piece of food stuck on it.

"Mama, you have something caught on one of your lenses."

"Are you sure? I don't see anything." She took her glasses off to look at them.

"It has to block your vision, it's big."

I took the eyeglasses from her hands. The lenses were deeply scratched and there was a piece of fish stuck to her right one.

"When was the last time you had your eyes checked?"

"I don't remember. But I've had these glasses forever."

The next day I hired two neighbors to carry Mama downstairs and put her into a taxi. Luisa came with us.

The optometrist looked at Mama's eyes. "She's blind. Completely blind in the right eye and the left one is not much better."

"Are you sure?" I asked, and then turned to Mama. "Have you been having trouble seeing lately?"

Mama didn't answer but he did. "Of course she knows she's blind, unless she's an idiot too. See, look." He moved his finger in front of her face. "See? She can't even follow my finger. Like I said, she's blind on her right side."

I prayed that when he went blind—soon, I hoped— he'd receive the same consideration he had provided my mother.

"How about prescribing a pair of glasses to help her see better from the left eye? Can you do that?"

"Of course. Let's take care of that up front."

I took Mama's arm and walked her to the front of the shop where she sat quietly on a chair.

"There's a difference in price according to the quality of the glass you decide to pick." He put two lenses on the counter.

"I can't see the difference. Which is the best one of the two?" I asked.

"This one, but it's double the price."

"Why?"

"Because it's a lot better to see through. The cheaper one is just that, a piece of crap and not as clear as the other glass."

"Why are you even showing me the crappy one?"

"I like providing choices to my customers."

"I'll take the more expensive one."

Luisa grabbed my arm and pulled me out into the street.

"What are you doing? You're wasting your money buying expensive eyeglasses. Didn't she tell you? Her doctor has given her three months to live."

My heart stopped, my head felt ready to burst. I reached for the wall to keep from falling. I tried to say something but my lungs had deflated. I just stared at her, my eyes bulging in disbelief. Then the flames exploded out of my mouth. "You are lying to me. What the hell are you saying?"

"I can't believe that she didn't tell you. Calm down!" She tried to hold my arm.

"You just told me my mother will be dead in three months and you want me calm down? You're lying to me. You are a cruel, nasty person." I began to cry.

"Her doctor's the one that gave her three months. Not me."

I pushed her out of my way and went back in.

"How long will it take you to have the eyeglasses ready—with the better lenses?"

"You can pick them up tomorrow morning."

"I'll bring her in to have them fitted."

"She doesn't need to be fitted. Just come by eleven and I'll have them ready."

I said nothing until Mama and I were alone on *her* veranda. I closed the French doors, and asked if what Luisa had told me was true. I felt better after she swore to me that it wasn't. She had made up the story, hoping that Luisa would be more patient and provide better care out of feeling sorry for her. Because Mama has always manipulated people to get what she wanted, I believed her.

That evening I was ready to leave their apartment when I saw Tania sitting on her parent's bed counting money. She waved a bill in the air and said joyfully, "Today was a profitable day."

Mama said, "She has a full time job begging on the streets as if she were disabled."

"Does Luisa know about it?"

"Yes, she encourages her."

Maybe I'm prudish, but to me, Luisa was teaching her ten year old to lie and steal.

The next day, I went to pick up Mama's eyeglasses. A young girl behind the counter showed them to me and then proceeded to put them inside a pretty colorful case. Just then the optometrist walked by, and when he saw what she was doing he snatched the case from her hands and slipped her a plastic brown one.

I'm a Taurus, which is most likely the reason I saw red. I lunged over the counter and grabbed him by the neck. I yelled, "You cheap bastard. Give me that other case now, or I'll kill you with my own hands!"

"All right, all right, you crazy freak American woman. Stay away from me." He backed into the counter and picked up the other case. "You don't have to scream like that, in front of my customers. Here." He put the case on the counter with the glasses.

"I'll scream if I want, you nasty pig! Someday you'll pay for the way you treated my mother. I curse you and your whole family!"

I grabbed the case and glasses and left the shop crying. When I got to the apartment, I found Mama sitting in the veranda, staring at the dead-end street. I gave the glasses to Mama and, dropping to my knees, lay my head on her lap still crying.

"Oh, Mama, I'm so ashamed of being part of the human race. I can't stand being a witness to their greed. If I could, I'd run away from this world and hide in a cave. Sometimes I wonder if God has had enough with watching men killing each other and left us all to our own destruction. I mean it, if I were God I'd have gone to another planet long, long ago."

"You have to think of your sons, Ralph and Steve, and your grandson, Jacob. You have a family now. And you have to finish school—so that I can be proud of you." She paused to take a sigh. "No matter how much you question it, God is always with us. He gave me you, didn't he, my daughter? And look at the beautiful eyeglass case you bought, just for me." She put the eyeglasses on and asked smiling, "How do I look with my new glasses?"

After lunch, Papa went to his room to take a nap and Luisa and the others left the room. I took Mama's arm and told her I'd like to sit on the couch with her. I put my head on her shoulder. We were both silent. I was trying to gather the courage to ask her why she hadn't loved me as a child. This quiet tender moment seemed to be the perfect time to get some answers. I sat up straight and looked at her. She turned to me and, before I could utter a word, very softly, "Veronica, tell me why didn't you love me when you were growing up?"

Did she read my mind? Had she felt the same as I did? What a mess.

"Mama, I always thought that *you* didn't love me. You sent me away, to America, to marry my cousin, a complete stranger."

"Sending you to America was a sacrifice I had to make to ensure your happiness. Here in Portugal, there was no future for you."

"You never hugged me, never said you loved me. And then you arranged my marriage with Al. I was sure you were trying to get rid of me."

"Of my three children, you were always my favorite."

"Me?"

"You were my little girl, Veronica. From the moment you were born I loved you more than anything else in the world, but I had to be tough, to make you strong. Veronica, I love you."

"I love you too, Mama." I wiped my tears with the back of my hands, feeling like a fool that she was also crying, but I had to let out all the hurt I had bottled up for most of my life. "I used to hate the way you treated me. I didn't know you loved me. You never said anything."

"I was afraid that if we had a strong bond between us, you'd never leave to America. I pushed you away on purpose, to make you independent. Remember the day you got married?"

"How could I forget? I looked for you when I needed you the most and you were gone."

"I was there for the ceremony but left to cry by myself. I knew I may never see you again but I wanted you to have a better life than me. I wanted you to go to America, the land of opportunity."

I shook my head in disbelief and said, "When I left, I didn't miss you or Papa. You were both strangers to me."

"I'm still not sorry for what I've done. Through the years, I've followed your accomplishments while you were married to Al and now that you're studying to be a doctor, it does my heart good. I'm so proud of you, Veronica."

"My goodness, I wish we had talked like this, years ago. Mama, let's embrace the future and not look back. Let's give thanks to God for this blessed moment. We love each other. What more can we want out of life?"

We hugged, laughed cried. It was indeed a miracle. After almost fifty years, we had finally broken through this invisible wall.

"Mama, let's do something together. Let's not spend the days locked up in this apartment. Tell me your wish. Of all the places in the world, where would you like to go? I'll take you there."

She looked away and sighed. I could see that she was thinking. She said, "Anywhere?"

"Yes, anywhere."

"Before I die, I wish I could see Sintra again. When I was young, my sisters and I loved going to Sintra, in the summertime. We would walk up to the Palace of the Pena, and take in the breathtaking view along the way. I wish I could see Sintra just one more time." And she took a deep sigh. This was the way she always had expressed herself, and I accepted it as who she was.

I told her that it was settled; I'd rent a car and drive her to the town of Sintra the next day.

Papa came in the room at that precise moment and said he was looking forward to going with us. When Luisa heard about it, she said she would prepare a picnic basket for everyone, herself included.

Early the next morning, I picked up a rental car. I paid a neighbor and Luisa's son to carry Mama down the two floors from her apartment. I had intentions of putting Mama in the passenger seat next to me, but Papa insisted on sitting up front so that he could give me directions. Luisa sat next to Mama in the back seat.

Oh my God! What a horrifying, experience. Papa, who drove a motorcycle forty years ago, could only recall the roads the way they used to be. When we drove the wrong way up a one-way road, he laughed and said, "Don't worry about that bus coming our way. Just wave at the bus driver and move over to the side of the road."

Getting in and out of two roundabouts during rush hour in downtown Lisbon gave me heart palpitations—most likely what a bull felt in the ring, trying to get the heck out with spears coming from all directions. Once out of the city and out in the countryside I became aware of having a driving-angel on my shoulder. There was no better explanation for having survived such death defying road experience.

Mama smiled the whole time. I believe her bad eyesight made her unaware of any road danger, but that also meant she couldn't see much of the scenery. She was just happy to get out of the house and be with me on an outing. Luisa filed her nails, oblivious of anything.

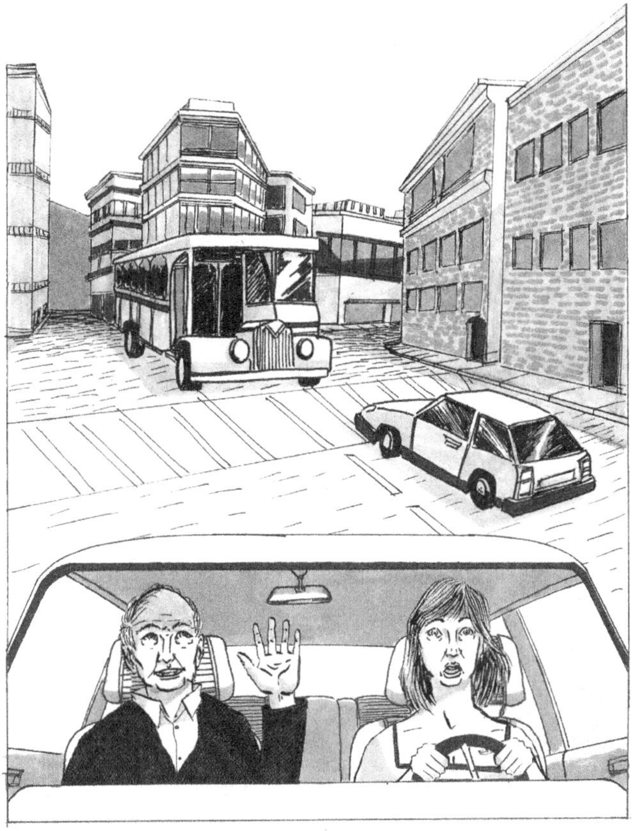

Backseat Driver

When we approached Sintra I saw a Brazilian Restaurant. Mama had been born in Brazil and always spoke affectionately of her native food.

"Mama, would you like some Brazilian food for lunch?"

She sighed deeply, followed by, "Oh, Veronica, I'd love it."

I hit the brakes and pulled the car off the road.

"I'll be right back." I told everyone.

I ran across the highway and asked the waitress for a platter of their most typical Brazilian food. We camped by the palace. Luisa covered the picnic table with a white tablecloth and after setting the plates and dinnerware put a large bowl of fish stew in the center of the table with a ladle and a bowl with sliced bread. She said, "I brought plenty of food for everyone. Why did you have to go and get more food for your mother?"

"Because I want to treat her to something that I know she will enjoy." I turned to Mama handed her the platter, and said, "Brazilian food just for you, green vegetables, with strips of meat, beans and rice."

"God bless you, Veronica." She picked some of the green vegetables with a fork. I waited for her approval. She rolled her eyes up and said smacking her lips, "Delicious, just delicious."

"Big deal," said Luisa. "My cooking is a lot better than that junk she's eating."

Papa smiled, winked at me, and said, "Your stew is great Luisa."

On the way back to Lisbon, Luisa asked me to stop at one of the villages so she could visit a cousin. We waited for her in the car for nearly an hour. Then Mama said she was feeling very tired. "I forgot to bring my heart medicine with me. But I'll be okay, don't worry."

On the way back to Lisbon, I looked in the rear mirror and saw Mama holding a hand to her chest. She looked pale.

"Are you okay?" I asked.

"I'm experiencing a heavy feeling on my chest." Then she went limp.

"Luisa, what's going on?"

"She passed out. Don't worry, she'll come to."

"My God, she passed out? Papa, where's the nearest hospital?"

Three hours later, they released Mama and gave her a prescription for nitroglycerin tablets.

We continued on our way home. At one point, Papa told me to turn right. I did. It put us directly onto a railroad track.

"Don't panic," he said. "If there's a train coming, you will hear the whistle."

"And then what?"

"Just remain calm and get off at the next opportunity."

Luisa crossed herself and yelled, "Jesus Christ, we're all going to die."

Mama put her arm over her shoulders and said, "Don't worry, Luisa. My daughter's a good driver. We'll be fine."

I got off at the next dirt road, which to my surprise, led us to a city street. Despite traffic, being back in the city made me feel more relax—until Papa gave me more directions, "I know a shortcut. Make the next left."

I should have known better than to listen to him.

The narrow street turned out to be a dead-end—unless I drove down a dozen steep steps to the street below. I was emotionally drained. No, I was terrified. I had two choices: drive the car down the steps in front of me or back out into the oncoming traffic.

"I don't know what's going on." Papa said. "When I used to drive my motorcycle, this street didn't have any steps. Sorry about that. Just back out."

I crept backwards along the narrow road, barely missing the parked cars. I reached the intersection and then pulled out slowly. Cars honked. Drivers cursed us as they their cars swerved away.

I learned the full meaning of a nervous breakdown on that daytrip. After I dropped everyone off, I took the car back. I had already paid for a week's rental, but one day of excitement had been enough for me.

Every morning, on the way to Luisa's apartment I stopped at a coffee shop. Coffee made me jittery and hyper, but I refused to be in Lisbon, where they had the best coffee in the world, and not have an espresso and eat my favorite *pastél de nata,* a fluffy crusty layered pastry filled with custard, still warm from the oven.

I went out with Papa only once, first to the German Embassy to pick up his monthly pension and then to the police station to see how things were progressing with bringing Alice to justice.

"I'm very frustrated about your mother not allowing an autopsy to be performed on José. But until she authorizes it, my hands are tied. As you can imagine, this makes it harder for me to prove Alice poisoned him. But I'm not giving up."

Papa carried a thick dossier under his arm filled with papers accounting for everything that had occurred while Alice was their employee. No doubt, the Portuguese legal system had more important concerns.

Papa encouraged me to spend the days with Mama instead of going out with him. He felt she needed me more than he did. Papa did love Mama; he just never told her. This is one of the things that bothers me about many marriages. While dating, most people will say *I love you,* but when they get married, they stop telling each other how they feel. One of the reasons I have no intention of getting married again.

Mama carried her medicine cabinet, from one room to the other—a shoebox stuffed with meds —in case she needed an "immediate" fix. I made up my mind to dissuade her from taking so many prescription drugs. As long as I remember, she took some kind of prescription every day of her life. Perhaps she would listen to me because of my status as a future doctor.

We sat on her veranda. I picked up the shoebox resting on the floor next to her feet. "Do you really have to take all of these?"

"That's what keeps me alive."

"Besides your heart, what else is wrong?"

"Every time I go to the hospital they find something else wrong and give me another medicine. I have problems with water retention, with my heart, liver, kidneys. My blood pressure goes up and down. Nothing is working right."

I read to her the side effects for some of the prescriptions. A few caused liver damage. Others were for the liver but caused high blood pressure. Some were for blood pressure but caused heart problems. Some went as far as stating, possible side effect: death.

Mama agreed but she wasn't going to stop taking them. Drugs were the only medical way of care she understood. I was only a chiropractor, not good enough to change her mind.

If I were living in Portugal, I'd throw all her medications away. Papa would brag that he went to the doctors only to learn the diagnosis. But on his way out of their offices, he would toss the med samples into the nearest garbage can. Papa didn't realize it, but he thought like a chiropractor, probably why he was so much healthier than Mama.

One evening, Papa put a tango record on and asked me to dance with him. I couldn't believe how well he still danced at his age. He held my right hand firmly in his and, with his other arm around my waist, guided me within the little space we had between the dining table and the couch. Mama's eyes filled with tears of joy, and Tania and Luisa clapped when we finished dancing.

I spent the days at home with Mama, but at seven-thirty, Mama would say, "I worry about you walking alone out there. You better leave now before it gets dark."

One evening it was eight o'clock and Mama asked Luisa to accompany me to the pensão.

Luisa and I had just walked down a block when she held my arm as if we were the best of friends and said, "My husband chauffeurs a young woman with multiple sclerosis. He's always telling me how nice she is to him. I know he's cheating on me. How can he love a woman that pisses on herself and has to be carried around like a rag doll?"

I just listened.

"The only one who understands and listens to me is Mario, my neighbor. He's unhappily married to an ugly bitch. Can you believe she came over to my apartment and charged at me like a mad rhinoceros, after accusing me of having an affair with her husband? I beat her senseless." She let go of my arm to show me how she had boxed Mario's wife unconscious. Once we were one block from the pensão, I said, "You don't have to take me to the front door; I can go on by myself now." We hugged and she left. I waited until she had gone around the street corner and took the subway to downtown Lisbon. This is the reason I don't like soap operas. They're a reminder of the miserable, dark side of humanity.

Mama asked me to visit Cousin Salomão, who was also her cardiologist. She implored me not to tell him—or anyone in our family—that I was studying to be a chiropractic doctor but instead say I was to be a medical doctor. Out of pride for my profession, I told everyone I met—especially Cousin Salomão—right away, "I'm studying to be a chiropractor."

In many ways I was still rebelling, even fighting for my independence, from Mama, but at least we had made peace with our pasts. Since we first talked about our feelings, Mama and I had many heart-to-heart conversations while Papa went out to do his daily activities. Mama cried when she told me that she couldn't stand the thought of a medical examiner cutting her son's body. "As long as I'm alive, there is no autopsy even if it means that Alice escapes from justice." She put her finger in the air as if pointing to the heavens and said, "God will take care of Alice in his own way."

As I was growing up, I remember Mama saying, "May God never show us how much we can endure." Mama was the living proof of how much one could suffer. She had lost most of her family and her children—one way or another. Papa was no longer there for her, as she was sure he was cheating on her. She had lost all her personal possessions, and their income went directly to Luisa. What was worse, Mama was in such bad health that she couldn't run away or even leave for a few hours. Her only escape was sitting in her rocking chair on the kitchen veranda facing the silent but familiar dead-end.

Mama, shared a secret with me. She liked being in the hospital. The staff in the hospital were aware that she was the author of three books and that her name and biography was in the *Dictionary of World Famous Women,* along with Mother Theresa and the Queen of England. In the hospital, they treated her like a celebrity. The nurses as well as the doctors would ask her to autograph her books they had bought. In the hospital, she had friends—and she was admired and loved. One particular doctor liked spending time with her. Their friendship began when he told her how much he admired her poetry. He began visiting her every morning. They had a lot in common and shared the same philosophy about life. They were friends. She missed his company. "Mama, given that you're good friends, why don't you invite him to visit you?"

"I could never do that out of respect for your father."

"Mama, are you lovers?" I asked mischievously.

She blushed like a schoolgirl, and I kissed her on the cheek as if asking her forgiveness for being so naughty.

"Veronica, all we do is talk, and sometimes he respectfully holds my hand. That's all."

"If you're only friends, what's wrong with him coming over an afternoon? You could invite him for tea."

"He's a man, and like I said, it would be disrespectful to your father to have a man visiting me."

"This is insane. Papa doesn't listen to you. He's the only one that speaks around here and most of the day he's gone. You live your days alone in this apartment. What's wrong with having a social life? I don't see what's so disrespectful about having a visitor. Who cares if he's a man? He's a friend." I was feeling very Americanized.

"It's true. Your father is too busy to pay attention to me. I'm so lonely when you're not here," she cried.

I prayed for God to give me an idea on how I could help her and then did what felt natural. I caressed her face and sang just for her to hear me, "You are so beautiful, to me. Can't you see?" Not remembering the rest of the lyrics, I hummed the rest of the melody. I wasn't going to stop until she smiled, so I continued with my own lyrics and hammed up on the vocals. "You have very soft skin. You're beautiful, on the outside as well as inside. And you are also a smart lady too. I should say a very intelligent lady. I'm so happy that you're my mother; you've done a great job as a mommy. I'm very proud that you are my mother. Mama, I love you." I tickled her under the arms and said, "C'mon let's see you smile."

We were both laughing silly.

"Veronica, you bring me so much happiness. Thank you for making me laugh. I feel alive and happy when you're here."

We hugged each other and there were no more tears.

That afternoon I witnessed a fight between Luisa and her husband. According to Mama, they fought often, and Luisa had a scar across her left breast as a result of one of those fights. She had tried to kill him with a kitchen knife, but the knife cut her instead when he smacked her into the new refrigerator Papa had bought.

Mama sat in the living room. Luisa and her husband fought in the kitchen, throwing objects, their cursing so loud that it reminded me of a Mexican cockfight.

I sat on the floor next to Mama's feet.

She whispered, "Shhhh, just stay with me, please. They're having one of their nasty brawls." She trembled. "The only way for me to get out of this miserable place is when I pass out and they call an ambulance. The hospital is my only salvation. In the hospital, I'm at peace."

"I'm going to stop them. This can't go on." I attempted to get up but she embraced me without letting go.

"No, Veronica, you don't want to go in there. They're like gypsies; they throw things at each other, including knives. Veronica, I don't feel good." She let go of me. "Quickly, open the sachet around my neck and place one of the tablets under my tongue. I feel like I'm going to pass out but I don't want to go to the hospital while you're here."

I slipped a tablet under her tongue. Her breathing returned to normal but she kept her eyes closed and reclined into the armchair.

I had to do something to calm her down, and asked God to help me. I stood.

Reiki was the only answer I could come up with. Dexter had performed it on me when I had the flu and it had helped me to relax. I had no idea of what I was about to do. I had never done Reiki. I only knew that I had to help Mama.

I asked Mama to keep her eyes closed and to let me treat her. I imagined gold sparkles from the heavens wrapping around her and protecting her from the emotional trauma she was being subjected to.

"Mama, try to relax. I'm here to protect you. Nothing can hurt you. You're free, Mama. You're happy again." I held my hands over her head, envisioning my energy like a protective field around her.

Weirdly enough, the sound of the fighting dissipated. Mama must have had the same reaction because she opened her eyes, smiled at me, and began singing an upbeat Brazilian song. She motioned for me to help her up, and, holding each other, she kept singing and we danced to her tune. Luisa came into the room with her hair in complete disarray and her shirt

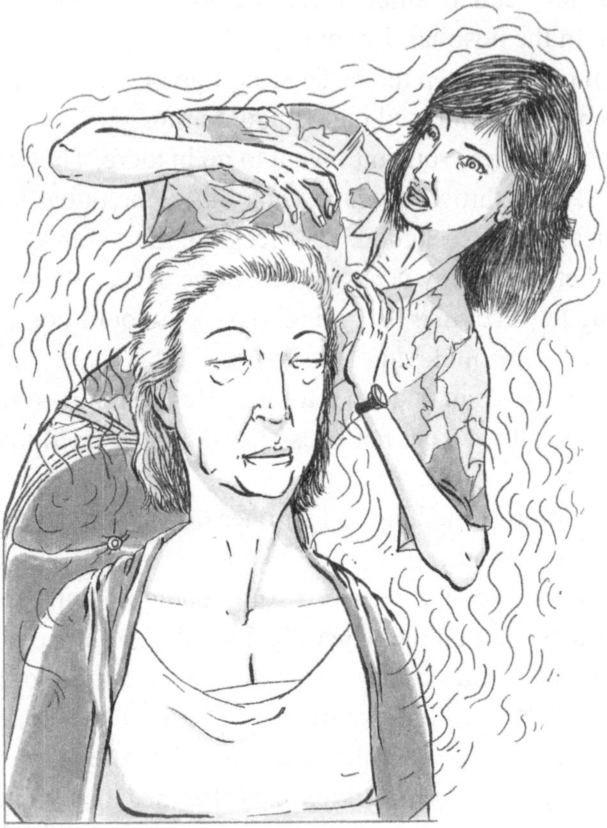

"Laying On Hands"

ripped opened. She sat on the couch, holding her head with both hands, and cried.

"The bastard dragged me by the hair. Filho da puta!"

Yeah, he was a son-of-a-bitch, alright, but Luisa wasn't much better.

Then she said, "One of these nights when he's sleeping, I'm going to cut off his balls."

I stared at Mama.

"Veronica, can you do to Luisa what you did to me? I feel like a new person. It helped me so much." She sat down, motioning her hands for me to go ahead.

"Luisa, will you allow me to take away your sadness?" I spoke calmly and slowly, in the same tone I had used during my theater productions in New Jersey when I had to ask a patron who had too much to drink to please behave or I'd have to ask him to leave.

"How you gonna do that?"

"She can treat you like she did me," Mama said. "See how relaxed I feel? It's a technique she's learned in her American medical college."

I wasn't going to correct Mama. "Luisa, sit back, close your eyes, and try to relax."

I put one hand over her heart and the other over her throat. Her energy bit me like a mad dog with rabies. To my surprise it worked to the point that when her husband came in the room she was completely relaxed, as if sedated. She looked up at him and said in the sweetest tone, "João, my dearest, would you be so kind as to bring me a glass of water? Please."

He looked at her in disbelief and said, "Sure. I'll be right back."

Mama's face glowed with happiness. She put her right thumb up and gave me a proud look.

When João came back with the glass of water, he looked at the euphoria coming from Mama's and Luisa's faces and said, "What's happening?"

Mama was on a mission. "Please, Veronica, can you do the same to João as you did to Luisa and me?"

I walked up to him.

"João, let me take your hurt away. Sit down and trust me to help you. You can close your eyes if you like."

He sat back in his armchair and closed his eyes.

Papa came into the room just then. Mama held her fingers up to her lips so Papa would not say anything. He sat down quietly on the couch next to Luisa, watching with a quirky look of disbelief.

Within a minute of holding both hands over João's head, I felt a dark, heavy feeling engulfing me, consuming what little energy I had. I felt like a drained battery and was forced to sit down next to him. He remained under whatever it was that kept him lifeless and with his eyes closed. Mama, Papa, and Luisa watched me with a look of, *now what?*

I shrugged my shoulders. I could see he was breathing, so I knew he wasn't dead. "You can now open your eyes and return to this room, without anger, calm and happy." I really didn't know what else to say.

What if I had fried João's brain when my energy collided with his? Would he ever return to normal? Would he be able to return to work as a chauffeur? It served me right for trying something that I had no idea how to do. His eyes remained closed and his breathing was shallow.

I touched his shoulder lightly with my left hand. "João, my friend. You need to come back and join us." We waited what felt like an eternity. Finally, to everyone's relief, he sat upright, took a deep breath, as if inhaling life back into his body, and opened his eyes. He then put his hands to cover his face and began to cry.

"Ms. Veronica," he said, "thank you. I feel like a new man." He wiped the tears from his face. "I want to apologize to everyone, and to you, Luisa, for hitting you. I'm going to do my best from now on to control my temper and be more patient."

Luisa jumped up and kissed him. They left the room with their arms around each other's waist.

"Go ahead, Veronica, do the same to your father." Mama said. "He needs it, too."

I felt burned out and didn't want to do any more *treatments.* The whole thing had gotten out of hand, but Papa flashed one of his condescending smiles.

"Go ahead, I'm your father and I should have a treatment, even though what I really need is a nap."

He eased into the couch and closed his eyes. I touched his head and said a few nurturing words, knowing he was just playing along with the whole thing. Soon after, I told him that he could open his eyes. He did, with a big smile on his face.

"Joachim, how are you feeling?" asked Mama.

"I feel great. That was very good, what you did to me, Veronica. Thanks, I feel wonderful." He winked at me. Then he whispered, "I cannot be hypnotized. A very famous doctor in Germany told me once, many years ago, that I'm not a good subject for this type of treatment. Only pathetic people can be hypnotized. I'm too resilient to be put under."

I had not hypnotized anyone, and I know nothing about hypnotism. I had done Reiki, or at least that's what I had tried doing. Perhaps what I had done didn't even have a name. Like Dr. Holdman, another chiropractor in New Jersey, once told me, the secret to being successful at helping people is the intention used. That's what makes it happen. I only knew that it worked with Mama, Luisa, and João.

I had no intentions of ever doing Reiki again. I was worried that I was getting into something that might be hazardous to my health. It had taken too much out of me, especially after I touched João. I'd do it again to help Mama, but no one else.

Mama asked me put my hand on her head and swear that when she died I would not cry. That was not the first time she had done that. She believed salty tears destroyed the eyesight.

"Mama, how can you ask me not to cry?"

"Veronica, I can't live forever. You have been a good daughter, the best I could wish for. There's no reason to cry. Swear to me that you won't cry."

Mama would never change. I had to accept her for who she was—a drama queen. I promised her I wouldn't cry.

When my friends returned to Lisbon, I learned they never made it to Coimbra. They had stopped at Eiriceira, the fishing village I had told them so much about, and fell in love with it.

Not long after arriving, they stood near a bridge overlooking the beach and talked about wanting to stay. A woman heard them and offered her house on the hill for five dollars a day. They followed the woman to her villa, which had a magnificent view of the ocean. Then she made an offer they couldn't resist. She would take them to the market daily so they could buy food, and then cook for them at no charge. They voted unanimously to remain in Eiriceira. Before returning to Lisbon, they gave her an extra hundred dollars for her hospitality.

I introduced my friends to my parents and Russell fell in love with my father who—amazingly enough—still spoke pretty good English. They connected like long-lost friends. My father was thrilled to have someone pay attention to what he said. Sara and Joyce felt more of a spiritual connection with Mama. I became the translator for Mama, who loved sharing with them the stories of her youth. Tania took a liking to Ruth and kept her busy playing in her parents' bedroom.

The night before Russell and his family left for the United States, Papa suggested we all take a walk through Alfama, the oldest part of Lisbon, and visit the São Jorge Castle, which sits upon the highest of Lisbon's seven hills. Mama couldn't come with us. She would never have been able to walk up those tortuous and steep narrow streets in that part of the city.

While we walked through Alfama, we all sang "Edelweiss," the song from the movie *The Sound of Music.* Papa could barely hold back his tears when he said, with a knot in his throat, "I love this life with my daughter and her good American friends. I'm very happy."

We took turns hugging him and then followed the sound of the *fado* music coming from the distance. It seemed to beckon us to find its source. The *fado* is the Portuguese blues, a very intense and emotional way of singing about love, and death. After walking up a few streets, we reached a large open plaza filled with tables and people drinking wine, eating typical Portuguese food, and listening to the singer that belted out successfully the sentiment of the *fado*. We took a table and joined the crowd eating freshly broiled sardines, black and green olives, and goat cheese, taking extra pleasure from dipping slices of rustic bread in olive oil. The *fado* singer maintained her passionate expression as she cried out one tune after another. My friends ate silently, mesmerized by the theatrical singer. Russell said to me, "I've never seen someone sing with so much emotion. Even though I have no idea what she is saying it grabs me right here." He pointed to his heart. Everyone agreed.

I explained, "The lyrics have a lot to do with the Portuguese word 'saudade' which means longing for someone."

I didn't translate the depressing lyrics. By the time we finished dinner it was too late to walk up to the castle; Ruth was tired and wouldn't stop crying.

The next day Russell and his family flew back to the United States. Sara and I would be staying in Lisbon two more days. Sara and I took a train to the beach of Cascais. We were shocked to see naked women sunbathing, but after a couple of them went back and forth we stopped staring and decided to eat our snacks and lie out in the sun in our one piece bathing suits like two old fuddy-duddies. At the end of the day we stopped to visit my parents.

I told them about the naked women on the beach. Mama said, "The last time I went to the beach, everyone was still using bathing suits." And Papa said, "They are young pathetic idiots, in a few more years they'll be ridden with skin cancer."

The next day Sara and I rode the trolley to the National Coach Museum located in Belem, a district of Lisbon. She was very impressed with the collection of antique carriages that had been used by the Portuguese royal families; some built as far back as 1716. Once the pungent odor of the old carriages entered my nostrils, I sneezed until we left the museum. We had lunch at a tavern and I introduced her to green soup and fried birds. On the way back, to see my parents, we stopped in downtown Lisbon. Sara suggested that we pick up a few loose cobblestones off the side of the road, to bring home as gifts. Each of us picked up six. I had to admit that as paperweights they were going to be very unique gifts.

That night, after Sara and I were in bed, I received a call from the pensão's manager. My brother, Max-Leão, whom I had not seen for I don't know how many years, was on his way up to our room. I jumped out of bed, but before I could get dressed, he was knocking at our door. Sara took a picture of my brother and me hugging, then he and I sat on my bed and talked until two about our lives and where they had taken us. Max-Leão lived with his British wife, Patricia, and their son and daughter in the south of Portugal. They kept a very private life. My parents rarely saw them. Now that Papa had taken upon himself to move out of his house and sell everything without consulting them, it had pushed them even further away. Thank God that Mama had called Max-Leão to tell him that I was in Lisbon and where I was staying; otherwise we would have missed each other.

The next morning, Sara and I were to be at the Lisbon airport by two o'clock for our three o'clock flight back to the United States. She said she would stay at the pensão and pack her luggage while I spent the morning with my parents.

When I left the pensão at seven in the morning, Sara was still sleeping. At noon I kissed my parents, Luisa and Tania, goodbye and found myself across the street from Luisa's apartment waving back at them.

At one window, Luisa waved goodbye alongside my mother who was slowly moving her hand from side to side, very much like the queen of England did when she was waving to a cheering crowd, but Mama didn't smile. Her eyes stared as if looking beyond the horizon. At the other window were Papa and little Tania.

Tania was laughing at Papa who was smiling and dramatically moving his right hand in the air as if he were conducting an orchestra with an invisible baton. Odd that Papa was doing that when Mama was the one who had wanted to be a maestro when she was a young woman.

I remained at the street corner for as long as possible, waving back and then, feeling like a coward running away from the enemy, I ran down the avenue and most of the way to the pensão. Sara was far from being ready, which made me frantic about catching the plane on time. By the time she finished packing and getting dressed, it was two in the afternoon. I didn't think it was a good idea to take a chance waiting for the bus and suggested a taxi.

The taxi driver must have thought that we were both foreigners and wasn't taking the usual way to the airport.

"Excuse me, but why aren't you using the avenue that will take us directly to the airport?" I asked him.

"I'm the taxi driver. How dare you question me?"

"Because I'm Portuguese and I know these streets well enough to know that you're taking us for a ride."

"You worry too much. You'll get to the airport in plenty of time."

"Yeah after you over charge us for a longer drive." I turned to Sara and said loud enough for him to hear me. "Portuguese taxi drivers are known for their dishonesty and this one takes the cake."

"Tell him that if we miss our flight I'll sue him." Sara told me.

The drive should have taken us twenty minutes, but instead took forty-five. We didn't tip him.

We both ran into the airport, but it was too late. The plane was getting ready for take off, and no matter what I said, they were not going to let us board.

Then Sara spoke—the personification of the rude American.

"How dare you tell us we can't board our plane, to the United States of America. How dare you tell us that we've lost our rights as Americans. How dare you refuse us to board our own plane? I don't care if it has taken off or not. You get that plane to return, now, and take us out of here. My wrist watch says five minutes to three, we still have five minutes." Her voice escalated as she added, "I will not remain in this forsaken country one more day because you've decided to leave five minutes early. Get that plane down, now!"

I instinctively stepped away from her, but her voice had been heard. They didn't even check our luggage. A man that looked like an airport security guard asked us to follow him. Sara kept going at him, and finally he said to me in Portuguese, "Please tell your uncouth American friend to shut up. I'm personally taking you both aboard the damn plane."

Indeed, the plane had been taxiing, but had stopped mid-runway, like a giant hen waiting for her two fledglings to get under her wings. There was a curious look from the passengers when we boarded.

As we both walked down the aisle to get to our seats a female passenger asked me. "Who are you that you can stop a plane from taking off?"

Sara answered, "We're Americans, that's who we are. And we're going home."

Sara and I buckled up and she wore a smile of accomplishment.

"Sara, only you could have pulled this one off." I shook her hand.

Sometimes it pays to be obnoxious.

~ *Chapter Four* ~

Choices

August 4

I'm back in school but it's hard to concentrate on my studies when my thoughts are with my parents. I need to get them out of Portugal as soon as possible. I spoke with Russell and Sara and they agreed that my parents are too old to wait months or even years for all the official paperwork to enter the US. We played with the idea that perhaps they could come over as tourists and "forget" to go back. We doubt the government is going to bother to deport two old folks.

I received a letter from Mama telling me once more that she was not allowed to write freely. Luisa was confiscating all her letters and then deciding which ones would be mailed. But Mama came up with a brilliant idea. She waits until Luisa is out of the apartment and then she puts her letter in an envelope and ties it to a string and lowers it out of the living room window onto the street. When someone goes by, she explains that she is too sick to go out and asks that person to put the letter into the corner mailbox. Mama is definitely a genius.

Yesterday I checked out a retirement home not too far from my apartment. I almost fell backwards when I learned how much they charged. For both my parents it would cost more than my yearly college tuition. The only way to make this happen was if they came for a visit and I hid them in my apartment. But how was I going to take care of them while in school all day? One thing was definite: they couldn't stay living with

Luisa. On my last visit, I mentioned to Papa the possibility of him and Mama going to a retirement home in Lisbon. His response was, "The day I go to an old folks home, I won't live much longer. I will kill myself."

The other option was to quit school and get a job. But if I worked, who would be home to take care of them during the day? Once I become a chiropractor I could—I hope—afford to pay someone I trust to take care of them, but I don't know if they would last that long. I planned to call Papa the next morning before going to school.

"Papa, I'm coming to Portugal on my next school break to bring you and Mama over here. You can live with me in my apartment while I go to school." I figured once they were here I'd come up with a solution.

"I'm like an old tree," Papa said. "My roots are deeply planted here. I can't be transplanted. It's out of the question. Besides, Luisa needs me; she depends on the money I give her every month."

When I heard that, I was upset but didn't say anything.

I bought a pair of scissors and chopped away at my hair. I looked like a punk rocker.

Nieght, one of my Vietnamese classmates, was impressed with my hair cutting skills and asked me if I'd cut his hair, too. I bought a barber's brush and a plastic smock.

While I cut Nieght's hair, he told me stories about Vietnam and how many times he and his family had tried to escape by boat. Even though he was only ten years old, he still wound up in prison with his family. He felt very lucky they had finally made it to the US. I admired how he had conquered our language. He is only twenty-four but very mature.

A few days ago, Steve and Diane offered to have my parents live with them in New Jersey, but last night Steve called to say they withdrew the offer. Given they both work, no one would be home to take care of my parents during the day. On top of that, the medical coverage they have in Portugal for drugs and emergency visits to the hospital would not be valid in the United States.

Robert and I bumped into each other in the hallway between classes and we hugged, but I remained cool when he whispered in my ear, "I was thinking about you last night. I miss you."

I gave him a gentle push and smiled. "Yes, we had a good time together, but I'm still very happy with my new boyfriend."

Robert didn't know that I was talking about my stuffed Teddy bear. Until I found the man of my dreams, Teddy would have to do.

Some of my classmates told me how beneficial group studies could be, so I joined one. I gave up after the second meeting at the library. My voice was too low to be heard, and I was too shy to speak up when I didn't hear something.

Ralph told me to stop saying that I'm deaf. According to him, I only have a hearing deficit because I still have one good ear.

It wasn't just my hearing deficit that was a problem with the study group. They wasted too much time talking about mundane things. It was nothing more than a social gathering. Josh, one of the students in the group, tried to talk me into working with him as a masseuse. He said that as a couple we could earn very good money. I told him that I needed my free time to study. Besides, I was doing well with my government loan. It would only take me away from studying.

I didn't tell him that when I was in New Jersey during one of my school breaks, I had an awkward massage experience. My son, Steve, who at the time was doing quite well doing massages, convinced me that I could make pretty good money, and he could even find me a client. I was at Steve's apartment when he received a call. He handed me the phone, after saying, "Mom, this guy seems to be a straightforward, honest person, and he's looking to have a massage this evening. It's one hundred dollars for one hour; do you want to talk to him?"

I picked up the phone.

"Hi, I understand that you want a massage this evening?"

"What's your name, honey?"

"My name is Veronica."

"Veronica, that's a very sexy name. You sound very young. How old are you?"

"Is that important?" I said, afraid to lose the job if I told him I was half a century old.

"Veronica, you have a very sexy accent. I like that. Veronica, do you use toys?"

"Not since I was a child. Why would I use toys now? I'm an adult."

"Put Steve back on the phone."

That was why I wouldn't do massages.

Just before I left for my morning class I received a phone call from Mama. "Veronica, I love you. I just wanted to hear your voice." Then she hung up.

Wouldn't Luisa or her husband be able to tell when they get the phone bill that someone in their house had made a five-second phone call to the United States?

Josh asked me again in school to go out with him after I have told him several times that I'm married.

"You don't look married. You'll have to come up with a better excuse than that."

"I have a picture of my husband and our older son. Would you like to see it?" I handed him the two pictures I carried in my backpack. I expected Josh to have a horrified look and ask me if they were for real.

Instead, he said, "Wow…this is your family, hum? Wow… Your husband and your son, hum? Wow…amazing…you have a very nice family." He was obviously lying.

I knew he would not ask me out again.

The pictures I showed him were part of a joke that Al and Ralph came up with, when I was still taking my pre-meds in Georgia. With lots of make-up including blackening their front teeth they were able to change their physical appearances to the opposite extremes and then took pictures of each other. The story was that they had taken ZZ compound, a drug name they made up, which supposedly reversed the aging process. The idea was to show that with Al the drug had worked, but with Ralph it had transformed him into an old, disgusting-looking man. I carried the *before* and *after* photos in my backpack to amuse myself before taking a test, it helps me relax.

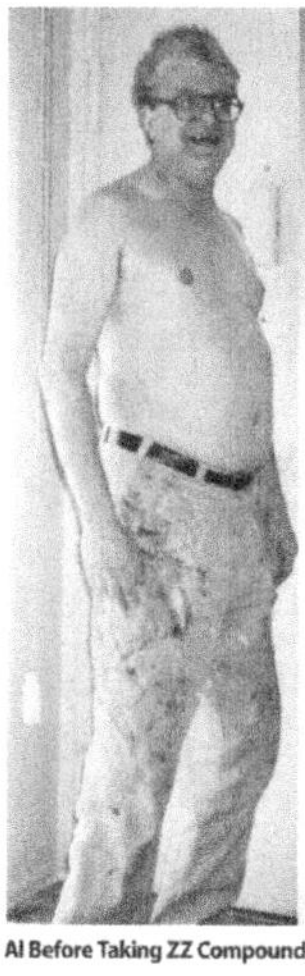

Al Before Taking ZZ Compound

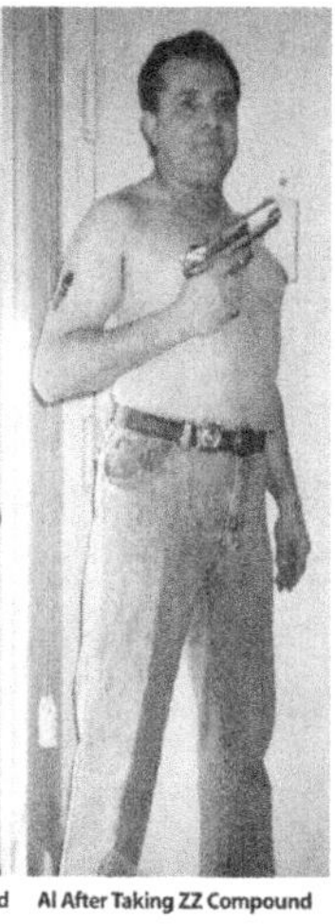

Al After Taking ZZ Compound

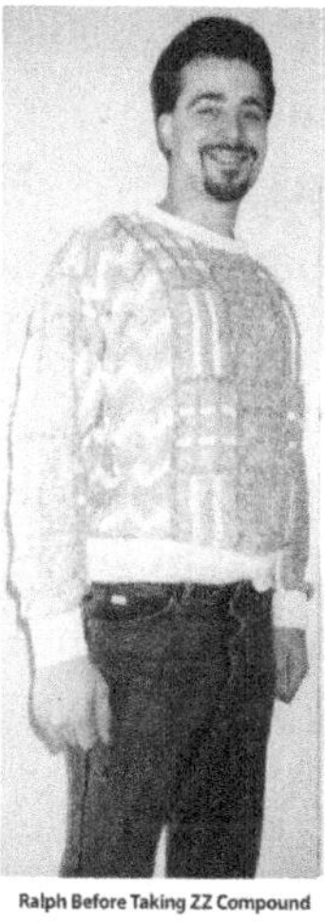

Ralph Before Taking ZZ Compound

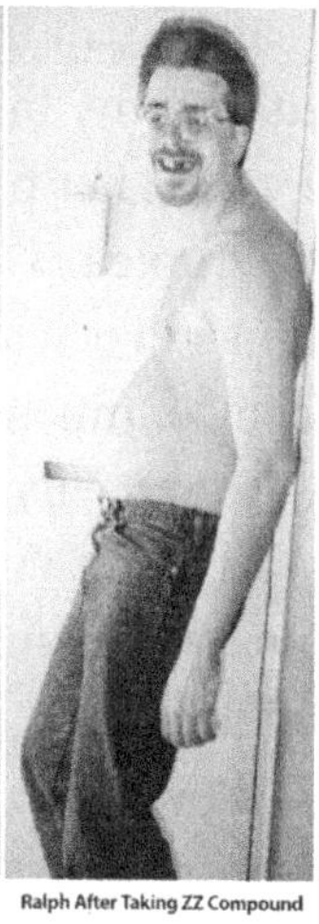

Ralph After Taking ZZ Compound

Harold the Hateful called. He needed to practice with the stethoscope and promised that it wouldn't take more than a few minutes of my time. I couldn't say no.

As soon as he entered my apartment, he began complaining about the Jews, the blacks, the gays, the other students, and the teachers. He hates everybody.

He took my blood pressure, listened to my heart and lungs. Gathering my courage I said, "Okay, now I need to get back to studying, by myself."

He looked like he had sucked on a lemon.

"Veronica, would you mind if I come over when I'm depressed? You make me feel younger." He gave a feeble smile.

"You're only forty-five. Of course you feel younger when you're with me."

"I know, but you have a young attitude that's very contagious. I need that."

Why I don't attract normal men, I'll never know. Yet I'm happy being single; I don't have to put up with anyone. Being single is the best thing that could have happened to me.

Mama did it again. She called and hung up. When I called back she said, "I just want you to know that I'm alone and it's safe to call me. If Luisa is here I won't be able to tell you what's on my mind."

I called her back.

"Veronica, I have a special favor to ask you. Will you promise that when I die you'll buy me a pink marble stone fifteen centimeter high to be put over my grave?"

"Mama, why are we talking about stuff like that…?"

"Oh, I don't intend to go anywhere for many more years to come, I just want to make sure that when the time does come, you know what kind of stone I want."

"Okay then…."

"I'd like my tombstone to have my name, followed by Wife, Mother, Author, Artist and Music Composer."

"I promise. I'll take care of it."

"Thank you Veronica. I know it's a lot to ask you to do but I give you my word that I will pay you back someday."

I could understand how Mama felt. She wanted a mark of some kind that showed her existence wasn't in vain. She wanted to be recognized. I wrote this diary, Mama wanted a stone. But neither a diary nor a stone could provide the true value of living. In the end, all that mattered was to be able to die without regrets. Friends and family are nice to talk to but when it comes to saying what's on my mind I find that writing is the best for me. Sometimes I wish I could disappear into the universe, but I would miss my grandson, Jacob. I want to see him grow up and become a man.

August 29

Lawrence, one of my classmates, was gay. It wasn't until we teamed up to study that we became friends. His apartment reminded me of an exotic Arabian palace. There was no furniture in his living room. Blue and gold curtains swept out from a small mirrored sphere in the center of the ceiling and draped down the walls. Below it, in the center of the room, live orchids hung over a rock formation. He had tossed about a dozen large pillows that he had embroidered, around the room.

"Those rocks…"

"It wasn't easy bringing them into the apartment but I made a special arrangement with the landlord."

"The room is very calm and relaxing, and if I may say, very sexual."

"It's seductive, my dear."

Sometimes we would hang in the hallway between classes, laughing and chatting about our taste in men and which guy walking towards us was the most handsome.

I found that cutting hair, feeding my friends Portuguese soups, and being available when they needed someone to talk to could be a very fulfilling experience.

Russell, who lived forty-five minutes from school, would come over when he was tired to take a pick-me-up nap on my Asian couch, which he swore was more comfortable than his bed. I gave him a key to my apartment and if I came home and found him sleeping on the couch, I would go about my business. Sara would come by once a week to check her two tomato plants growing in garbage containers in my back patio. Where she lived she only had room for three containers. Leila loved my bathroom décor and found it so luxurious that every time she was over for a psychotherapy session, she took a shower. My weakness as a good psychotherapist was that I couldn't keep my mouth shut while listening to her complain about her mother not loving her enough.

I told her what had happened during my last visit to Portugal, and how my mother and I had discovered that we did love each other.

"You say that because your mother listens to you. My mother doesn't. She is very hard to talk to."

"If you keep saying that, then that's what it is. You need to put a piece of tape over her mouth and make her listen to you."

We laughed.

"Veronica, you're a funny psychotherapist."

"Look, being a parent doesn't make people automatically accredited from some kind of Parenthood University. It only meant that they had sex and procreated. You need to visit your mom during the next school break and make peace with her or you'll have to live the rest of your life crying over it."

"Okay, I'll do it even though I don't expect any miracles."

I was already in bed when Mama called but this time didn't hang up. Luisa's sister, Rosa, was there. She had just been diagnosed with muscular dystrophy. Mama wanted me to treat her over the phone, like I had done for Luisa and her husband. My first reaction was, are these people out of their minds?

"Tell me what to do, Veronica, and I'll pass your healing energy to Rosa. She's very sick."

"Mama, you're kidding me?"

"Yes, Veronica." She paused. "I can help her; just tell me what to do next."

"You know that this is ridiculous, right? How can I help her over the phone?"

"Yes." She paused again. "I understand and I'll do the best I can. Just keep guiding me. And now what is it that you want me to do next?"

"Mama, it's good to hear your voice. Are you doing okay?"

She hesitated. "No, Veronica. I didn't get that. You want me to hold my hand over Rosa's head?"

I sat up in bed and took a deep breath. "Mama, if you're answering my questions, tell me so with a yes."

"Yes. That's a good idea Veronica. You keep telling me what to do, and I'll carry on with the treatment."

"Is Luisa hurting you? Can Papa help you?"

"Yes, Veronica," she answered. "No, Papa can't help me with the treatment, you know how he is."

"Why don't you and Papa leave Luisa's apartment and go live at the pensão where I stayed? It's clean and the people are very nice."

"That's very hard to do." Again she paused. "My arm is getting tired from keeping my hand over Rosa's head. Even my ribs hurt, for no reason, of course. I love you, my daughter, Veronica. Thank you for guiding me with the treatment. You really think that Rosa needs another treatment tomorrow? Oh, okay. I'll let Luisa know. I'm sure she wants her sister to get better. Bye-bye my love."

Mama missed her calling as an FBI agent. She was a truly amazing woman.

I received a letter from Mama. She still spent the days alone at home. When she had spoken to me on the phone, her ribs were hurting because she had fallen. She believed she had broken several, but they would not take her to the hospital. Luisa was not feeding her properly and wouldn't help her wash.

Trying to keep my head clear over all this madness and keep my studies going, I wrote to Aunt Coty and asked her to please visit my parents and check out their situation. Perhaps she could put some sense into my father's head to come to the US or move to England with my mother, since his cousins in London had offered them a place to stay. If they don't want to leave Portugal, then they should move to the pensão, where I had stayed when I visited them. Something had to be done immediately.

My letter to Aunt Coty resulted in a phone call from Portugal at four-thirty in the morning. It was a very angry Luisa. Aunt Coty had spoken to Papa, who in turn told Luisa that I had advised him and Mama to leave her place.

"You! Come over right now and take your parents to America!"

"How is your sister, Luisa?" I used the same subdued voice I had used during her Reiki treatment.

My parents must have been in the room because she spoke away from the phone. "Your daughter is crazy. I tell her to come and get you both and she asks me about my sister."

Mama came to the phone.

"Veronica, Luisa is like an angel, the way she treats me."

"Yeah, Mama, I know, more like the angel from Hell."

"Yes." She paused. "I cannot ask for more than that. The whole thing has been a misunderstanding. As you know, Luisa is the kindest friend I could ask for."

"If I come over to get you will you and Papa come back with me?"

"No. Your father doesn't want to go to England or America and I won't go without him. We're both perfectly happy living here with Luisa. She treats us very kindly and there's no reason for us to leave. The whole thing has been a misunderstanding, that's all."

I hung up, feeling as though I were going out of my mind. I climbed into the shower and stood under the hot water until I stopped shaking. I needed to come to terms with the fact that my parents were lost. They wouldn't listen to me and I couldn't help them.

September 7

We were almost at the end of the quarter when Lawrence's mother died. He sewed a dress for his mother and was actually looking forward to combing her hair and putting makeup on her face. I admired his strength to be able to do all that. He left me in charge of watering his houseplants while he was in Connecticut. His orchids were to receive an ice cube each on Tuesday.

I received a letter from Papa saying that he and Mama must leave Luisa's house at all costs. They were being emotionally and physically abused and he had enough of it. He asked me to send my letters to Aunt Coty's house and then he would stop by her house to pick them up. There was no reason to wait any longer I was leaving immediately to get them.

I called Papa to make the arrangements and his answer was, "Nothing can be done for us."

"Papa, you wrote to me telling me what you need to get out of there. Let me help you."

"I changed my mind. I can't leave Luisa; I can't abandon her."

I tried to remain focused in my studies.

Aunt Coty called to tell me that she visited my parents once again. Now she understood why Papa had not paid her back what he borrowed. He gave the money he received each month to Luisa. Aunt Coty started arguing with Luisa, and Papa told Aunt Coty to butt out of their business and the apartment. I could no longer count Aunt Coty to help them. They were not speaking to each other.

Between studying for finals that week and worrying about my parents I was feeling depressed and very frustrated.

When Sylvia, passed out hand-made invitations for her famous end-of-the quarter party, she skipped my desk. I called her as soon as I got home.

"I'm very hurt you didn't invite me to your party."

"I meant to, but I didn't see you in class."

I pulled out a dry laugh from my inner guts and said, "You gave an invitation to the person on my right, to the one on my left, the one seated in front of me, and the one seated behind me. Are you telling me I'm invisible? Or are you telling me you hate me because you still think I stole Dexter from you?"

"I know you didn't steal Dexter. I just didn't see you, I swear. I'll give you an invitation, tomorrow, at school."

"Thanks, but I can't come to your party unless you apologize for having accused me wrongly and obviously still holding a grudge against me."

"Okay, I apologize." Her voice rose slightly.

"Thanks. I feel a lot better now. See you tomorrow."

The next day, I was standing in the hallway with Leila and Sara, after one of our finals. Sylvia was giving out more invitations. When she saw us, she walked over and handed an invitation to each of us, saying, "These are for you guys. I hope you can make it." She walked away.

Leila said, "Such a snob. She's never invited me before."

"She thinks we are too old for her crowd of friends," said Sara. "I'm not going. Are you?"

"Are you kidding? I can't stand her," said Leila. Then she walked to the trashcan and dropped in her invitation. We followed her and did the same.

I had ten days off before next quarter. Not much time to do anything. Maybe I was getting lazy, but I opted to stay home. I planned to touch up the paint on my apartment walls, clean my desk, and hang out at the pool and hot tub. I'd cook a bunch of meals and freeze them, enough to last me through the beginning of next quarter, which promised to be very demanding with a lot more diagnostic classes in preparation for being an intern at the college's chiropractic clinic.

~ *Chapter Five* ~

The Teacher's Pet

September 21, 1994

Classes had just begun but I was already feeling apprehensive about the next quarter when as a clinician I would be adjusting patients at the college's chiropractic clinic under the supervision of a staff doctor. My anxiety, increased significantly when my classmate Maryann had a meltdown prior to performing a manual adjustment in class.

"Please, Dr. Lawson, don't make me do it." Tears rolled down her face, along with her mascara, giving her a dark gory look.

"You're being silly. You know very well what to do." Dr. Lawson had little patience with whiny students, especially Maryann whose voice always had a whimpering tone.

"But I'm scared I'll break her neck. Sally is my friend." Maryann sobbed.

Dr. Lawson pulled a few tissues from her coat pocket and handed them to Maryann. "Clean your face. You're scaring the crap out of Sally." She then smiled and added, "I understand how you feel, but you have to trust me when I say I wouldn't allow you to adjust her neck if you weren't ready. You need to let go of your fears, Maryann, relax. Take a deep breath. Let your Innate Intelligence guide you and, for Pete's sake, adjust Sally's neck."

Maryann regained her composure and, under the teacher's guidance, adjusted Sally's neck without any problems.

After the dramatic episode in class, I eagerly began exchanging spinal adjustments with other students. Josephine, a student, who was two quarters ahead of me, warned me about such practices. "You'll be sorry. I did that and now I'm suffering from ligament instability. My neck and back are trashed. I'm telling you, as a friend, stay away from unskilled students that want to practice on you."

I knew she was right, but that was the nature of the beast, I couldn't expect students to let me practice on their spine and not return the favor.

September 23

I finally called a hemorrhoid clinic and made an appointment. What convinced me wasn't the pain from the hard chairs at school but the bright red blood I'd found in the toilet that morning. I was terrified when the doctor I spoke to on the phone said that from my description it sounded like I had external hemorrhoids and they were best treated by strangulation. That night I barely slept but at three in the morning, it suddenly hit me—if the saying was true that we were what we ate, my symptoms had to be the result of something I was ingesting.

I canceled further lunches with Leila at the Korean restaurant and started a non-spicy diet.

My only experience with hemorrhoids had been thirty years prior, after giving birth to Steve, my second son. During my check-up with the gynecologist, I was shocked to learn that I had two hemorrhoids.

"It's impossible. It doesn't hurt and there's nothing sticking out. How can that be?"

"That's because they're internal. It's normal for women to develop them after the serious straining they go through with pushing during the birth process."

I was sure Dr. Wanker had misdiagnosed me, but after three decades of hiding in the dark, the darn things had obviously escaped.

Within a week, all my symptoms vanished. I canceled my appointment at the hemorrhoid clinic and called Leila.

"You ain't going to believe this. I had a serious case of painful bleeding hemorrhoids and guess what? They're gone." I stopped myself from jumping up and down, but my voice was singing.

"Gone? How did you do that?"

"You've noticed I stopped eating at the Korean Restaurant with you."

"Yes, I know. But why…"

"Their food is tasty but too spicy. I've also stopped using pepper or hot spices in my food."

"That's it? Are you sure?" And then she lowered her voice. "I've the same problem."

"You mean hemorrhoids?"

"Yes, and they bother me a lot. Do you think if I stop eating spicy food it will help me?"

"If what you eat burns your lips, and mouth and throat, what do you think's going to happen when it comes out your anus?" I stared at the ceiling, the floor, anything to keep me from laughing.

"My God, it makes sense. I'm going to watch what I eat, too. I'll keep you posted about my, you know what."

"Leila, hemorrhoids are just veins that went bad, like varicose veins, nothing to be ashamed of."

"My mother has hemorrhoids. It's too much for me to admit that I have them too." She chuckled in the same distinctive tone as Muttley, my favorite cartoon dog.

October 1

I was walking in the college hallway when a teacher standing by the door to his office waived at me.

"Good morning, Veronica," he said.

"Good morning, Doctor." I couldn't remember his name and kept walking.

He called out, "Veronica, wait a second." He signaled with a finger to follow him into his office, where he handed me a VHS tape. "Take this home and watch it. It will help you study the Diversified Adjusting Technique for next week's exam."

I read his name tag, Dr. Smith. Then I remembered him. Last quarter, I was practicing a manual sacroiliac adjustment on Lee, a fellow student, when my contact arm and hand slipped off his back and I fell face down on top of him. That's when Dr. Smith entered the adjusting room and stood at the doorway with a look on his face as if we were doing something indecent. "What's going on in here between you two?"

"This is not what you think. My hand slipped." And I quickly got up and so did Lee who felt as embarrassed as I was.

October 4

Donna called from California. About a year ago, she and Cody, along with Dexter moved, to the chiropractic college in California, because they didn't like the academics at this college.

"Why you are still there when *our* college is so much better? They even sell brown rice at the cafeteria!"

Her enthusiasm made me smile. It was nice to have friends who cared, but I wondered if Dexter, my ex-boyfriend had something to do with her trying to lure me into moving. I'm into healthy food, but I'm not a nut over it.

October 6

When I arrived with Bryan, my colleague and *volunteer* patient for my test on the Diversified Adjusting Technique, my instructor, Dr. Lewis was missing. In her place stood Dr. Smith, looking sternly at me from behind a small desk. He would be my examiner. The room was colder than I expected. There was nothing attractive about the white walls, a desk on the corner and an adjusting table in the center.

Dr. Smith wasted no time. "Show me how you perform a right posterior to anterior move at T7."

I instructed Bryan, to lie face down on the adjusting table. I demonstrated my stance and how I'd position my hands and fingers during the move but I wasn't to use any thrust. Dr. Smith watched with a serious look. He asked Bryan to leave and told me to stay and sit down. He pulled the black curtain room divider behind him. I figured I had failed and he wanted to talk to me in private.

"I could tell you were nervous. Don't worry. I'm going to pass you anyway."

"Thank you. You're very kind." I stood, ready to leave. He stopped me by putting a hand over my shoulder, and then he put his arms around my waist and held me in a close embrace. He whispered on my right ear, "*We* admire you and *we* like you a lot. *We* will look after you."

I wanted to ask who the heck are *we,* the teachers? Why wasn't he straightforward about being *him* that liked me?

Maybe I was reading too much into it. Maybe he felt sorry for me and hugging me so intensely was his way of showing he cared. I pushed him away delicately. "Thank you, doctor, for being my friend." I left the room.

It wasn't every day a teacher showed interest in me. That night I couldn't sleep. I tried to make sense of what had happened at school, but had no luck, so I turned my thoughts to Mama. Cursed by a family full of medical doctors, she was used to their philosophy that, if there was no pain, there was no problem. But as a future chiropractor, I knew better. Drugs were nothing but a temporary bandage. If Mama's doctors took a proper history and followed up on her living conditions, they would realize that they needed to move her and my father out of Luisa's house even if taken by force, in order to save their lives. Instead, they kept her sedated. Mama's health was a direct result of her living conditions and the prescriptions she took. The drugs were no different from those that Alice used to murder my brother José. The more I thought about it, the clearer it became that I had to stop school and go live with my parents for as long as they needed me. I could open a chiropractic office in Lisbon and, with luck make enough money to take care of them. My background as a music teacher and theater producer wouldn't provide a decent income; I would need to practice chiropractic in Portugal without a license, if that were possible.

Life Chiropractic College had helped to introduce chiropractic all over the world and Dr. Smith was on their teaching staff. He had given me a passing grade when I had failed the test, maybe he would know a way for me to practice in Portugal illegally. I made an appointment to see him at school.

Dr. Smith listened patiently and then said, "You need a chiropractic degree to practice in Portugal and there's no way around that. How can you even think of quitting school and giving up everything you've worked so hard for all these years, you're making a big mistake. And like me, your parents will be very disappointed with you."

"They would. You're right. I won't be much help if I don't have a way of making a living." I was thinking out loud, but then said directly to him, "I should tell you, I'm not happy you passed me the other day. I didn't deserve it."

He stared at me. I had hurt his feelings, I was sure. Perhaps he was more of an ally than I gave him credit for. My mind was racing, and I said, "I really could use help practicing the Diversified Adjusting Technique. If I were to gather a few other students, would you consider supervising us once a week?" I knew I was asking a big favor, but I had nothing to lose.

"Veronica, I don't have the time to do that, and besides the college would not go for it. How about if you come to my office and I teach you there? You can practice on me—all you like."

He stood, walked toward me, and handed me his business card. Then he lifted me by my hands and held me close to him. *My goodness he's so tall and his face reminds me of a stuffed frog. Definitely not my type. But if hugs are all he needs in order to help me, so be it.*

He kissed my neck, then my ear. I turned my face away, so he kissed me on the corner of my mouth. I wasn't fighting him off, but I wasn't encouraging him either. He let go and said, "Call me."

If the way he kissed was merely a sign of pure friendship, I needed mental help, because I saw it as more than that. But he was the only teacher I knew that was willing to go out of his way to help.

When I arrived, Dr. Smith was the only one in his clinic. He locked the door behind me and gave me a tour, turning lights on and then off, as he proudly showed me around. We walked through the spacious reception area, down the hallway, past the two bathrooms, and five adjusting rooms. Then he opened the door to his office. "This is where I provide my patients with a report of findings."

"It's very nice. I like the wall colors." I pointed to the framed portrait of a woman hanging on the wall behind his mahogany desk. "Who is that lady in the picture, your mom?"

"My wife."

"Oh, I'm sorry. It's kind of dark in here, makes it hard to see." I felt bad, but knowing he was married helped me relax.

I followed him to one of the adjustment rooms, and he laid down supine on an adjusting table. "Go ahead. C5 on the right side needs to be moved." He crossed his arms over his large abdomen.

His head felt like a bowling ball, and his short neck made it hard for me to find the vertebral segments. My hands shook from the weight of his head.

"Veronica, when you open your practice, don't bother getting malpractice insurance. You're too gentle to injure anyone."

I didn't take that remark as a compliment. I put his neck into position and thrust without fear. The distinguished sound associated with a manual manipulation was heard, loud and clear.

"Very good. You did it, girl." He sat up and smiled. "You may not realize this but I purposely requested to be your examiner during the midterm exams. I'm very attracted to you."

I grabbed my backpack and slung it over my shoulders.

He stood. "I like you a lot. Will you stay with me tonight?"

I moved backwards out of his reach and walked out of the room trying, not to show any fear even though the hallway had grown darker and double in length. He followed me as I tried to open the front door. It wouldn't budge.

"Can you please unlock the door? I want to go home." I knew my voice was trembling.

"Is this it? You're leaving?" He put a hand on my right shoulder.

I flashed him a look that could have struck him dead. Being in theater for ten years, I could show a lot of emotion without words. He removed his hand, took the keychain from his pocket, and unlocked the front door. My instincts told me to act calm and walk normal until I was in the safety of my car. A few blocks down the road, I pulled into someone's driveway, turned off the engine, and waited to stop shaking. (I can't believe how naïve I used to be. That and my constant quest for adventure and excitement took away a lot of my common sense. Whenever I recall these types of episodes in my life, I wonder how I escaped unharmed. My mother used to say, "I already went through that and I'm trying to save you the heartache." I would answer rebelliously, "Mama, I have to experience my own blunders, so that I can make my own deduction if it's good or bad for me." Even today everything I do has to be hands-on if I'm going to grasp the whole concept.)

As soon as I got home I called Leila. Leila wore many hats. She used to be a sex therapist, a psychotherapist, and a caterer, not all in that order.

"Veronica, don't go back to his clinic. He's married. Sooner or later he will get his way, and that's bad karma."

I had no intention of going back to Dr. Smith's clinic.

Dexter called. He started seeing a psychologist a week prior and he was very excited about it. "Veronica, I'm responding well to the treatment." I told him to keep me posted.

~ *Chapter Six* ~

Life's Lessons

October 7

I mailed a letter to Aunt Coty to give to Papa. I knew Luisa confiscated Mama's mail and couldn't be sure she wasn't confiscating his. But a week went by and I didn't hear from him. If I didn't hear anything by that afternoon, I would call the house. Papa called that morning.

"Veronica, my daughter, I will never leave Luisa. Please forget about us going to America. As I've said before, I'm like an old tree. I can't be transplanted. I must stay here. Please, stop asking us to leave and thank you for respecting my feelings."

I do not give up easily, but I took his request as being an official statement. He was not leaving Luisa, and Mama had made it clear, that she was not leaving Papa. I had to accept their destiny and go on with my own life.

Mama had done a great job convincing Luisa I could treat her family over the telephone—for whatever ailed them. At least I was guaranteed to hear Mama's voice once a week and that was as good as it was going to get.

October 8

Dexter called. "I have great news. I've been seeing the psychologist I told you about and it's already making a marked difference in my life."

"How's that?" Holding the phone against my right ear since I'm deaf on the left side I did my best to stir the oatmeal with my left hand.

"I'm no longer afraid of showing emotion. Listen, are you ready?"

"Yeah…"

"I love you. So…what do you think?"

"Impressive." I tried giving meaning to the word and added, "Really impressive."

"My psychologist is doing a great job teaching me tricks on how to show affection and deal with my insecurities. She believes that if you attend a few sessions with me, it will be even more beneficial towards my recovery. Would you consider coming to California during the Christmas break?"

"I already made arrangements to go to New Jersey, but I wouldn't mind including a trip to California since I don't have to be back to school until January fifth."

"You make me so happy. Let me know the dates you'll be here and I'll make a few appointments. Veronica, I'm a completely changed man. There's no reason we should be apart anymore. You can move in with me, and we'll go to school together. You know what, we should get married. What do you say?"

If that was a marriage proposal, it had a lot to be desired. Did he actually expect me to say, yes to his casual proposal? The oatmeal was sticking to the bottom of the pan.

"Hello, are you there?" he asked.

"I'll see your psychologist with you, but living together or getting married is out of the question."

October 12

I got a phone call from New Jersey. Steve and Diane were expecting another baby. I couldn't wait to see Jacob, my grandson, now seventeen months old. How time flew. I always thought Ralph would be the first to get married and have children, since he was the eldest, but I had assumed too much. He would never get married. He was too busy dating.

"Why buy a cow, when you can get the milk for free?" One of Aunt Heydee's favorite proverbs.

October 13

Sometimes I wonder if Michael ever married or if he's still living with his mother. Michael was the first man I ever loved, and I can't allow myself to forget him. I like the idea that I can love someone forever, even if I'll never see him again. It's probably my Portuguese melodramatic way of feeling like a complete woman. I have a *real* love, an extraordinary treasure hidden deep within my heart, and no matter how much time goes by, it lives on and on.

Ralph called from Oregon. Every weekend we exchange anecdotes about our experiences in college. He told me about the IQ test he had taken a few days ago and, just for fun, asked one of the math questions. After a few struggling moments, I said, "Sixty-four pounds?"

"That's right, mom. Congratulations! But how did you know?"

"I multiplied the number you gave me by eight."

"That's amazing, because that's not the way to get the answer. But you did it."

"Yeah, tell me about it. The test proves I'm not smart, just lucky."

"Mom, you need to stop being so hard on yourself. You answered correctly and that's all that matters."

Ralph has always been very supportive of everything I do, but when it comes to numbers I have a well-deserved inferiority complex confirmed by my ineptitude to even dial the phone without pressing the wrong number.

October 20

On the way to my morning class, I noticed a black-and-white flier on the hallway wall with a picture of a young Asian woman, a student at our college, who had been missing for a week. Below her picture was a phone number for the campus police department. Before going home I stood in the hallway staring at her photograph. There was no smile not even in her eyes.

Before falling asleep, I wished I could *see* what had happened to the missing girl. I believed I could be clairvoyant if I concentrated on it.

I woke at five in a cold sweat and my heart pounding. My dreams were usually in color, but this one was dark and made of several shades of gray thick with clouds that drenched me with rain and soaked my flannel pajamas. I wasn't wearing shoes, and my feet were like ice. I took refuge in what looked like a farmer's house. A family of seven sat at a large wood table in the kitchen eating fried chicken legs, green beans and mashed potatoes. I asked them if they had seen the girl I was looking for. They refused to acknowledge my presence. I left through their back door and walked along a dark riverbank, where I almost stepped on a flat tombstone. I sensed that she had drowned and the stone symbolized her need to be buried.

I dressed and rushed out to talk to the campus police.

Mr. Johnson, the officer in charge of the case listened briefly, took no notes and asked no questions. Finally he said, "We're already working with a psychic, but your information could be valuable, so I'm taking you to talk with Ms. Natasha. Let me call her and tell her we're coming."

"I really don't have the time for that. I have a class starting in an hour." *I felt disappointed, and frustrated. I had just given him a complete description of the house and the river site, all he had to do was to go there. What was his problem? What kind of a cop was that?*

He insisted I follow him.

Ms. Natasha lived in a small cottage, a five minute walk across the campus. When I entered her house, I inhaled a lungful of stagnant tobacco, and let loose a series of loud sneezes that continued until my sinuses adapted to the environment. Ms. Natasha sat propped up by half a dozen dark purple pillows on a beat-up red velvet couch. Dark antique furniture and an abundance of ceramic knickknacks cluttered the tiny room. A table lamp next to the couch glared with a dull yellow light that complimented the red curtains covering the window behind her. *So this is how psychics live!*

She was in her mid-to-late fifties and wore a long, dark purple, baggy dress with a yellow and green flower pattern that was quite flamboyant. Several long strings of brown beads covered her chest. She possessed a wacky look in her eyes and I wondered if all clairvoyant people had that same stare. I must have also made an impression on her because she looked me up and down before she stood from the couch. She was shorter than I had thought, and her shoulder length black curly wig needed combing. I wondered how long she had been a psychic.

"I'd rather hug you," I said, opening my arms when she put her hand out to shake mine.

She hugged me stiffly, and then pulled away. It crossed my mind that like Dexter she had the same issues with touching. The cop remained by the front door watching us. She walked with a slight limp back to her couch and said, "Mr. Robertson tells me that your name is Veronica. Come. Sit next to me and tell me all about your dream."

I did, including what the family was eating.

"Are you telling me she's dead?" She watched me with skepticism.

I had never seen pupils like hers, one was green, the other brown. I stared at one eye and then the other, and nodded my head.

"You're wrong. Lisa is alive."

"Really? The dream felt so real."

"I know her personally and feel she ran away from her husband and is hiding. She's safe where she is."

"If you think that she's alive, that's great." I wasn't going to argue with a psychic.

She scribbled her phone number on a piece of paper and slipped it into my hand. "If you have any more dreams about Lisa, give me a call." She gave me a stern look. "When you came in, why did you hug me, instead of shaking my hand?" Her tone demanded an immediate answer.

"I'm a chiropractic student, hugging seems a natural thing to do." What I wanted to say was that it was more sanitary. A lot of people don't wash their hands after going to the bathroom.

"You're a liar. Hugging is for people who want to feel each others chi."

I didn't have the courage to ask her what a chi was. I was more than glad to get the heck out of there. I hate it when someone says I'm lying or think they can read my mind.

October 24

Laura, one of my classmates, returned my stethoscope set with one piece missing. When I asked her about it, she said I lent it to her that way. When am I going to learn not to lend my personal stuff? I once loaned a microphone to a friend. She dropped it right in front of me and didn't even apologize for denting the mic head. More than once I've lent out a book, and never got it back. When I lived in New Jersey, I let a friend use my favorite evening dress to a wedding and afterwards she asked me if she could keep it. I couldn't say no. I wished I could be more assertive. Like when Howard, the school hugger, called last night.

Leila had introduced Howard to me a few quarters back. He was famous for his hugging technique. But he lacked any sex appeal, and all my female classmates, when we saw him in school, welcomed his hugs without worrying about being attracted to him. But that was as far as I knew him.

"Hi, Veronica. How are you?"

"How did you get my phone number?"

"I asked our friend Leila. Is it too late for me to come over?"

"You know where I live?"

"Leila gave me your address."

I guessed he was too shy to say he wanted to borrow my notes like everybody else did or look at my wall where I had written the adjustment techniques on a plastic board. He arrived within fifteen minutes. My instinct told me not to hug him. Instead I pointed to the living room. "Have a seat." I went into the kitchen. "Would you like water or milk? I don't have anything else to offer." I spoke over the kitchen counter overlooking the living room. I felt protected behind it. Why did I say it was okay to come over? Why did I open the door to him?

Howard sat on a dining room chair with his head down and his back slightly curved forward, twirling his fingers on his lap. He reminded me of a weasel.

"No, I don't need anything to drink. Would you like a back massage? Would you like that?" He was the personification of *Count Dracula* just before biting his victim.

"My roommate will be home any moment." I should run into my bedroom and grab my handgun from under my pillow. Better safe than sorry. But then I thought it might be overreacting. Feeling bad for my negative thoughts and not wanting to hurt his feelings, I added courageously, "I have a lot of studying to do but if it doesn't take too long, I guess it's okay."

He asked me to sit on one of my dining room chairs and he pulled his chair behind me.

He massaged my shoulders softly without saying a word. My mind was racing, I didn't trust him behind me, yet I was afraid to act scared. Obviously my roommate was going to be home late. I lasted about two minutes, then stood and said, "Howard, that was a wonderful massage. Thank you, but I've a lot of studying to do. So… thanks for stopping by."

He left quietly. I never asked him why he came by. Leila had no right to give Howard my phone number and address. I intended to give her hell the next day, at school.

October 27

They found Lisa's body, the girl that disappeared a few weeks back. She had drowned in the river close to her house. I wished I had been wrong and had never seen that flier on the wall. I promised myself never to mingle in the spiritual world. It was a world of darkness and pain— not very different from reading the news. One of the reasons I stayed away from newspapers unless it was about art or a musical event.

October 28

Cida, and I were having our usual fun at the school cafeteria, jabbering in Portuguese, about school, teachers and students when she said, "I want to ask you a big favor, if you introduce me to anyone, don't tell them that I'm from Brazil!"

"Are you kidding? Why would you ask me to do that?"

"Brazilians are known all over the world for having no morals and I don't want to be associated with them."

"I don't know about that. The Portuguese admire the Brazilian's zest for life, and love them as if they were their own family—which in many ways, they are."

"The Portuguese may love them, but I don't. Don't forget that I was born in Brazil and lived most of my life there. They're not to be trusted. They'll steal from you and then kill you if they can."

When I was twelve, my parents contemplated on moving to Brazil until a cousin that lived in Rio de Janeiro wrote to my mom, warning her not to move to Brazil because crime was rampant. But that had been more than forty years ago. I couldn't believe things were still that bad.

Later that day Cida called. "There's a guy I want you to meet. He's not only handsome, but also very intelligent. I know you'll like him."

"Does he drink alcohol?"

"No. He's perfect for you. If I weren't married, I'd snag him in a heartbeat. You ready for this? He's very rich!"

"Does he smoke?"

"Yes, who doesn't?"

"I have no interest in him if he smokes."

"Are you out of your mind? Veronica, at least meet him and see if you like him."

"If he smokes he has an addictive personality. Sorry, not interested."

"You'll never find a man if you keep thinking like that. You're too nitpicky."

"I'm not in a hurry. I know what I want, and a smoker isn't in my future."

Being able to say *no* without worrying about someone's feelings was a great achievement for me. I was finally growing up and becoming a more mature woman.

November 2

Cida invited me to her house for lunch. I couldn't wait to check it out. A day didn't go by when she didn't brag about it.

Saying her house was big was an understatement. With six bedrooms and three bathrooms, it was more like a palace, each room an interior designer's dream. Her impeccable kitchen had two gas stoves with ten burners. "Wow Cida, you could bake a flan in one oven, a cheese cake in the other, boil water for spaghetti, make pasta sauce from scratch and brew up a variety of soups and stews—all at the same time. You can cook every three months and get away with it."

"I don't cook. It would get the kitchen dirty."

I prided myself in having a spotless apartment, but her house was *Snow White* perfect, as if no one lived there. To make matters worse, she lived under constant surveillance. A motion detector alarm system set throughout the house was controlled from her bedroom upstairs. I couldn't live like that. What if I had to go downstairs to get a glass of water in the middle of the night? Turn off the alarm every time I left my bedroom? The poor thing lived in constant fear of being assaulted.

For lunch she served a tomato salad and small tuna fish sandwiches without the crust. I was very careful not to drop any crumbs. When we finished eating she said, "Veronica, what I'm going to tell you is just between you and me." Her hands shook and her eyes filled with tears. "I was in my third floor apartment, in a very nice neighborhood of São Paulo, Brazil when a man from the floor above slid down a rope onto my balcony. He robbed me and raped me and left me for dead. I have no desire to return to my homeland. I love my country but I don't trust the people." I finally understood why she talked so much and so fast. She was trying to cover her thoughts with the sound of her words.

Cida and Raul, her husband, first came to the U.S. to work for a Hollywood movie star in California. Cida made me swear that I would never tell anyone the star's name. I was very impressed that she knew all the intimate details of *her* life and I was very disappointed to learn that *she* was not a nice person and very demanding. Raul, chauffeured, gardened, and took care of the mansion's maintenance. Cida handled the shopping, and was in charge of organizing the banquets. They worked for *the star* for seven years. Because they had a place to live and no expenses, they saved every penny they made, paying cash for their house, Cida's college tuition, and a new car for each of them. Raul now worked for a restaurant chain. Financially they were doing well.

Cida's success story was a good example of how the U.S. is truly a land of opportunity for those willing to work hard enough.

December 12

Sylvia and I sat next to each other in the hallway, waiting to be called to take our final neurology exam. "I'm worried." She took a deep sigh and added. "I'm scared that I'm not going to pass."

"Don't worry. It will all come to you."

"I didn't have time to study." Tears filled her eyes.

The old teacher in me came out.

I knew my strength in understanding a subject came from teaching, like when I used to teach guitar many years ago. The more I taught the better I played. So I was happy to go over the dermatomes and reflexes with her.When she came out of the exam room, she smiled, winked, and gave me a thumbs up.

With each final exam I took that week I felt more confident about January, when I'd be entering chiropractic clinic as an intern.

I owe Ralph for urging me to be academically self-sufficient. He was the one who that encouraged me to study on my own when we started chiropractic college together.

December 15

By seven in the morning, I had packed my car. I forced myself to eat a slice of raw, red onion. Someone at school told me that red onions helped to get rid of a runny nose due to a cold. After three slices my nose was running even more and so were my eyes. I cheated and put the rest of the onion between two slices of toasted bread.

Normally, my drive to and from New Jersey was lonely and tedious, but this time my friend, Sara would join me. I was thrilled when at eight o'clock she showed up with her luggage.

~ Chapter Seven ~

A Change of Heart

Winter of 1995

Today is January 13. I'm back in school, but everything in my life has changed since I took off for Christmas break.

After leaving Sara with her daughter in Philadelphia, I drove to Steve's apartment in Brick, New Jersey. Thank God I remembered my wool leg warmers; the winters in New Jersey were freaking brutal.

Diane, my daughter-in-law, now three months pregnant, worked at night and slept most of the day when Jacob was in daycare. Steve spent the days managing his music store. I saw Al only once, when he treated me to lunch at his favorite German Restaurant. After I had visited all my friends, the days began to drag and I couldn't wait to leave for California.

I was driving by a restaurant and decided to stop. I don't know what possessed me, but I asked the owner if he needed a waitress. He said a waitress had quit the evening prior, and if I could come back that afternoon, he'd be happy to hire me. He didn't even ask if I had any experience.

I had always wondered what would be like to wait tables in a diner, especially after having watched, the TV comedy sitcom *Alice* a few years back. Alice worked in a diner in Phoenix, and had a great time with her co-workers. This would be a rare opportunity to find out how much fun it could be.

I arrived an hour early and was fitted with an apron. My training consisted of the restaurant owner telling me to add one dollar to each bill.

"What if they ask what that is for?"

"Don't worry. Most of them don't even look at their bill, and if they do they're not going to question one dollar."

I would be working with two waitresses. When I met Meryl, she popped her gum at me. When I said hello to Rose, she ignored me. It was no better after I introduced myself to one of the cooks.

He was overweight, dripping in sweat, his clothes heavily stained. "Great, another idiot for me to work with." He pointed to the counter. "See that pin? Take the customer's order and stick the fuckin' paper on it. When the bell rings, grab the plates from the counter and deliver them to the table. And stay out of my way."

Loud elevator music played in the background. With that, and the customers chatter, I was concerned my hearing loss would be even more of a problem.

I smiled at the first couple that walked in and led them to a table. Before they even asked, I brought them water and took their order. When I walked into the kitchen, all I could hear was the two cooks cursing at each other.

I finished waiting on the couple. Before they left, they handed me a five-dollar tip. I shoved it in my pocket.

"What do you think you're doing with *our* tip?" Meryl yelled.

"Yeah, give me that," said Rose, reaching to pull the bill out of my apron.

I slapped her hand. "Stay out of my pocket."

"Until you work here for a month, you get none of the tips, missy. Or else you're gonna get one from me." Rose made a fist.

The restaurant owner showed up just in time. "You girls can go at it when we close tonight. Right now, just do your jobs." He headed for his office. I followed.

"The energy here is too negative for me. I quit. But I'm keeping the five dollar tip." I walked out of the restaurant. Being *Alice* for one night had been enough.

On Monday I flew to San Francisco.

I planned to spend a week with Dexter and then visit Ralph in Oregon. After that I would fly back to New Jersey, say goodbye to my family, and pick up Sara in Philadelphia.

When I landed in San Francisco I felt as though I had traveled back in time, three hours earlier. I had just picked up my luggage from the slow-speed conveyer belt when I saw Dexter waiving at me from among the crowd. We ran towards each other and hugged and laughed with delight.

As soon as we stepped outside the terminal, I noticed that the air was different. I felt high on sunshine.

He drove through the city, pointing out the different neighborhoods. "I'm taking you to Castro," he said, "famous for being one of the largest gay neighborhoods in the world. I think you'll enjoy all the unique shops."

I couldn't help staring at the people in their outlandish garb. Young men posed along the sidewalks wearing undersized shorts and see-through tee-shirts, leaving little to the imagination. They reminded me of prostitutes looking for a trick.

Dexter was having just as much fun as me, checking out the quirky assortment of gifts at the small shops and boutiques. Everything about the West Coast fascinated me. I had never seen anything like this, not even in New York City. At one shop, we took turns reading the humorous cards to each other.

Time flew. He treated me to dinner at a vegetarian restaurant. The ambiance had a careless hippie feeling that made me feel at home. The food reminded me of my Aunt Heydee's cooking, with lots of garlic and fresh herbs. As always, Dexter's company was a delicious treat. We talked for hours and were the last patrons to leave the restaurant. We had a lot to catch up on. It was pure intellectual pleasure being together again. When he acted *normal,* no man could compare to him.

After dinner, we drove to Hayward, where he lived. The San Mateo Bridge became my favorite bridge in the whole world. Its narrowness gave the illusion of driving on water and kept on going and going as if it would never end. Several times I asked whether we were still on the bridge.

Dexter rented a house, with a couple who also attended Life West Chiropractic College. They had gone east to visit family for the holidays. The place was all ours.

He opened the sliding glass door in the living room and walked out into the narrow terrace. He called out, "Check out the view from here. Have you ever seen anything like it?"

I followed him out. I saw a deep cliff below us and what looked like a canyon that ran like a river along the pathway below us. "It is breathtaking." I tried not to look down again, since heights made me lose my balance and focused on the cliff across from us. "It's like we're standing in midair!"

"Basically we are. This part of the house stands on wood stilts," Dexter said. "That's why we have such a panoramic view."

I stepped back. I smiled heroically and said, "Getting a bit chilly out here."

We headed inside and sat on the oversized couch. I sat at the end opposite him, trying to show no signs of affection. We had hugged at the airport, but I would go no further until I was sure he wasn't going to freak out on me. The months we had dated in Georgia had taught me well. He couldn't handle any affection but sex.

He showed me his bedroom upstairs. He had made space in his closet for my clothes.

I took a shower and returned in my pajamas.

He went to take a shower and returned in his pajamas.

"Do you need an extra pillow?" He stood at the foot of the bed.

"No. This one is perfect. Where will you be sleeping?" I was sprawled across the mattress.

"I thought we would be sleeping together."

"That can't happen. It's been months since we've seen each other. We're practically strangers. I need time to get used to our relationship once again."

"I guess I can sleep on the sofa."

"That would be great. I don't know if I can handle making love to you after being…"

"Oh, you don't have to worry about that. It didn't even cross my mind. I'm only planning to sleep. You know… sleep!" He held his hands at the side of his head, as children do when they are tired.

"Are you telling me we'll just sleep, like good friends?"

"Of course." He shook his head as if I were nuts.

"In that case, forget the sofa. You might as well be comfortable in your own bed." I moved to one side.

He lay flat on his back and pulled the covers up to his neck, looking like an embalmed mummy.

"Goodnight," I said softly.

"Goodnight." He turned over.

He had not changed. He was still scared of human contact. What kind of a man lies next to the one he loves and curls into himself like a snail in its shell?

No problem, I'll enjoy my visit to California and let things run their own natural course.

I slept and then woke up. I slept again and woke up again. The sexual tension I felt next to him and the excitement of being in California for the first time was equal to drinking a large mug of coffee. I was awake more than I slept. When the sunlight hit my eyes, streaming in through the thin, sheer, white curtains, I could not go back to sleep and lay pondering what to do next. I would take my chances and see if I still had what it took to turn him on. The worst that could happen was that he would kick me out of his bed.

His back was turned to me so I curled myself into his body, wrapped my hands around his body and waited for a response. It was soon obvious he wanted sex as much as I did. He was on top of me so quickly, we rolled out of bed. Thank God he was under me when we hit the hardwood floor. We laughed heartily over the unexpected, but that didn't stop us, if anything it seemed very appropriate.

Mama had told me several times that sex was a human necessity for maintaining one's health. It made a lot of sense. We felt energized and ready for a full day of activities.

That morning, Dexter drove to San Lorenzo, not too far from where he lived and gave me a tour of Life West Chiropractic College. It was located in an old middle school, in what seemed to be a lower-income residential community. Though it didn't have the grand new look of my college in Georgia, Dexter brought up some important details about the school. "The president of the college experienced the healing power of chiropractic when he was a child. It saved his life. He understands our profession better than anybody I know. He values our education and goes out of his way to meet with every student and make sure they are doing well. The teachers carry the same passion for chiropractic that he does. You are not a number here, like larger colleges. We're more like a family."

After Dexter's passionate description I began considering my transfer to that college. My one year scholarship at the other college was over, and I took that as a sign to move on.

That afternoon, we drove to San Francisco to meet with Dexter's psychologist. Except for Leila, I had never been to a shrink. I believed that a psychologist or psychiatrist could tell within two or three questions if someone was mentally unstable, which made me somewhat apprehensive since I'd never professed to be normal.

Dr. Sherman was younger than I imagined, but she was apparently able to help Dexter. He trusted her and seemed relaxed in her presence. He didn't lie on a couch like I had seen in so many movies. Dexter and I sat on a loveseat. She sat with excellent posture on a wood chair across from us.

"Veronica, do you love Dexter?"

"I…"

"You must love Dexter very much. You came all the way from the East Coast during your school holiday, just to be here with him, huh?"

"I…"

"Dexter, do you realize that this woman loves you enough to stand by your side at a time like this?"

"Yes, and I want to spend my life with her." He took a deep breath and smiled at me.

"Veronica, are you willing to continue to support Dexter through some difficult times ahead?"

"I…"

"Dexter, you are a very lucky man. Tell me Dexter, why did you ask Veronica to come to California? Do you love her?"

"Of course I love her. Just look at her. She's like sunshine, bright and cheery and we get along great. I'm hoping that I'll get well soon, so that we can get married and open our practice jointly. What more can I say?"

"How's your sex life?"

"It couldn't be better." He smiled.

The next appointment with Dr. Sherman was scheduled for when I returned from Oregon.

Dexter and I spent the day walking through the city and found ourselves at Fisherman's Warf. When we came across a young street musician playing a romantic tune on the saxophone, I reached for Dexter's hand. He pulled his hand away.

I could barely keep from crying. I wanted to tell him, that he was wasting his time and money seeing Dr. Sherman. I lacked the courage to speak my mind. Instead, I went into my mode of self-preservation and focused on enjoying the moment without any further expectations from him.

He introduced me to sourdough bread filled with clam chowder. I didn't like the bread, but I enjoyed the soup. When he offered to buy me chocolates, I said, "Thank you, but I'm allergic to chocolate. But I could go for some strawberry ice cream instead." Being a chocoholic, I was proud of my self-control.

Later that evening, we walked by a bathhouse and he told me that he had always wondered what it was like inside.

"Let's check it out." I said.

"You don't mind?"

"When Ralph and I visited Morocco we didn't get a chance to visit their bathhouses. I'd love to see what it's all about."

He gave five bucks to the guy at the front desk to let us take a look inside. The guy gave us a disdainful look. I knew what he was thinking, *freaking tourists!*

I sat on the bed checking out the mattress for comfort but the mattress lacked any softness. The metal tub wasn't inviting, either. "I wonder why they have a bed in the room. Isn't that kind of odd? People go to sleep after taking a bath?" I was a bit disappointed with the lack of luxury. Considering that it was a bathhouse, I expected some kind of Middle Eastern sultan like décor.

"These bathhouses are designed for gay men so they can have sex—in privacy. That's the reason for the bed."

We spent the next three days touring Berkley and San Francisco's Chinatown, walking across the Golden Gate Bridge, and visiting friends from Georgia who had transferred with Dexter to the school here.

I was absolutely delighted when Dexter offered to drive me to Oregon. I had planned to take a train, but traveling by car would let me stop at interesting places along the way.

Traveling up the coast I couldn't get over how the West Coast was so much like Portugal, with pristine beaches and stunning views from the top of rock cliffs. Truly spectacular. *Another good reason to move to California.*

The sun disappeared right after we passed the "Welcome to Oregon" sign, and it rained the whole two days we visited Ralph, in Troutdale. I will never be able to live in Oregon. I love sunshine too much to give it up.

I missed Ralph and it felt great to see him again. He gave us the full tour of Western States College, showing as much pride in his school as Dexter had shown with his. Then Ralph introduced us to Sandy, his girlfriend, who invited us to stay at her home for the two nights, since Ralph didn't have space at his apartment. It was my first experience at sleeping on an air mattress. I would not recommend it to anyone with a bad back.

That evening Ralph offered to take us to see a historical house not far from where he lived in Troutdale. But Dexter was going through one of his down moods and said he'd rather not go. I felt bad about his refusal, especially after I saw how much he missed. The place was called McMenamins Edgefield and had been built around 1911. It had served as home and a farm for the poor, elderly and disabled in the days before Social Security, Welfare and Medicare. It was a huge mansion, now renovated into a hotel and restaurant and once I started walking through the hallways somehow I lost Ralph and Sandy. I found them seated at one of their bars, talking. It did my heart good to see that Ralph had found someone special and he was happy. I left them and went back to investigating my surroundings. I'd always wanted to go on a treasure hunt or an archeological expedition, and this place was a mixture of both. The walls, doors and every possible niche spoke to me through the original artwork by local artists depicting the people who supposedly had lived there. Some of the satirical paintings made me smile. Others made me think and grab my heart. One mural showed a large empty green ballroom with a lone old lady seated in a corner, mending a dress. The memories of her youth projected across the room, like a hologram. She wore a pink evening gown and her dancing partner wore a black tuxedo. The artists painted the couple dancing at three different levels, giving the feeling they danced to the sound of a waltz. I had worked as an activity director three years prior at a Senior Retirement Home in New Jersey and that experience had made me aware that no matter how old one was, love lives forever in our hearts and so do memories—unless, of course, one went senile, and then it no longer mattered. I finally joined Ralph and Sandy for a cup of tea.

When we returned Dexter was sleeping.

The next day, Ralph took Dexter and me to the famous Portland Saturday Market. On the way there, they talked about relationships and age differences. I sat in the back seat listening.

"Older women have more experience with life." Dexter said. "They have it more together."

"Absolutely, Sandy is fifteen years older than me, and I'm very happy."

"I understand how you feel. Your mom is ten years older than me, but it's like we're the same age, physically and intellectually. I've no patience for scatter-brained younger girls."

I smiled, happy to know that as women aged, some men valued their mature charm and wisdom.

That evening, Dexter and I were seated in the living room couch and he said, "Veronica I need to know what you plan to do. Are you planning to move to California and live with me?" I said yes because that's what I always say when I can't handle confrontation or hurting someone's feelings.

Back in California, we saw Dr. Sherman once more. That time she was interested in what I had to say.

"I feel like a flower when I'm with Dexter. I get a lot of water and good soil, but there's no light to keep me alive."

"You're a very visual person but can you clarify what you mean?"

"Dexter feeds my intellect and we share the same views on life, but when it comes to a simple action of holding hands or holding me in his arms he freaks out."

"Your description is very valuable. Tell me, Veronica, are you happy having sex with Dexter?"

I couldn't believe it. Dr. Sherman not only asked me questions but also waited to hear my answers.

"For me, sex is not good by itself. I need affection, and as you know, Dexter can't handle that. We had sex the morning after I arrived, but later that evening he reminded me that he didn't like to have the woman initiating the act because that was a man's job. I stopped making the first move and nothing more has happened."

"Dexter, what do you say to that?"

"She's right," he said sheepishly, not looking at either one of us.

I took that as encouragement to continue.

"Dexter, I know I can't live with you the way you are. We already tried it when we lived in Georgia, remember? I have to be honest, if I'm not happy, I'll either leave or look for someone else."

"I will stay under Dr. Sherman's care for as long as it's needed, and do my best to get better. You have to give me at least a chance to prove myself."

"Veronica, what do you say to that?"

"I'm thinking of taking the advice of a mutual friend of ours. She advised us not to move in together and instead to date each other before getting into a serious relationship. I like this idea. It will give us an opportunity to see if this is what we really want to do."

"Sounds like a very good idea. Dexter, how do you feel about that?"

"I'm not sure. I was hoping we could live together. But if you think it's better that way, I'm fine with it." He wasn't fine and the rest of the day he was moody and barely spoke.

The next day I boarded the plane to New Jersey. I looked forward to changing colleges, but felt uneasy about my situation with Dexter. I pulled my notebook from my backpack and started to write a letter to Dexter. "Dear Dexter," and then my mind went blank.

"You look like Janine Turner."

"What?" I turned to the passenger sitting on my right.

"Janine Turner, from Northern Exposure, the TV show..."

"I look like her?"

"Yeah, you have the same haircut and a lot of spunk." His name was John Murphy and he was an insurance auditor. We chatted about chiropractic versus medical treatments and, insurance fraud.

Steve picked me up at the airport.

"Mom, what did you do to the restaurant where you worked? Plant a bomb?" He laughed.

"What do you mean?"

"The whole building went up in smoke the night you left."

I couldn't believe it, so he drove me past it. The building had been leveled.

Before leaving the next morning, I took a snapshot of Steve and his family seated on the living room couch having breakfast. Steve held a cup of coffee in one hand, with Jacob sitting on his lap, drinking from his bottle, and Diane drinking a cup of tea.

I picked up Sara in Pennsylvania and described everything that happened with Dexter.

After listening to my sob story for a good part of the trip, she yelled, "You're some dumb broad! Can't you see that the man is batty? Don't you have any common sense in that head of yours?"

"If you love someone, you try to help them."

"He can't be helped. He's nothing but a loser! You are out of your mind to even consider him as part of your life. Veronica, he's using you to lift his own spirits. I met him when he was in school with us, don't you remember? I saw the way he acted when you had that little gathering at your apartment. There's nothing that you can do to help him. He's a grown man. Can't you get that through your thick head?"

"He's seeing a psychologist..." I paused. "You're right, it's not helping him."

"You better believe I'm right. He isn't good for you or anyone else. If you move in with him, you'll stop growing. I'm telling you, he's damaged goods, and he's going to hurt you. That's all I have to say."

She spoke like Aunt Heydee would have if she were still alive, and that gave me the strength to call Dexter as soon as I got home.

"I'll be moving to California at the end of next quarter, but I hope you understand that I do not intend to live with you. Let's wait and see where we stand when it comes to our relationship."

"I understand. Veronica, you have done a lot for me, coming over and supporting my efforts, so I'd like to do the same for you. How about if I fly over and keep you company while driving here?"

I liked his offer. Our talk had gone better than I imagined.

I also called Mama to let her know about my decision to move.

"Are you out of your mind? Everybody knows that it's just a question of time before the Pacific Ocean swallows the State of California."

I would take my chances.

~ Chapter Eight ~

The Internship

January 10, 1995

I began spreading the word around the college that I was transferring to California, at the end of the quarter. I made colorful fliers describing what I wanted to sell and posted them everywhere. I had about three months to dispose of anything I didn't want to take, so there wasn't any rush to settle for less than what I had paid.

Practicing in the chiropractic clinic at the college didn't turn out the way I had imagined. I was in trouble after seeing my first patient, Ms. Lacey Jones. She was a thirty-seven year old disheveled blonde that was overweight by twenty pounds. I followed everything by the rule. I took her history and did a detailed physical that included orthopedic and neurological exam, but I had never been told I couldn't use common sense when treating a patient.

Lacey worked in an asylum, and occasionally patients would get so violent they had to be restrained. It wasn't the first time she had been attacked and beaten. "It comes with the job," she said. This time, she was in a lot of pain, with bruises covering her back and upper extremities. A prominent welt covered the back of her head, the reason she couldn't comb her hair.

"I'm concerned about your safety." I said. "Are you happy doing this kind of work?"

"No. I hate it."

"What would you rather be doing?"

"I'd love to be a taxi driver, but I can't leave my job at the hospital. I get paid well there."

"A good paycheck won't help if you get beaten to death."

She covered her face with her hands and cried. "This time it almost killed me. I really thought I was going to die. I was just walking in the hallway when the patient attacked me. After pushing me into the wall, he threw me on the ground and began jumping on my back. These types of unexpected assaults happen all the time."

"I'm your doctor and as such I want you to think about what's more important, living your life the way you deserve or getting buried with a good paycheck. If I were you, I'd tell my boss I'm quitting and then get myself a taxi."

I took Lacey to the radiology department to have neck and back X-rays done and asked her to return Friday for a Report of Findings and treatment plan. Meanwhile I would be meeting with Dr. Sphinter, my supervising doctor to talk about my findings and how I was going to treat Lacey.

When Dr. Sphinter heard about my advice to the patient, he got up from his chair and yelled, "How dare you tell your patient to quit her job."

"The job is harmful to her health…"

"Who are you, her mother? Your only business as a clinician is to adjust the spine and get rid of subluxations. That's all. Do you understand?"

"Yes, I understand."

I thought that would be what he wanted to hear, but he still wasn't happy. The jerk took me to Dr. Baltam's office, the clinic director, who lectured me without even knowing any of the particulars about my patient.

My philosophy about chiropractic would remain unchanged. Everybody needed to get their spine adjusted to rule out nerve interference, which, could not only cause pain but could also ruin overall health. So what if patients felt great after getting adjusted? If they returned to the same environments of emotional or physical abuse, if they smoked, took drugs to excess, and ate junk food, the symptoms would return, no matter how good a spinal adjustment. That was as clear as night and day and I was sticking to my beliefs.

Screw them, with their analytical, closed minds. I couldn't ignore the emotional and physical pain my patient had been put through with her awful job. From that day forward, I kept to myself what went on between my patients and me. I would give Dr. Sphinter only the results of the history, the exam findings, and my treatment plan.

January 12

Ralph called. He planned to look further into Judaism.

"I'm sorry I didn't provide you and your brother with a Jewish education while growing up," I said.

"Don't worry, Mom. I was too young to appreciate it, anyway. Now I can learn about it because I want to. In fact, I've already applied for a grant to go to Israel this summer. I want to learn more about it."

With his inquisitive engineer's brain, by the time he finished researching he would probably have found all the answers. I felt proud of him.

Marie, a third quarter student and one of my patients at the clinic, called me at one in the morning crying. Her boyfriend of two years had broken up with her. "You're lucky to find out now that he's no good for you," I said, "instead of when you get married. When you least expect it, the right person will come your way." I encouraged her to call me every day, until she was over the depression.

Marie must have told Sara about our phone conversations, because Sara came over Saturday morning and said, "You're definitely sick." She pointed to her own head. "Why are you constantly trying to help everybody? All that does is consume you. What's the matter with you?"

"Sorry, but I can't help myself. I'm happy when I'm able to provide solutions."

"No. It's none of your business if Marie, or any other jerk, jumps out of their window. It's their choice, not yours. You should be concentrating on your own life. Stop butting into other people's lives. When you get to California, promise me that you tell Dexter to go fly a kite."

"Okay, I promise."

"Don't give me that. You're just saying okay, to shut me up. I swear it's like an addiction with you, always trying to fix people's lives. You need to start taking care of yourself."

She was my friend and I knew she was trying to protect me, but it annoyed me that she saw me as defective. Only I have the right to think of myself that way, no one else. I also found it a bit ironic. When we first became friends, she had shared some of her own issues with living in her brother's house. I helped her resolve her problems by teaching her how to set up a budget and encouraging her to get her own apartment with the money she saved. She needed to become independent and I provided her with a strategy. She had been so happy she even gave me a bucket of fresh tomatoes.

Unless someone asks me to act as a psychotherapist like Leila does, and keep my mouth shut, I'll always give my two cents when requested.

January 22

Stewart, my roommate announced that he was leaving at the end of the month.

"Why? I'll be here for another two months. Once I leave you can rent my room to someone else."

"Too much work to find a roommate. Besides, a friend has a room for only $150 per month."

Afterwards, I stopped at the front office for the apartment complex. When I gave my notice the manager said, "If you stay, I'll give you two months of free rent and a ten percent discount for one year."

"It's a great deal, but I'm not leaving because of finances. I'm transferring to another college."

"Why? What's wrong with your college here?"

I'm probably the only tenant to paint her apartment during school breaks.

January 25

As part of a class assignment, we had to perform a urine analysis in the lab. Out of curiosity, I put my own sample under the microscope. It showed positive for a urinary tract infection. Oddly enough, I didn't have the usual painful symptoms associated with it. I felt extremely lucky. No symptoms meant I had caught the infection in the very first stage. Still, I had to get an antibiotic and that meant having to see a medical doctor. As a chiropractor, I couldn't dispense medication.

I made an appointment to see my gynecologist the next day. Dr. Lawoski knew I was a student on a budget. With luck, she would give me free samples without an exam.

While waiting to see Dr. Lawoski I made the mistake of picking up a newspaper. Al used to make fun of me when we were married because I only read the entertainment section. I don't do well with bad news. I get frustrated because I can't do anything about it. So I should have known better than to pick up that paper, but I already had gone through all the magazines in the waiting room and had cleaned my backpack of undesirables, such as receipts for gas and groceries, little notes with reminders, and tissues that have been used over and over again.

At the bottom of the third page was the picture of a young man lying dead on the pavement, surrounded by four bystanders who had witnessed a robber sticking a knife into the victim's chest.

The receptionist opened the glass window and said, "Ms. Esagui, the doctor is ready to see you."

I told Dr. Lawoski that my lab test at school showed I had a bladder infection and I needed an antibiotic. I saw Dr. Lawoski once a year for my usual gynecological checkup. She was about my age and I always felt like we could talk. This time she was in a hurry and didn't seem to be listening.

"We still need to test your urine. Wait here." She left.

The receptionist came in and gave me a small plastic cup and asked me to go to the bathroom and pee in the cup.

I knew exactly what was going to be done. Her office girl would dip a swatch into the cup and if it changed to a specific color, I had an infection. My test under the microscope was not valid enough?

I handed the half-full cup to the office girl, and she took me back into the exam room. I was asked to gown myself and remove my clothes from the waist down.

Twenty minutes later, Dr. Lawoski came in, put her rubber gloves on and had me lying on my back with my legs up in stirrups. I wondered what she could be looking for. I had enough experience to know that a gynecological exam was not needed.

"Everything looks fine." She removed her rubber gloves. "I'll be right back."

She returned to the exam room with a prescription for the antibiotic. "Here you go. Your urine test shows that you have a urinary tract infection." She left the room.

When I returned to the reception area, the girl at the front desk said, "It's going to be $150 for the physical exam and the lab test."

I'm a Taurus and as such I tend to put my emotions on hold until I can't take it anymore, and then I only see red.

"I'd like to speak to the doctor."

I sat down and picked up the same newspaper and went back to staring at the picture on the third page.

"Dr. Lawoski will see you now," the receptionist announced, waving for me to come in.

Dr. Lawoski met me in the hallway. "What seems to be the problem?"

"I told you I had a urine test done at school and it was positive for infection, but instead of giving me the antibiotic I needed, you gave me a gynecological exam and had me pee in a cup. If I give you $150, I won't have the money to buy the antibiotic."

She didn't answer me. Instead, she reached in the hallway closet, which was packed with prescription samples.

"Here is the antibiotic you need. Take it for a week. That's all I can do for you." She walked away.

I paid the $150 and drove as fast as I could to the college clinic, crying the entire way. Leila sat in the waiting room, waiting to be seen by her clinician. I sat next to her, weeping.

"Leila, my doctor just robbed me! Just like the murdered young man I saw in the newspaper today, killed over the couple of bucks in his pocket. The crowd just stood there, doing nothing to stop it. The reporter, too, more interested in a photo than the guy who lay there, so he could make a lousy dollar. What kind of beast is the human race? I hate humanity!"

"Now, Veronica, you need to take it easy. Breathe deep." Her psychotherapist background, coming across in the honey-covered tone of her voice, frustrated me even more.

"I hate humanity!"

She held my hands and kissed me on the cheek. "I'm your friend, Veronica. From now on, I want you to have dinner with me every Friday night, until you leave for California. Promise me."

"What does dinner have to do with what I just told you?"

"Not all human beings are bad. You, of all people, should know that by now. I'll expect to see you this Friday night."

God bless Leila and all my friends at school. They kept my life balanced. Leila, made me laugh, she fed me and was nurturing. Sara was a solid friend, straightforward. Nieght was my inspiration when it came to showing how strong the human spirit could be, I admired how much he had achieved at such young age.

I had already fallen asleep when Nieght called one night. He was emotionally devastated by the callous attitude of some chiropractors and he felt that some of our classmates were just as callous as them.

"I made a mistake in wanting to become a chiropractor. I don't want to be associated with a profession where making money is the main priority."

"I used to feel that way, when I first came to this school, until I realized that it's up to us to make a difference. As long as we do well by our patients, *that* is what's important. There are good and bad lawyers, and good and bad presidents. If we quit because of the bad ones in our profession, then the world would be prey to them."

"I understand what you mean, but what about the bad reputation they give our profession? A lot of them are only out for the money."

"As long as we are honest and do our best we can prove that one bad apple doesn't make the whole bunch a bad crop. I'll never forget when I was taking a pre-med class in New Jersey and a student came into the class and made fun of another student and me because he heard us talking about how we couldn't wait to be doctors so we could help as many people as possible. He told us disdainfully that he was becoming a medical doctor with only one intention, to make money." I knew I sounded preachy but I couldn't stop my train of thoughts. I was scared that he was going to quit. "Swear to me that you are not going to quit." I said in a dramatic tone, sounding just like my mother.

"I promise not to quit. I will treat those that can't afford care, while still making a living from those that can pay."

He promised to visit me in California when he graduates.

February 1

Stewart, my roommate, moved out yesterday afternoon. When I walked into his bathroom I almost passed out. Mildew encrusted the walls around the bathtub. If someone had told me before I entered the bathroom a dead body had rotted in the tub I'd have believed it. I gagged from the foul odor and taste that I unexpectedly took in through my nostrils as I ran out the bathroom and closed the door behind me. I waited a few minutes to clear my lungs and went back in to evaluate the situation. I pressed the handle to flush the toilet and all the contents from the stinking clogged toilet came pouring out into the floor. I ran out of the bathroom in time to close the door.

Stewart had not given me his phone number, so I had to track him down at school. He needed to come back to our apartment and clean his bathroom.

Stewart turned out to be a real jerk. He said he was too busy preparing for midterm exams, to help, so I was stuck having to clean his miserable bathroom. I should have suspected this devious side of his character, when he told me a few months prior he didn't intend to pay his student loan after he graduated. He was just the type of loser that Nieght was talking about. People like him were the scum of the earth.

I spent three paper towel rolls to pick up all the crap off the floors and put a bunch around the toilet to absorb the spill when I used the plunger. By cursing at Stewart while using the plunger worked well. I hoped the bastard got a shitty grade for midterms. Afterwards, I rushed to my bathroom to take a hot shower and then went back to scrubbing the bathtub with a cleanser, but the mildew was dry and hard. I pulled down the moldy plastic curtains, and tossed them out. Then I filled the tub with hot water and half a bottle of bleach. I closed the door and let the bleach sit for two hours. When I got back into the bathroom, I cried. I had to stick my arm into the water to pull the plug. I felt my skin crawling and I ran out again, to take another shower. I sat outside breathing in the fresh air before going back to finish my work. It was late at night and I had classes early the next morning. I sprinkled the tub with more cleanser and scrubbed harder than ever. I had to keep going in and out of the bathroom, to catch my breath. I couldn't believe this guy had kept his bedroom and the kitchen so spotless. When it came to his personal hygiene, he was a filthy slob.

The next day I woke sneezing and coughing. The bug lasted two days. I blamed it on a reaction to the bleach, or worse, from breathing the bacteria left from Stewart's body.

February 5

When Lacey, my patient, came in for her next adjustment, her eyes glowed with happiness. Her family agreed to help her financially, while she prepared to become a licensed taxi driver. She brought me a bouquet of flowers and hugged me. I felt proud of myself, my job as a doctor was to teach and I had taught her well. More than ever I couldn't wait to transfer to the college in California, where I could flourish with the support of other doctors. I had no intentions of sharing those feelings or the good news with the supervising doctors. They would not understand.

February 7

Because Leila was my best friend, I wanted to give her a Reiki treatment before her midterms. She was far from being a good student and had to repeat most of her classes. We'd met for the first time when we were starting our first quarter. Now she was three quarters behind me. She struggled with all her classes but excelled in chiropractic philosophy, yet even that class she was forced to repeat last quarter. I'd found her at the library studying for a pathology test when she had a philosophy test in five minutes. She didn't make it to the testing center in time.

My intention for the Reiki treatment was for her to be more organized, concentrate better on her studies, and then recall enough to pass the exams this quarter.

February 16

Friday dinners at Leila's apartment were always a conglomeration of festive homemade dishes. She used lots of fresh herbs, but didn't use pepper or hot spices. Like me, she no longer had hemorrhoid problems.

Leila practiced the Jewish religion and as such she celebrated the beginning of Shabbat on Friday nights. She lit the candles according to tradition and took her time reading the Bible, while my stomach growled from all the delicious aromas coming from her kitchen.

I didn't practice any Jewish rituals, but I found comfort with Leila. It brought back memories with my childhood in Portugal.

The first night, she offered me a glass of wine to sip during prayers.

"Leila, I'm sorry but I can't drink wine. It makes me sick."

"Really? What happens?"

"I'm allergic to chocolate and wine. Chocolate gives me bone pain and wine speeds up my heart and makes me dizzy to the point that I feel like I'm going to pass out."

"You're not allergic Veronica. You're pure."

I laughed. "You must be kidding. Leila, I'm far from being pure."

"Let me explain. Your system is so healthy and wise that when you put something offensive into it, like alcohol, it tells you by making you sick. That's what I mean by saying that you're pure."

One of the things I admired most about Leila was her unique approach to life.

February 18

I had an eye-opening experience at the clinic after adjusting Mrs. Thompson, a new patient. She used to see Laura, another intern who had graduated the previous quarter.

"I miss Laura," she said. "She was the only chiropractor able to *pop* my back."

I felt like the woman that married a widower, who could talk about nothing but his wonderful, deceased wife. How could anyone compete with a dead saint?

Then she said, "After Laura adjusted my back, I always burped. That's how I knew that she had done a god job."

She lay face down and waited for me to adjust her back.

Shit! I reached for the power above and prayed, *Dear God, please guide my hands*. I put my best effort forward.

"I didn't hear a crack," said the disappointed patient.

"It doesn't have to make a cracking sound to work," I said, a bit unsure of myself.

"If it doesn't crack, I won't burp." She sat up, shaking her head.

Suddenly, she let out a brash and smelly belch from deep within her bowels. I almost keeled over. She had a joyous look on her face.

"My goodness, you barely used any force, yet you moved it. I like this type of adjustment, better than the way Laura did it. How did you do that? Remarkable, that's all I can say. I'll be seeing you again, on Tuesday, that's for sure."

This proved that gentle spinal adjustments worked fine and I didn't have to use brute force. I couldn't be happier.

February 19

Cecilia, a chiropractic student in my radiology class, told me in class her parrot was sick and she was afraid he might die. I made the mistake of giving her my phone number in case she needed someone to talk to.

Listening to her on the phone the last two nights took me away from studying, but I didn't have the courage to tell her to stop calling me unless the bird died.

"Thank you for listening. Carrion is my baby. I don't want to lose him." She cried loudly.

"I've never had a pet. I do remember one of my aunts having two parrots from Brazil, they had beautiful colorful feathers."

She cried even harder. "My Carrion is losing his feathers. He has serious diarrhea and is skin and bones. I've spent $275 between his meds and visits to the veterinarian and nothing is helping. Can you come over this Saturday? You are the only one that cares. I'd like you to meet him."

Cecilia's bedroom was disgusting. I wondered if her two roommates were aware of the mess. It couldn't be healthy for anyone living in the apartment. Feathers were scattered across her bed and floor along with seeds and bird poop. At the corner of the room close to the window, Carrion stood shaking on a long wood perch that hung from the ceiling like a swing. The few green feathers he still possessed stuck out as if he had been electrocuted. Cecilia was right, there wasn't much left to him. He stared back at me. "Nice to meet you, Carrion." I was being polite, since some parrots are able to talk. He didn't answer.

They say pet owners tend to look like their pets. I wondered if the unhygienic conditions of her bedroom had contributed to Cecilia's warts around her eyes.

Sunday night I had my pajamas on and was about to get in bed when she called.

"Veronica, I don't know if Carrion is going to make it through the night."

I recalled what my mother used to give my brothers and me when we had diarrhea. "I have a suggestion. Boil some rice and then give him only the rice water. Then get your Activator instrument and adjust Carrion's neck."

"I can't adjust my Carrion. I might hurt him."

"What's the difference between his spine and ours? Doesn't he also have a nervous system? Get his neck adjusted and give him the rice water. And do it tonight, for goodness sake!"

After two days of rice water and neck adjustments, Carrion was as good as new. No more diarrhea and back to eating fresh fruit, nuts and seeds. Cecilia gave me a heartfelt hug at school.

She was contemplating becoming a veterinarian chiropractor after she graduated.

February 21

Leila passed all the midterms. Hurray for the power of Reiki!

After I settled in California, I would look further into Reiki and see how practitioners did it without getting burned out at the end of a treatment.

Slowly, but surely, I'd been selling everything. I even sold the four dresser drawers I used as a bookcase after my real dresser had been delivered in broken pieces by a non-reputable moving company. This happened when Ralph and I first moved from New Jersey to Georgia to attend school. In order to get all our belongings he had to call the FBI. The moving company was collecting the delivery fee from dozens of customers and keeping everything in a warehouse. It took about three months to make the bust but the FBI made sure we received everything that belonged to us and we were compensated for the damaged dresser, the microwave, Ralph's computer, and my mattress.

I sold the drawers for five dollars each to a student who thought it was the most original bookcase she had ever seen. Another student bought all my houseplants, including the dead ones. Leila bought Joe, the dummy, for what I had paid. I took her picture as she carried him out. She slung it over her shoulders, like a sex trophy, while insinuating she intended to use him for more than just practicing adjustments. I couldn't part with the two old wine barrels I used as theater props in *The Playboy of the Western World.* They were a sweet reminder of my life as a theater producer in New Jersey. They were too old and fragile to be sent UPS. I would wrap them carefully in towels and set them in the back seat of my car with my other family heirlooms such as my acoustic guitar, Grandmother Rica's antique evening dress, Grandmother Mutter's crystals, the stamp collection, my Japanese kimono and Japanese doll.

One student bought my adjusting table. His school buddy bought the plastic wall panel I had nailed to the wall of the living room, under the condition that I didn't wipe the charts I had drawn for the various techniques of adjusting. My next-door neighbor bought my dining room furniture. I had the amazing feeling that everybody was purposely buying my stuff just to help me out financially. I felt blessed.

~ *Chapter Nine* ~

Weeping Tears

February 29

The day was one of the darkest of my life. The phone rang as I was leaving home to see my morning patients. It was Papa.

"Mama died in the hospital last night." He was crying.

I pulled the phone away from my ear and then out of disbelief squeezed hard against it, hoping that what I had heard was not true. "I talked to her four days ago and she didn't sound sick. What happened?" I knew it was just a question of time before one of my parents died, but hearing my father crying made me realize that I wasn't ready to face it.

"They said she had pneumonia, but I doubt they know for sure."

I drove to school and parked, still in shock. An overwhelming numbness covered my body. I wanted to cry but couldn't.

I turned on the radio. Music always told me what to do. It was my communication to the Universe.

Beethoven's Piano Concerto Number3 *Allegro Con Brio.* I closed my eyes and imagined Mama in heaven. She had a baton in her right hand and was smiling. The maestro of her own orchestra, happy and without pain. I wished hard for that to be happening, I wished with all my heart that what I was imagining was true, my profound wish that her wish had come true. When I entered the clinic, one of the clinicians commented that I didn't look right and asked what was wrong with me.

"My mother died last night."

"And you're here in the clinic? Go home."

"Portugal is too far."

She must have said something to one of the clinic directors because within ten minutes Dr. Norman called me into her office. She sat next to me and put her arm over my shoulders.

"Go ahead, Veronica, go ahead and cry."

"I'm not allowed to do that. I promised my mother I wouldn't cry when she died."

"That's not healthy. Let go of your emotions and cry for your mother."

"My chest feels heavy and I can't breathe. Still, I can't cry."

"Tell me about your mother."

"My mom died without really living. Except for having my two brothers and me, she was a prisoner of her times, when a woman had no rights to do or be what she wanted. I'm angry with that. I'm angry that she was never a part of my life until the last time we saw each other and we understood what we had missed all those years. She was a victim of preconceived, old-fashioned ideas throughout her life. She was a concert pianist but was not allowed out of her country by her parents, and later her artwork disappeared from her house, when my father sold all their possessions. She suffered in silence, believing that was the only way to be strong. Except for her poetry, she had no way of expressing her most intimate feelings. I'm sorry to say, but I never understood her way of thinking—or most of her actions."

I began to cry feeling sorry for myself more than anything else. I had failed to save my mother, and inside of me, I blamed Mama for not allowing me to do that. I cried out of anger and despair. And then I cried extra hard just to make Dr. Norman happy. She was a psychologist and I didn't want her to feel she had failed as a doctor. And the crying did feel good. *Sorry, Mama. I know that I promised you, but Dr. Norman insists.*

They sent me home and told me not to worry about classes or my patients. They gave me two days off for mourning.

I didn't know it would hurt so much to lose my mother. Part of me was gone forever. No more memories to be created, just an empty space that could never be filled again. I couldn't send her any more pictures. I couldn't call her every week. I couldn't write to her again. She no longer lived there.

Three days later, I received a letter from my brother Max-Leão. His letter was brief but the words cried from a broken heart. He truly loved Mama. How pathetic that it's not until someone dies we realize how wonderful they were. I count my blessings that Mama and I made peace the last time we saw each other.

Russell came by with his pickup and helped me transport my boxes to UPS. When he lifted the box with my new electric typewriter out of his truck bed, he dropped it on the ground. "I'm sorry. I hope you don't have anything fragile in there."

"Just an old typewriter. Don't worry."

Perhaps breaking a brand new electric typewriter was a good omen.

March 4

Before Ralph left for Oregon, we used to refer to Doug, one of our classmates, as "Doug the Degenerate." Everything that came out of his mouth was sexually offensive. This day was different. When he saw me at school, he gave me his condolences and a long heartfelt hug. He cried silently, his tears wetting my face.

"I'm okay, Doug. I feel terrible you're crying."

"I lost my father a year ago." He began sobbing loudly.

"I'm sorry Doug."

"I still grieve him. Would you go out for dinner with me, this Saturday night? I could use a friend."

On Saturday night, Doug not only took me to an expensive restaurant, but also insisted on paying for dinner. He talked about his dad the whole time. When he cried, I did too. Like laughter, crying was contagious.

"Thank you for being my friend. You understand what it's like to lose a parent." He reached across the table and took my hands. The tears continued.

Doug was probably in his mid-thirties, but because he was my height and heavy set with a prominent belly, he seemed older to me. His salt and pepper beard face and matching thin hair, which he tied back with a rubber band, would have made him look like a biker if it wasn't wearing a white shirt and a Donald Duck tie. I'm glad we sat in a dark corner. No one could see two grown people crying.

He offered to tape a few cassettes of my favorite rock bands and an audio copy of Michael Adams's book, The *Hitchhiker's Guide to the Galaxy.* "It will help you and Dexter stay alert while driving to California," he said.

Singing in the rain, what a beautiful feeling, I'm happy again... I love dancing and singing when it rains, particularly if I found a few puddles. Then I could jump up and down on both feet, making sure I splashed extra hard to the beat, just before singing *happy again.*

I didn't care if someone saw me playing Fred Astaire as I crossed the school parking lot. To me rain was nothing but liquid sunshine. And if that wasn't enough to make me dance the thought of going to California made me feel even more euphoric. Life was beautiful!

Thank you Mama for sending me to America to marry Cousin Al. If you had not done that I wouldn't be here today, *Singing in the rain, what a beautiful feeling, I'm happy again…*

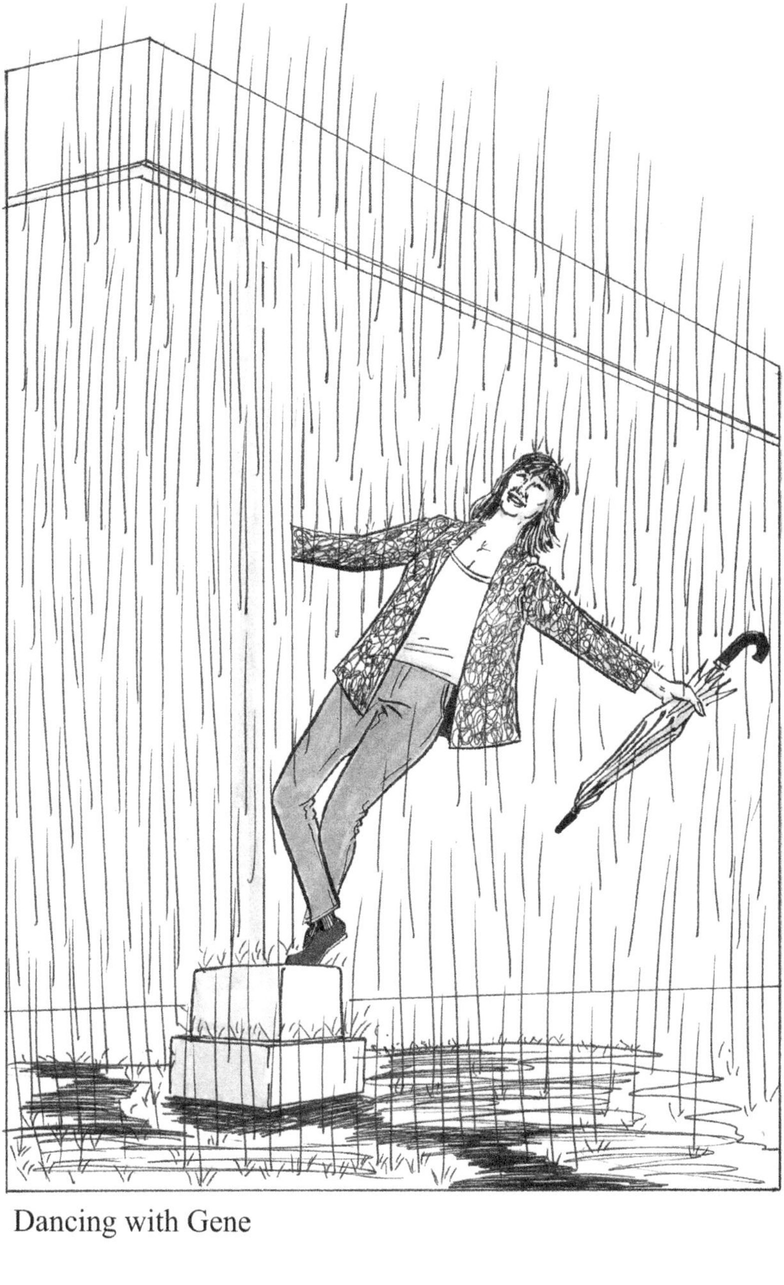

Dancing with Gene

~ *Chapter Ten* ~

The Blues

I changed my mind about selling my gun to Harold. When I asked him what he was going to do with it, he said, "I'll sell it to someone when I get back to New York."

Just what I needed—my gun being traced to me after some street punk shot someone in a dark alley.

Lucia, my Brazilian patient, invited me to a party for her twenty-eight birthday.

She wanted me to meet Rodrigo, her cousin who was thirty-seven and single. I told her I was leaving the end of next month, but I'd still stop by to give her a birthday hug.

March 7

I found Lucia's party easily, despite becoming lost in her housing development. I followed the sound of Brazilian music, and there she was, waving at me from her second floor balcony. She was dancing with a few of her guests, who joined in the waving. I wouldn't be able to just give her the wine and leave. Music pulsated through the apartment, and soon I became wrapped up in the festive sounds of the Samba and joined the dancers in her living room that were delighted that I spoke Portuguese.

Not a half-hour had gone by when I discovered Lucia crying in a corner of the room.

"My boyfriend just broke up with me. He couldn't wait. He had to spoil my birthday. All I wanted to do today was to dance and be happy."

She stopped crying and looked past me at someone who had just entered the room. She grabbed my arm. "C'mon Dr. Veronica. I want you to meet Rodrigo."

"Lucia, I really have to go."

"You can't. *Pleeease* stay." She hugged her cousin. "Rodrigo, this is my doctor and good friend Veronica, who I told you so much about."

He was my height, with short brown curly hair, brown eyes, and in good shape.

"It's so good to meet you," he said, looking at me while kissing my hand.

He took my hand and led me to a small couch at the far end of the room, where the light eased into soft shadows. I felt a slight tightening in my chest. I wanted to dance, and he wanted to talk.

With the music playing so loudly, and everybody chatting and laughing, the Portuguese language had taken on a distorted experience of meaningless sounds. I could barely hear him. And he wouldn't let go of my hand. He talked and talked and I nodded yes to whatever he said. When he stood and gave me a signal he would be right back, I left.

The following day, when Lucia arrived at the clinic, she requested someone other than me to treat her. Now I understood why doctors didn't have personal relationships with their patients.

"Lucia, I'm sorry about this weekend. I didn't mean to hurt your cousin's feelings."

"Rodrigo is very upset. He asked you if you wanted to go out to dinner with him, you said yes, and when he asked to wait while he changed, you also said yes. When he returned, you were gone. That wasn't nice."

"Lucia, you know I have a problem hearing, I'm basically deaf on the left side. I couldn't hear a word he was saying, with all the noise around us. Please tell your cousin I was just being polite by saying yes. I'm very sorry."

"He was very hurt."

"Lucia, I already have a boyfriend, and he would be very upset if I went out with someone else."

"In that case I understand."

She didn't. She cancelled all scheduled appointments with me.

March 15

On Sunday, Leila treated me to a tour of an art museum in Atlanta. At one point she stopped before three small frames, one black, one yellow, and one green, with absolutely nothing inside them.

"This is so creative, so unique."

"Are you joking?"

"I'm very serious. I appreciate the artist's sense of uniqueness."

"I'm no art expert, but this is pure rubbish. The artist that came up with these empty frames is playing a joke on us."

She pointed at a large canvas that covered one of the walls across the room. "Look, look, over there, the artist used two black splashes on that one." She walked up to it and then took a few steps back. "Very intense, the black against the bright white background. I wonder what the artist is trying to convey."

I walked to the window and stared out at the real world outside.

March 17

Papa called. He was still living in Luisa's house. I did not to bring up the subject of Mama. I was afraid he would start crying.

He was a ninety-one-year-old man with the mind of an idealistic youngster, stuck inside a body that was breaking down day-by-day. I asked God why human beings had to die without dignity and with a worthless body. Was this the only way that our souls could be set free? Why couldn't we just drop dead?

I missed Mama's voice on the phone. I missed the long letters she wrote and I used to take for granted.

My last Saturday night in Georgia would be followed by a week of finals, so going to the movies was imperative.

I arrived at the theater an hour early so I took off to explore the surrounding businesses. I hit the jackpot—a blues club right around the corner. When growing up in Portugal, the sorrowful sounds of Fado, a type of Portuguese blues, was one of our few options, but could never compete with American music. The club's showcase windows showed a full line-up of, black performers. Even the man sitting behind the ticket window was black.

"Lady, you don't want to come in here. This is an all-black-folks club."

"I don't mind."

"Sure, you don't mind, but I could get into a lot of trouble."

"Please, I'll be very quiet. Nobody will know I'm there."

"You're kidding me, right? No I guess you're not."

"All my life I've been in love with American-style blues. All I want is to hear some real music. Is that a crime?"

"The show doesn't even start till eleven."

"That's perfect. I'll go see a movie and then come back, all right?" And then I used the Brazilian supplication method. "Pleeeease?"

"Okay, but make sure you get here exactly at eleven so I can get the hostess to sneak you in."

Groundhog Day with Bill Murray was hilarious. I waited patiently on the street corner with an eye on my wristwatch. At 10:59, I crossed the sidewalk. It was exactly eleven o'clock when I smiled at the ticket man and handed him a twenty-dollar bill. He whispered something to himself that sounded like, "I hope I'm not going to be sorry about this."

A young black woman opened the front door to the club.

"C'mon, honey. Follow me."

I entered a long narrow room filled with smoke. She led me to a small table at the farthest corner from the stretched out bar.

"You just stay seated here. Ms. Lily is running late. What possessed you to come to our club, of all the places? You're a very white girl."

"Why does it matter what my skin color is?"

"Do you see any white folks in here?"

"No, but I'm Portuguese. And even though I look white, my mother's ancestors came from Azagui, a small town on the Ivory Coast."

"You're very sweet. What would you like to drink?"

"Club soda, a twist of lemon, and no ice, please."

"Except for no ice, I had a feeling that's what you were going to order."

I counted ten people, mostly men seated at the bar and the three small tables. I felt a bit disappointed about the simplicity of the club. Nobody was looking in my direction, so I relaxed and pulled a book out of my pack.

About half an hour later, the hostess asked me to follow her to another room. I was pleasantly surprised when she sat me at a small, round table facing the foot-high stage. That was more like it. The room was barely lit and not too crowded. I focused my attention on the stage. A man was seated at a baby grand piano. Then Ms. Lily entered. She was a big lady, full of confidence, and I knew from the applause she was good.

I thanked God for giving me the opportunity to be in blues heaven.

I had not yet finished my drink when the waitress came by and pointed to two men seated at another table along the wall.

"Those two gentlemen would like to buy you a drink. What would you like?"

"I'm not finished with my soda, and I don't drink alcohol, so please tell them that and that I said thank you." I waved at them to acknowledge their kind offer.

I felt I had handled the situation like a pro, but then the one with a mustache and looking a lot like Sammy Davis Jr. came to my table and, crouching by my left side, the side I have difficulty hearing from, mumbled something about my table.

It sounded like he was asking permission to sit at my table with his friend Roy so they could hear the singer up close. I said okay.

I soon realized my mistake. So I kept nodding to the one on my left with the mustache and answering Roy on my right as politely as I could while hoping they would go bother someone else.

"You're a very beautiful lady," said Roy.

"Thank you."

"I really like you a lot."

"Thank you, that's nice… Ms. Lily sings great, doesn't she?"

"I'm single." He looked at me attentively.

I maintained my focus on Ms. Lily.

He went on, "I've been looking for a lady like you. I'd like to have a family and at least two children."

"I can't have any more children. Do you mind backing off?" I put both elbows on the table and my hands to the side of my face, staring at Ms. Lily. Marriage proposals must been the latest pick-up line at bars.

The one sitting on my left stood, walked around the table, gave Roy an encouraging tap on his shoulder and then announced, "I have to get going. I'll leave you two young people alone."

In the blessing of a badly lit room, I had become ageless.

"Roy, how old are you?" I said.

"I'm twenty-four."

"I'll be fifty-one in May."

"I don't care how old you are."

"Roy, I'm not here to find a man," I said slowly with a steady beat, "I'm here for one thing only, to listen to Ms. Lily sing. For goodness' sake, can't we just enjoy her music?" I added the magic word *pleeeease.*

"I respect your request." He remained quiet for the rest of the performance.

When the show ended, I stood. "Goodnight Roy."

"It's almost two in the morning. Did you drive here?"

"Yes. My car is in the parking lot."

"For your safety, I'll accompany you to your car."

"Thank you, Roy." Because he was so polite, I believed he could be trusted.

We walked slowly across the almost empty parking lot. He told me he was from Jamaica and worked at Applebee's and wanted me to know that he meant everything he had told me inside the club.

"Roy, I also meant everything I said. Thank you for walking me to my car. I appreciate that."

"I never met anyone like you. I envy the lucky guy you'll love someday."

We shook hands and, as I drove away, I waved goodbye. I liked him.

March 20

Marie came over to look at my bed and paid what I asked without blinking an eye. She had a new boyfriend. She was happy.

"I don't know why you're going to California. I used to live in the Bay Area, you know?"

"I'm looking forward to changing colleges. My friends there brag about the curriculum."

"You're going to a school that's across from San Francisco. So let me tell you, forget about meeting a straight man. They're all gay there."

People are so prejudiced. It's pathetic. I could've cared less about the population's sexual orientation. The furthest thing from my mind was dating. Matter of a fact, I didn't even count on Dexter to be my boyfriend again. I preferred not to make any plans until we were both sure about how we felt about each other.

When I left the testing center after my last final, my feet barely touched the steps out to the front lawn. "I'm done, finished. Yippee hurray!" A group of students heading the stairway stared and then smiled.

I couldn't wait to see my old friends from school, make new ones, and start a new life.

~ Chapter Eleven ~

Hello California!

I picked Dexter up at the Atlanta airport early the next morning. The idea that he had flown all the way from California to drive back with me made me feel loved. I was glad to see him. We planned leaving for California that same morning. Russell came by to pick up the couch and told Dexter that he'd better take good care of me, or else. Russell was smiling but I knew he meant it. I took extra precautions when loading my car. I wrapped the wine barrels with my thickest bath towels and placed my acoustic guitar inside its case in the trunk, I had loosened the strings so weather changes wouldn't affect the neck. I then set the two boxes of breakables, also in my trunk. My clothes and Dexter's duffel bag went into the backseat in case we needed to get to them. I've heard that driving light can make for better mileage, and we did have a long trip ahead of us.

Spring was in the air and since we were traveling west I wore only shorts and a t-shirt in keeping with the freedom of the road. Dexter warned me that some places might still have snow, but I was prepared. I had taken my green, goose-feather coat I used for winter visits to Jersey as well as my old but very warm Pittsburgh Steelers knit hat I had found ten years earlier on the sidewalk of a snowy sidewalk in Freehold, New Jersey.

Dexter and I planned to take our time driving and see a little of the country. We gave ourselves five days on the road, taking turns driving every three hours. Classes would be starting two days after we'd arrive. I felt we were cutting it close, but Dexter felt confident that five days was more than enough time.

We didn't have a chance to listen to Doug's tapes. There was too much to see and talk about. Sometimes that was good and other times not so good. Like when he came up with the idea of trying to explain the chiropractic philosophy to the first person we met to show how comfortable we were talking about our profession to a complete stranger.

When we reached Arkansas, we stopped at a small convenience store in a desolate little town. He bought beef jerky and waited for me by the door. I grabbed a bag of chips. When I was paying for them, the clerk asked about my spine keychain, so I told her that I was studying to be a chiropractor.

"I'll wait for you in the car," he yelled.

When I climbed into the car, he ignored me.

"What's the matter?"

"I saw the way you went on in there. I'm not as comfortable as you and feel very inadequate dealing with the public."

"She asked questions and I answered them. I didn't even do a good job."

"You're just saying that to make me feel better. You did fine in there."

"How do you know I did fine? You left when I was talking to her." I turned off the radio and opened the window.

"I'm not a people person like you. It comes natural to you. Besides that I have no patience listening to patients complaining about their health. I'll never be a successful chiropractor."

"So why are you studying to be one?" *What a lost soul, he just professed what's going to happen to him.*

"I used to think I wanted to be a healer. It sounded like something I'd like to do. But the thought of touching people to adjust them grosses me out."

Three days into traveling, he yelled, "Can't I share anything with you without you telling me you've had the same experience? It's very annoying. "

"Sorry, but that's how I fix things, by sharing solutions that worked for me."

"Who said I want solutions? I'm just telling you stuff that bothers me. Stop giving me advice. My last girlfriend was the greatest when it came to listening. Why can't you just listen?"

"Okay, go ahead. I promise to listen." *What a jerk! What a waste of money on the psychologist! My goodness these interstate roads are long. Boring!!!*

He enjoyed feeling sorry for himself, and I listened to him for hours, complaining about his childhood, his mother, his failing relationships, and how miserable he was with his depressing life. Good thing I had some practice treating Leila. I just nodded.

My trip to California had turned into a fulltime therapy session. No wonder his last girlfriend would just listen to him talk. She knew there was nothing she could say to help him.

We were headed down a mountain road in Arizona, with Dexter driving, coming around a corner. Suddenly, like an apparition, the scenery opened into a wide and phenomenal fiery red sunset, matched only by the surrealistic red of the rugged mountains.

"Oh my God, Dexter, have we landed on another planet?"

"That's Sedona. Some people believe the area is a vortex of psychic energy, releasing power from the Earth."

"I believe it. It's unreal. Let's stop and take a look."

"It's getting late and we need to find a place to spend the night. We can't afford a motel in this town." We drove right through, but I swore that one day I'd return to enjoy the vortexes and take in the energy I could feel summoning me.

The next morning we followed a nearly-deserted highway that led us toward the Grand Canyon. Slight vestiges of snow covered the stark landscape. When we stopped at a lookout point and stepped up to the rim I could see how it got its name. It truly is one of the most amazing natural wonders of the world. It was God's grandest creations.

We stood by one of the canyon lookouts, taking pictures of each other, but there was no romance. We had sex the night before; or, I should say *he* had sex, as he stated after the quickie that it was for his benefit only because I had been nothing but a flirt all day and didn't deserve any satisfaction. That statement made me very sad. In other words, he was punishing me. His perception, or, should I say his *reality,* was way out of whack. If anything, sex was the furthest thing from my mind after driving all day. I saw him as a lonely man suffocating in his own misery. I felt sorry for him and decided that all hope of being a couple was gone.

"We are so close to California how about if we stop in Las Vegas? I have always wondered what it's like." I asked.

"We'll drive through it. I really don't want to stop and waste time looking for a parking spot."

My mouth dropped open when we drove through the Vegas Strip. It was a man-made Grand Canyon of outlandish hotels, people, lights and sounds, another awesome place to visit someday on my own. It was midafternoon when we crossed the Nevada desert, a vast open field of nothing but sand color landscape when I noticed close to the road a purple cactus that looked a lot like a cabbage, with nothing growing near. I had never seen anything like that before. I pulled the car over and told Dexter that I wanted to look at it up close.

He stayed in the car.

I sat next to the cactus. It was as though Mama had put it there, just for me to see that even in death there was life, a different kind of life. I wanted to share those feelings with Dexter, but he said, "I'd rather you don't tell me anything about it." Then he withdrew into his own world.

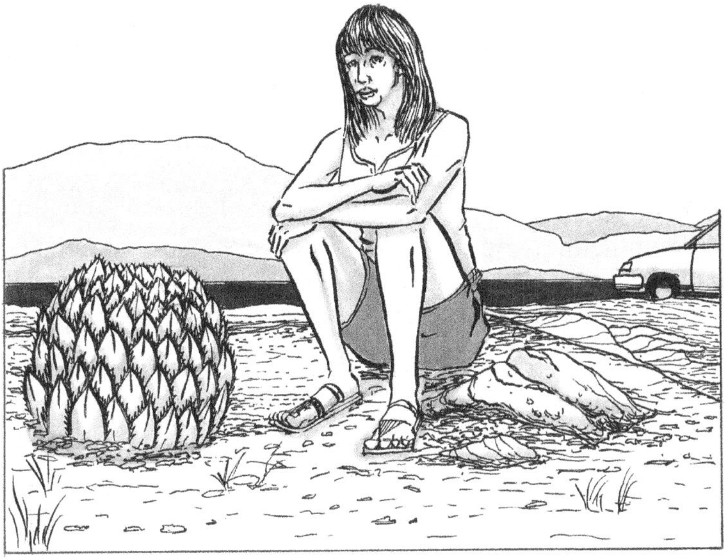

Desert Rose

After we arrived to California, we found ourselves on a tight curvy road in the mountains. Dexter was driving. I realized how pale he looked when he stated, "I can't breathe. My chest is closing down on me."

"What's the matter?"

"It's these curves, I can't take it." He stopped the car in the middle of the road and insisted I drive. It was a miracle that we didn't get rear-ended.

When we arrived at Dexter's apartment he told me he loved the trip, and more than ever, he was sure we were meant for each other. I felt the opposite. If anything, the trip had driven me further away from him. I would live with him only long enough to find a room to rent.

I walked into Life West Chiropractic College, waiting for the earth to swallow me. A radio psychic had predicted on our drive to California that, without a doubt, in his mind, California would be in the bottom of the Pacific Ocean, April 5.

Obviously the psychic was just another wacko looking for attention. I would hate to have crossed seven states, played psychoanalyst for five days, eaten breakfast and dinner every day at Denny's, and greeted all my old friends, only to be gobbled up after a quick but agonizing goodbye.

When I was walking to my first class, I saw an ad on the school bulletin board that said, "Room for Rent." I immediately called the number. A woman answered. Her name was Terry. "Yes, we have a room available, but you need to know that Marcy, my roommate, is a lesbian. Do you have any issues with that?"

"It's none of my business what her sexual preferences are. All I want is to rent a room, and I'm ready to move in today."

"Don't you want to look at it first?"

I did, during my lunch break. It was too good to be true, a house only two blocks from school. The room was small but it was furnished with a twin size bed and even had a built-in closet. I couldn't ask for more. I gave Terry four hundred dollars for the first month's rent and made plans to move in Saturday morning. Dexter didn't show any emotion when I told him I was moving. "Don't count on me to help you move. I'm busy." He is smart enough to know that it's over between us but we'll always be friends.

The next day, I found a bank, where I opened a checking account and rented a safety-deposit box to store my gun.

"Have you ever been in an earthquake?" I asked the bank manager.

"Oh yes, several times. We have tremors every day."

"Every day? I haven't felt any."

"They are little ones, not enough to bother anyone. Even the bigger ones aren't a big deal. You get used to them. Except for the last one, it brought down a few houses in San Francisco, including the bridge a few blocks down from here."

"What did it feel like?"

"Not bad. Not *really* bad, just the usual shaking. But I could tell this one was a bit stronger than usual because while driving home my car was weaving in all directions. I just kept driving and half way home everything settled down."

I was more relaxed after he said most earthquakes were just slight trembles, *healthy* trembles, needed for the earth to vent out from having a big one.

After a week in my new place I knew I had made a huge mistake. The San Andreas Fault ran through the middle of my room, next to my bed. It gave me the creeps every time I had to step over the crack. I hadn't noticed it when I checked the room because they had a throw rug over it. Having the fault, in my room was affecting my sleep.

Unfortunately going home meant locking myself in my room. My roommates had failed to mention they had two dirty, hairy, large dogs that made me sneeze from the moment I walked into the home and gave me a terrible sinus headache at night. The mildew in the bathroom was gross, but the kitchen made me gag. I couldn't bear to set my food on the counters. One evening, I scrubbed and cleaned one of the counters so I could make a salad. Marcy came in and reached into the salad bowl with her hand and stuffed her mouth. "Tasty stuff you have there." She grabbed another handful.

"It's all yours." I headed to Pizza Hut.

Besides the dirty kitchen and bathroom and two smelly dogs, Marcy turned out to be a female flasher. The first time she caught me by surprise. She looked like a man with tiny boobs, and I couldn't stop myself from busting out laughing. She looked so disappointed that I said, "Sorry, I didn't mean to laugh."

I knew I had it with her behavior, when I came out of the bathroom after taking my morning shower and caught her coming out of my bedroom.

"What were you doing in my room?"

"Oh, sorry, I thought it was my room." Once again she opened her robe in all her nakedness and went into her bedroom. If she were a man, I would have labeled her action as sexual harassment. Because she was a woman I acknowledged it as a clear case of identity crisis.

Aside from my deplorable living conditions, I loved my new school. The classes were small and the teachers enjoyed teaching, welcoming questions and staying after class if a student needed help. I had never been exposed to anything so wonderful in my life.

I spent the weekend looking at ads for another room to rent that would fit my meager student budget. Everything in California was double the price in Georgia, not only rentals, but also food and gas.

The main office informed me that I had to re-take a few classes that weren't transferable, so I couldn't do my clinical internship until the end of the year. I didn't mind. It was a small price to pay for a good education. I felt nurtured in my new environment and wasn't in any hurry to graduate. I saw Dexter at school and we were back to being good friends. I felt that like me he was content with our relationship.

I found a room at the home of Dr. Roberta Stuart, a chiropractor in San Leandro. I told my roommates that their dogs' hair was making me sick and I'd be moving out at the end of the week.

I bought a new twin-size bed that included a fancy black metal frame and had it delivered to my new place. I also bought a beautiful wood desk and matching chair for fifteen dollars at a garage sale. I couldn't wait to move into my new nest.

My bedroom window faced a gorgeous backyard with two lemon trees and a large avocado tree in the center. Three hundred-and-fifty dollars a month included utilities, my own bathroom, and lots of fresh lemonade.

Dexter called to ask if I wanted to go shopping at Costco, a new store where only members like him were allowed to shop. I found some very unique crates to put together. They came in flat metal square pieces and connected with plastic corner slip-ons. The crates were sturdy, but very light, and had a snazzy modern look. I stacked them against the larger wall in my bedroom to store my clothes and display some of my possessions. I figure that if an earthquake came along, I wouldn't have to worry about getting hit in the head with a dresser. For the final touch, I pulled out my creamy color lace bedspread and matching curtains that I had brought from Georgia. They had been used as stage props when I produced Veronica's Room a murder mystery, at the Simy Dinner Theater, in New Jersey, many years ago.

Roberta, the landlord and my roommate, was forty-nine years old, six feet tall, and had never been married. She had given up fighting the battle of the bulge, and even though she was a practicing chiropractor, she didn't lead a healthy lifestyle. Neither did her obese dog. She kept him tied to the avocado tree where he lay around all day and ate avocados. Roberta also had two cats, but they spent the day roaming the neighborhood. At night they slept on her bed.

My new found nest was a happy place to be. At the end of the day I was always glad to go home.

~ *Chapter Twelve* ~

Patrick

Transferring to Life West Chiropractic College had been a good decision on my part, a very satisfying experience to say the least. Wherever I turned for help, someone was always ready to show and tell. When Patrick the supervisor at the computer lab, noticed my frustration at the computer, he took me under his wing and wouldn't let me leave until I proved I knew how to use the computer. He worked part-time at the lab but was also a chiropractic student, one quarter ahead of me. He was very young, probably in his mid-thirties but he knew everything about computers. I was also very impressed that he was able to work and still keep up with his studies. Being a student was already a full time job for me and I felt very fortunate to have a government loan that covered not only tuition but also living expenses.

Dexter and I were not in the same classes, and at the end of the day we each went our separate ways. We still enjoyed talking to each other and a day didn't go by we didn't talk on the phone, but he didn't pressure me into going out with him. It was understood we were friends and could count on each other but our love for each other as a couple was no longer feasible. I had the freedom to date anyone I wanted. The last time I had seen him at the cafeteria, he said, "I spoke with someone at the finance office and if we get married we'll get a pretty good discount on our tuition. What do you think?"

I wanted to say, "Are you nuts?" Instead, I said, "I'm fine on financial aid. But thanks anyway."

As soon as I was done with lunch, I headed to the computer lab. I was determined to finish as many assignments as possible, even though we were only three weeks into the quarter. Some of my classmates called me anal-retentive, while they played shamelessly on the Internet. I imagined the small lab looking like a zoo during midterms and finals.

I sat in front of a computer. Patrick looked over my shoulder. “I admire your strategy,” he said, and then whispered in my ear, “I do the same.”

He helped me get over my fears about computers. He showed me how to browse the Internet, cut and paste text, and print my documents. I felt very computer literate.

One evening Roberta asked me to take her blood pressure. It was high—180 over 90. I said, “I’m worried about Span, being tied to a tree all day, eating avocados and not getting any exercise. He isn’t going to live long.”

“Are you talking about my dog or me?”

“Span.”

“My lifestyle is a lot like Span.”

“It doesn’t have to be that way.”

“I know. Having you here and watching how healthy you eat, makes me want to change.”

We did the pinky swear and she promised to start working out and eating healthier.

I was working on a class assignment at my usual computer station when Patrick stopped by. “Are you saving your work to a floppy disk?”

“What’s a floppy disk?”

“A disk storage medium to keep your work saved until you need to use it again. They sell them at our bookstore. Go get yourself a couple of them and then come back and I’ll show you how to use it.”

I ran down the hallway and was back in a jiffy.

He taught me how to insert the disk, and save my work to it. After I finished my next project and saved it successfully I glanced at Patrick. He sat at his desk on the other side of the lab smiling at me. I stood and walked over to him. "Thanks Patrick for all your help, I really appreciate it."

Just then two students approached his desk to talk to him.

"If you have a few minutes, have a seat next to me, and we'll talk after I help them out," he said. I sat down but I felt a bit uncomfortable, not sure what that was all about, since I already had thanked him. I took a good look at him for the first time as he helped the students. He had a beautiful smile, and his dark eyes seemed to sparkle every time he spoke. With thick curly dark hair and outdoorsy type of tan, he had a typical Mediterranean look. I presumed he was about ten years younger than me, but his demeanor projected tremendous self-confidence. He was in great physical condition and when he told me he worked out daily, I wasn't surprised.

"Are you a runner too?" he asked.

"No, but I enjoy speed walking. I do it every time I have a chance, like when I walk from my car to my classroom or when I go shopping." I laughed heartily, appreciating my own sense of humor.

But he was very serious. "I work out every day at the gym, but running is still the best for staying fit. You have a great figure but you need to start running if you want to maintain what you have."

"I don't like running. I get out of breath. I've never been able to handle it."

"You need to try harder. You want to run with me this Saturday?"

"I'll stick with speed walking. It's more my speed, get it?" Once again, I laughed about my keen sense of humor.

"I'm running this Saturday in San Francisco. Come run with me."

Wasn't he even listening? He was a bit pushy.

"I gotta go. See you another time." I left.

April 27

I had finished my last class and was heading to my car when I heard Patrick calling me across the parking lot.

He asked what kind of car I had and I showed him my Saturn.

"You keep it so clean. It looks brand new. I like it when a woman takes good care of her car. Would you like to see mine?"

I followed him.

"This is my 300ZX Nissan, five speed, manual."

"That's a very nice white car. Does it have good mileage?"

"No, but I don't use it every day. I save it for special occasions, like when I want to take a beautiful woman like you for a ride."

He took the top off and then opened the passenger door for me.

"C'mon, get in. I'll take you for a spin." I climbed in.

He drove around the parking lot, doing lots of sharp turns while shifting gears. I laughed while trying to hold on to my seat. The idea that he was trying to impress me with his driving skills made me feel special.

"So what do you think?" He flashed a dazzling smile.

"You're a very good driver."

"It's a very expensive sports car."

"Oh, wow! Well… it drives really well."

I didn't know what else to say. He probably thought I was an idiot and wouldn't help me at the computer lab anymore.

Roberta had begun walking her dog. She also bought a treadmill and set it up in the living room. I noticed she was more careful choosing what she ate. I just had to watch out she didn't eat my *healthy leftovers*, as she called them. I counted on them through the week. But considering she adjusted my spine every other day without charging me and she was such a pleasant roommate, I didn't mind. Like me, she was totally sold on the Activator Technique, a small handheld spring-loaded instrument that delivered safely an adjusting impulse to the spine and that was the only adjusting method she used.

Over the weekend, she attended a chiropractic seminar in Texas and left me in charge of feeding her pets.

Breanne, a student in one of my classes, invited me to study for midterms with her. We had a chance to talk one day when we sat for lunch at the cafeteria. She told me that she didn't like any of our classmates who seemed to ignore her, possibly because she was overweight. I didn't have the courage to tell her that she was the one that had created an invisible wall when she sat quietly at the back corner of the classroom and disappeared like a chameleon. Being overweight was not the problem, her clothing was unkempt, her hair would do well if she combed it, and her body odor yelled bad hygiene. I felt sorry for her and didn't have the nerve to tell her that I'd rather study by myself.

The house where she rented a room was in Hayward. It looked like a small house from the outside but it opened into a gigantic modern kitchen that was part of a living room and dining room with lots of geometric polished metal furnishings. The house smelled of deodorizer.

"We have to study in my room," she said. She was restricted from using all the other rooms including the kitchen. A twin size bed against her large bedroom window and a small desk with one chair filled her bedroom. She stood on top of her bed to pull open the white bedroom curtains. "How do you like this great view?"

I climbed on the bed, saw a deep ravine with a river below and quickly moved closer to the desk. “It looks like this room is standing in midair. It makes me feel unsafe.”

“It’s a California home. That’s the way they build them, on cliffs.”

“If there’s an earthquake, I hope you’re not in here. Your bed will be the first thing to slide out the window.”

“I never thought about that.”

“I would. Is there a part of the house standing on firm ground?”

“The whole house stands on posts.”

“I’m sorry, but I can’t concentrate in here. It makes me nervous.”

We made plans to get together the next day at the school library. I added earthquakes to my phobia list of bees and roller coasters.

Thanks to Patrick I now have an email address. I like the idea that he pays so much attention to me. Every day I make sure that I find something to do on the computer, just so I can see him.

Roberta brought me a beautiful abstract watercolor from Texas.

“I love it. What do you think the artist was trying to capture?” Abstracts have always puzzled me, just like poems, it’s all about individual interpretation.

“I don’t know, but the blue and gold colors reminded me of an angel. I just thought it fitted you.”

I hung the watercolor on my bedroom wall and thanked her by making dinner, my very special salad of fresh kale, lettuce, tomatoes, grapefruit, walnuts, avocado, garlic, olive oil and lemon juice.

April 30

During my lunch break, I stopped at the computer lab to see if Patrick had won the race on Saturday. He was all smiles and hugged me exuberantly.

"I love country-western music," he said. "How would you like to go out with me Friday night to a country dance club?"

My first instinct was to ask whether he wouldn't rather go with someone his own age, but decided he only wanted to take me dancing. *Stop making a mountain out of a molehill and enjoy the night out.* We exchanged phone numbers.

When I got home I called my sons to get some manly advice about going out with someone much younger than me. Steve said, "Most likely he wants to have sex with you. Why else would he ask you out?" Ralph said, "It's only a date, just have fun."

The night of the dance, I wore my old leather miniskirt with my favorite cream-colored lace shirt, which Mama had made for me many years ago. To give myself the final touch of a country-western girl I put on my tight knee-high dark brown boots. These boots were very special, because when I wore them I knew I looked sexy. When I opened the door, he smiled. I had chosen the right outfit. He wore a cowboy hat and shirt, jeans and his belt displayed a large silver belt buckle that couldn't be missed. The western pointy boots completed his outfit. He was very handsome.

On the way to San Francisco, we talked about earthquakes. He knew a lot about them and gave me all kinds of ideas on how to cope with *the big one.* When we walked into the country bar, I felt very special when he put his arm around my waist. He wasn't afraid of showing affection, and that made me very happy.

We sat at a small table by the dance floor. It was easy to hear him because we were the only ones. He had been married twice. I figured that was normal for California people. He had a son and a daughter from the first marriage and they lived in Sacramento with their mother. He had been born in Sacramento and decided to be a chiropractor, because it provided a good living. People started arriving and a small band of musicians began playing country music. I couldn't wait to dance since I could no longer hear him anyway.

He said something and stood. I knew he wasn't asking me to dance because he was very serious, looking around him as if he was scared.

I got up. "What did you say?"

"I'm not comfortable with the look of things here. Let's get out of here."

"What's wrong?"

"I can't explain. We need to leave." He walked towards the exit and I followed him.

I felt disappointed. Then I reasoned, perhaps he had detected an earthquake coming and he didn't want to scare me. As we walked down the street, we passed by a pool hall. He asked if I would play.

"I'd love to. But I warn you, I'm not good at it."

"I never met anyone so wild and yet so ladylike."

"Thank you, but I consider playing pool far from being wild. I used to have a pool table in my house in New Jersey when I was married. My sons and I played it all the time."

As soon as we walked in, he said, "I can't handle the smoke. I can't stay here."

It was a chilly night. I should have brought a jacket. I held on to his arm, taking in some of his body heat.

He said, "My father is the cause of my asthma. He used to hold me on his lap when I was a toddler and smoke. I hate him for ruining my lungs."

"In the old days, people didn't know about the dangers of smoking. My mother used to pretend to be smoking when we would go to the theater. In those days smoking meant you were sophisticated."

"Ignorance is no excuse. My father should have known better."

It was an irrational statement, but I felt I should stay away from his family issues.

When he dropped me off at my place, he didn't try taking advantage of me. We hugged briefly and said good night after I invited him to my birthday party next week.

I guess I'm slow but it wasn't until the next morning that I begun wondering why Patrick had left the country bar in such a hurry. Maybe he did say the reason but I had not heard him because of my hearing deficit, when there's noise around. I decided not to question him.

May 7

Patrick arrived on Saturday with a bouquet of pink roses. He was the first to arrive and offered to put the chicken pieces on the grill. When he saw I had used a whole bag of briquettes, he said, "I can tell you've never barbequed." He laughed. So did I, but I felt humiliated. Then the doorbell rang and he said, "Don't worry, I'll take care of the grill for you, okay?" And he gave me a quick hug.

Donna, Cody, Sean, Brian and Isabelle had arrived. I made believe I didn't see Donna hiding a cake box behind her back. She said, "So where's the kitchen, in this lovely place?" A few minutes later Dexter showed up.

I served barbequed chicken, corn on the cob, and potato salad. We ate at the picnic table on the back patio. We had a great time talking, mostly about school and chiropractic.

After a bit, Donna disappeared. When she returned with the birthday cake, I acted surprised. They all sang and I blew out the one candle. Dexter gave me a delicate pair of silver earrings. Sean brought a jar of incense, Brian and Isabelle, a bottle of red wine. In addition to the roses, Patrick gave me a card with the illustration of a donkey jumping off a cliff. Inside it said, "How does it feel to be this old today? Let me know what to expect when I get to be your age." He was surprised I didn't laugh when I opened the card.

Everyone left except for Sean and Dexter. They remained seated in the living room. I stood by the doorway to the kitchen. "I need to clean up the place and get back to studying." Dexter stood, walked to the front door and said, "It's late. I'm sure Veronica wants us to leave now." He waited for Sean to respond.

"Go ahead, if you want," Sean said. "I'm staying a little longer."

Sean helped me clean up, and then we sat on the living room couch. "How do you know so many people in school?" He said.

"Except for you and Patrick, I knew everybody else from Georgia. They used to attend school with me."

"Are you and Patrick dating each other?"

That was none of his business. I remained silent.

"Do you know Karolyn McCarter in eighth quarter?"

I shook my head no.

"She's Patrick's ex-girlfriend. They lived together for a month before she left him. She was afraid for her life and she has a court order against him. He isn't even allowed to be in the same classroom."

"Thank you for telling me all that, but I don't have any personal problems with Patrick. We are only friends." I stood to show him the door.

Dexter called me the next evening. "I'm very concerned about you being involved with Patrick. Karolyn told me to warn you about him."

"Warn me about what? My goodness, Patrick and I have gone out on one date and the whole school is up in arms."

"She's certain that he has some kind of mental illness and isn't to be trusted."

"That's a terrible thing to say about someone. What did he do to her?"

"She told me he's very possessive and it was hell living with him. He wouldn't allow her to even talk to her family or friends. He wouldn't let her out of his sight, and the only way she could talk on the phone was to come up with a good excuse to leave his apartment."

"I will not make a decision based on Patrick's past relationship with someone else."

"You know I'm your friend and just want what's best for you. You need to talk to Karolyn and hear what she has to say."

I didn't appreciate his intrusion into my private life. It sounded as though Karolyn was trying to get back at Patrick by destroying his future relationships and Dexter was going along because he was jealous. People can be so mean, making up stories like that just to destroy someone's happiness. I was shaking when I hung up.

Roberta and I sat in her living room after dinner and I told her about the first date with Patrick and my birthday party.

"Is he handsome?" She asked.

"Yes, very good-looking."

"Is he a student? How old is he?"

"Patrick is a chiropractic student, one quarter ahead of me. He's twelve years younger than me." I added quickly, "But he looks older. We actually look about the same age."

"Age means nothing. What's important is that you get along and have a lot in common."

"We get along great and we have a lot in common. But don't worry, Roberta. I'm just enjoying his company, that's all."

Patrick and I began meeting every day during lunch break. The weather was always pleasant and sunny but not harsh on the eyes. We didn't need sunglasses. We sat on a bench by the school's parking lot eating our homemade sandwiches and talking. He shared some of his chips or pistachio nuts and I would give him half of my fruit. He liked making games out of everything, like throwing a chip in the air and catching it with his mouth or juggling the grapes I shared with him. He enjoyed entertaining me, and being with him was pure fun.

I felt very special when he asked me to go to the school picnic with him that weekend.

The picnic was sponsored by our college and held outdoors. It took over a quarter of our parking lot. There was a festive feeling in the air, teachers and students mingled together, a music band composed of four students played some light rock music, the picnic wood tables were covered with bright red plastic table cloths, and decorated with red, white and blue balloons. Patrick and I stood in line at the Western Style buffet and filled our plates with fried chicken, baked beans, mashed potatoes, corn on the cob and some fresh green salad. He didn't want to sit with the other students and asked me to follow him to the middle of the empty field behind the parking lot. "Isn't this a lot better, just the two of us?" he said as we sat on the hard granular ground. When he asked me if I had anyone special in my life, I told him about my past involvement with Dexter and assured him that were just friends. We exchanged funny stories about our past and took turns feeding each other bits of food while laughing at the mess we were making. When we stood, he used his paper napkin to wipe the side of my mouth. Then he said, "You're so beautiful." He caressed my face. I responded by touching his face. We drew closer. We kissed. It wasn't a simple or even average kiss. It was probably the longest kiss I ever had. "Will you be my girlfriend?"

How could I resist such simple request?

"I want everyone to see that you're my girl."

We held hands as we walked back to the school picnic. He wasn't afraid to show his feelings towards me and I felt the same towards him.

The next day he surprised me during our lunch interlude with a daisy inserted in a plastic mini green bud vase.

"I bought two of these vases just to keep your flowers alive. Tomorrow bring me the vase back so I can use it again. And every day I'll bring you a new flower."

The following day he gave me a pager and on a small piece of paper he had typed numbers that referred to a letter of the alphabet.

"This will be our secret code for sending messages to each other," he said.

I learned a lot about Patrick during our lunch dates. Before he decided to become a chiropractor, he had worked for the CIA and been trained in various skilled techniques of self-defense. At one point he told me what had happened less than a month ago but made me promise I wouldn't tell anyone. When he was running in Castro Valley, where he lived, two Mexican men with knives had attacked him. He beat them so badly he believed he killed them. The next day he checked the newspapers, but found nothing about them.

I put Patrick's small framed picture on top of the desk in my room. It was just a head shot but his smile and the way he seemed to look directly at me made my heart beat faster. I was in love. When my birthday flowers began to dry up I tied them to the curtain rod on my bedroom window. My bedroom looked like a love nest.

One Saturday I attended an all-day Parker Chiropractic seminar with Dexter. Dexter and I had already paid for the seminar tickets and Patrick knew about the event before we had started dating. He showed no sign of jealousy. He was running in San Francisco on that day.

When I got home there was a message in my answering machine from Patrick. "I ran seven miles and my feet are killing me, but I'm hoping I can come over and spend some time together. Call me." I did.

We sat in the porch swing in the backyard. Roberta brought us a blanket. "It's cold out there. You guys need a love blanket to wrap yourselves with."

Patrick and I couldn't get any closer. I wound up on his lap. We kissed.

"Let's make a game of it." He said. "I'll kiss you on the lips first and then you kiss me back, but it has to be different from the way I kissed you."

The kissing *game* was more than interlocking lips or French kissing. Romance and creativity went hand in hand. We did our best to outdo each other.

"How about going to my room and I'll give you a foot massage?" I asked him.

"Can you do both feet, though?" He laughed.

He lay on my bed and I propped him up with pillows. Massaging his sparkly clean feet became a sexual encounter, fueled by all his sweet-talking. Chemically speaking, we brewed well together, and if fireworks were to be the metaphor, one could say we lit up the sky that evening.

In less than twenty-four hours I came down with the honeymoon curse, a urinary-tract infection that had me curling up in pain during the afternoon classes. Roberta came to my rescue. She called her sister-in-law, a veterinarian, and asked for an antibiotic for her dog. No doctors' bill and the price of *dog antibiotic* was one-tenth of *people antibiotic.*

I was back to normal the next day.

While we were having our usual lunch in school, Patrick told me he had dedicated a wall in his bedroom for the love notes I was giving him, and he would be thrilled if I would do the same. It was a brilliant idea. That evening I decorated the wall above the metal crates with all his love notes, using a long string and two thumbtacks. He was the magician of romance and I enjoyed being under his spell.

I invited Roberta to see my bedroom wall, but she left without saying a word. I found her seated on the living room couch.

"I thought you'd be happy for me. Patrick and I are in love and he wants me to move in with him."

"If you don't mind me saying this, you're both going too fast. Give it some time. Besides, I'll be very upset if you move."

"Patrick and I are in love. You've seen my bedroom. All his love letters and little notes are hanging on the wall, like a tapestry. We can't live apart from each other."

"I don't want to alarm you, but there's something about him that scares me. I don't trust him. Don't ask me why."

"Roberta, you're wrong. You've seen him only once. If you knew him like I do, you'd realize he's a very nice person."

"It's only been a few weeks since you met each other. Besides sex, what do you like so much about him?"

"He's the opposite of Al, my ex-husband. Al never made any decisions. Patrick has everything planned all the time. And he's full of surprises, every day."

"Do you mind if I look into your future with him?"

"How are you going to do that?"

"I have ways."

"Are you kidding me?"

"Just trust me, will you?"

"Okay, sorry…."

Roberta held my hands and closed her eyes. I waited patiently until she opened them and sat up straight.

"Veronica, please listen. He's going to ask you to marry him. It would be a big mistake."

"I have no intentions of getting married again."

She held up her hand. "Stop right there. He's going to change your mind. Believe me when I say he's a very persuasive man. Veronica, promise me you won't change your last name to his. You must keep your last name."

She saw my disbelief and picked up my right hand and put it on her chest by her heart. "Don't ask me any questions; just promise me you'll do what I'm asking you. You'll be much happier later." She sounded like my mother.

"I promise."

Before I went to bed I knocked at her bedroom door. "Roberta, are you sleeping?"

"Almost..."

"Don't worry, I'm not moving soon but when I do I'll give you at least one month's notice. Good night."

She didn't answer.

On weekends, Patrick and I had dinner at his apartment. It always consisted of a salad and a small portion of grilled chicken and potato or rice. He prided himself in preparing garlic bread with every meal. I was in charge of making the salad, but there wasn't much to do. He had the salad already pre-washed and sliced inside two sandwich size bags. He had the amount down to a tee, it all fitted exactly into two small salad bowls.

When he ran out of his pre-packed veggies one day, his instructions were very precise. "For each of us, use two thin slices of green pepper, one slice of tomato, three small lettuce leaves cut into bite sizes, one slice of cucumber, and one thin slice of onion."

Mincing the garlic I was allowed to use my judgment, since he loved fresh garlic.

Patrick invited me to spend the weekend in Sacramento at his parent's house. He wanted me to meet his family, who he described as being very unusual, yet simple, country folks. On the way to Sacramento, I mentioned that I would like to pick up a melon or a watermelon at one of the vegetable stands on the road to share with them.

"My family doesn't like melon or watermelon." He then added, "They're settled in their old ways and are not sophisticated like you."

"I'm far from being sophisticated. I'm just a regular person like you."

"No, you grew up in Europe. My folks have lived most of their lives in Sacramento. I'm a bit nervous, hoping that you'll like them."

"They're your family. Of course I'll like them."

"Yes, they're my family, but they're also a bit bizarre."

How bizarre could his family be?

He didn't take his eye off the road. "You need to be prepared. I'm going to describe to you each member of my family, so you'll have a better understanding of who they are. I asked my parents not to invite Christine, my first wife, but they insist she's part of the family. She has shoulder length dirty blonde hair, is five feet tall, and weighs over a hundred and fifty pounds. She doesn't take care of herself, one of the reasons I asked for a divorce. I don't talk to her and you shouldn't either. And she's spoiling my kids, but they're going to love you, I'm sure. I already told Paul, who's fifteen and taller than me, that you play guitar, and he can't wait to meet you. Lauren, is a year younger. You'll recognize her because she looks a lot like me. She's also a lot smarter than her brother. I hate to say this but I have no hopes for Paul. He's lazy, like his mother. My sister, Nancy, is the tallest of the family. Too tall for a woman, it's really pathetic. I should have been the tall one, not her. Her husband makes a lot of money and she doesn't have to work. They spend all their money on antiques. I can think of better things to do with all the money they waste on junk. My mom is my mom. You'll know her as soon as you see her. She has curly white hair and is always in the kitchen cooking for everyone. My father has no education and acts crazy sometimes, very embarrassing when we go to a restaurant and he comes out of the bathroom wearing the toilet seat paper around his neck like a bib. He thinks it's funny. Would you like to see how fast my car can drive around the curves?"

"Faster than this?"

"Just watch."

He drove like a professional racecar driver—or what someone else might call a suicidal maniac. I maintained my confident smile while psyching myself not to show fear, except for holding on to my seat with both hands while trying to relax my shoulders.

Finally, at fifty-one, I find someone that's wild and fearless like a superhero, yet, he loves me enough to want to introduce me to his family. If the car goes over the abyss on my right, I will be dying with the man I love, someone as cool as James Dean.

I could see the sheer drop on my side. Straight down. He was a great driver and very precise in everything he did. There was no way he would lose control of the wheel and run off the road. I relaxed. If this was my last day on earth then it was meant to be. I would enjoy the moment.

When he stopped the car in front of his parents' home, a retired mobile home community I took a deep breath of relief. Patrick's family welcomed me with opened arms. I recognized everyone from his detailed description. Bonnie, his mom, was the matriarch of the family. She didn't wear make-up or color her naturally snow-white curly hair, and she didn't talk much, but I was immediately attracted to the warmth and kindness that seemed to radiate naturally from her. Roger, his father, was a real down-to-earth funny character. He was tall and skinny with dry leathery skin, most likely from years of smoking.

I also took a liking to Christina, Patrick's first wife. She spoke softly, and like Bonnie, gentleness seemed to radiate from her. Her son, Paul, was a happy-go-lucky kid that was determined I was going to teach him how to play guitar the next time we got together. His sister, Lauren, kept putting her head on my shoulder and then hugging me. Nancy reminded me of a young Native American, with her beautiful dark features and silky long dark hair. Sean, her husband, had a contagious laughter and they both looked like a happy couple. Their son, Mark, was very tall and extremely quiet, but his sister, Susan, made up for it by being bright and cheery. She reminded me of a young hippie.

Josh, Patrick's brother, had his latest girlfriend with him and her two small youngsters. According to Patrick, his brother was a ladies' man and had more children than fingers on his hands from two ex-wives and unlimited ex-girlfriends.

I felt loved by everyone and there was a sense of family unity in the air that made me relax and feel glad to be there.

They all seemed very normal until Patrick said, "In order for you to be part of my family you'll have to go through a family initiation process. Stay here in the kitchen until we ask you to come into the living room."

I could barely hear what they were saying. It crossed my mind that maybe they were cannibals or into some kind of witchcraft ritual and soon enough I would be sacrificed on the altar possibly hidden behind one of their living room wood panels. It would do me no good to cry or show fear. Most likely the front door was bolted shut. My goose was cooked, and there were too many of them to fight my way out.

Patrick came into the kitchen and announced, "Come on! We're ready for you."

I walked in the living room to find the whole clan standing in a circle, holding hands. Most likely a Satan ritual and I was about to be indoctrinated into some kind of blood exchange. If I left that house alive, I was done with Patrick and all future dating.

"C'mon Veronica, don't be scared. Stand in the middle of the circle," said Patrick's brother.

I did and waited for further instructions. *They look so ordinary and yet they're the strangest people I ever met. Patrick was right when he said his family was kind of weird.*

"Okay, now, these are the rules. You're to do something special that will make us all clap our hands at the same time, but you can't speak. If you're successful, you'll be accepted into our family."

I didn't even pay attention to who had spoken. My goodness, they were so lovable in such a creepy way! I began humming the theme song to the television show, The Addams Family. They hummed along. I finished the tune with the famous double handclap. My indoctrination was a hit.

Patrick bragged to his mother, that he'd found the woman of his dreams. "Veronica didn't show any signs of fear when I

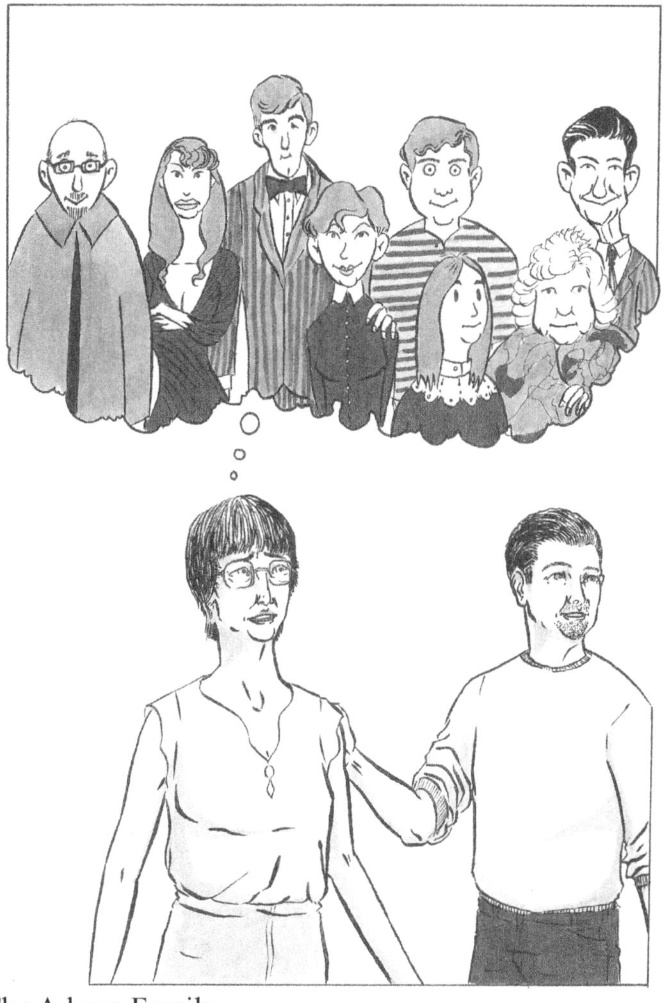

The Adams Family

drove a bit enthusiastically around some steep roads on the way here. She trusts me completely with her life." He hugged me and put his arm over my shoulder as we sat next to his mom.

"Son, you shouldn't take a chance driving crazy just to make a point. You could have lost control of the car."

"Veronica, tell my mother how good of a driver I am."

"He drives great."

"See? Nothing to worry about." He kissed me.

Dinner included lasagna, salad and cherry pie with ice cream. There was no formal seating arrangements, there were too many of us, some sat in the dining room with the plate on their lap others at the kitchen counter. Bonnie insisted I sit at the kitchen table with her, Nancy and Christina. I felt like a very special guest of honor. They wanted to know everything about Portugal, where I was born, and why I came to America. I told them about my pre-arranged marriage. I had lots of stories to tell them.

By ten, everyone had left and Bonnie showed us the room where Patrick and I would be sleeping. The room was small, just big enough to fit a full-size bed and a side table. The bedspread was covered with cowboys riding on horses. Three antelope antlers hung on one of the walls, and the ceiling lamp was made of what seemed to be cowhide.

The next morning we planned to stop at the old part of Sacramento, before heading back to the Bay Area. Bonnie made us pancakes for breakfast. Before leaving, Patrick said, "Mom don't you agree that Veronica and I make a perfect couple?"

"Yes, honey you do."

He grabbed me by the shoulders. "Veronica, let's get married."

"I'm sorry, but we haven't dated long enough." I looked at his mother, waiting for her to put some sense into his head. She read my mind.

"I agree with Veronica. You need to spend more time together before jumping into marriage. Besides, you've already been married twice, son, and it didn't work out. Why do it again? "

"Oh, I shouldn't have asked your opinion. Okay we're leaving." He kissed her goodbye.

When I hugged Bonnie, she whispered, "I like you a lot. Please don't take personally what I said."

"What you said makes a lot of sense. And I like you a lot, too." I gave her a kiss on the cheek. She smelled of apple pie with a hint of cinnamon.

Flowers, love notes on my car window, walking hand in hand, looking onto each other's eyes, kisses—lots of kisses—sex every night. I was hardly ever going home. Sex was different each night; I never knew what to expect. He must have read the book of positions, because he was an enthusiastic expert on the art of lovemaking. No place was out of limits; even his kitchen counter was christened. He insisted on making dinner and always had two lit candles on the table and the extra plastic bud vase he kept with a daisy, by my plate. Sometimes we danced after dinner, in his living room, but we always made love.

He was moved to tears when I brought my guitar to his place and played the classical piece Romance Antigua.

"I'm the luckiest man in the world to have a woman like you in my life. You're everything I ever wished for."

He asked me to leave the guitar at his apartment so I could play for him every time I visited.

The next evening we were in his bedroom when he turned on his message machine and I heard a woman say, "Hi, Patrick, thanks for asking me out. Give me a call. I'd love to go out with you this Saturday."

I left the room crying and ran downstairs to get my coat. He ran after me. "Are you upset about what you heard?"

"What do you think? I like to cry for no reason? Yes, I'm upset. You told me you loved me and asked me to marry you. How do you think I feel after hearing that message? What's going on?"

"This was just a test. I wanted to know if you really love me. Now that I see you're upset and crying, I know you really love me. Look, I'm going to call her back right now and tell her I only have one woman in my life, you." He grabbed my hand and took me back upstairs to his room so I could hear him tell Susie I was the only woman in his life and not to call him again.

I forgave him.

Supposedly, Patrick had a young couple renting the bedroom next to his, but I never saw them. "They work evenings," he said.

The first night I went to use the bathroom he stopped me. "You have to use the bathroom downstairs. This bathroom belongs to my roommates."

"What about a shower? There's no shower downstairs, only a toilet."

"You can shower upstairs but that's it."

"I hate having to go all the way downstairs to use the toilet when there's one up here. Besides, if I'm using their shower, I'm using their bathroom already. Can you talk to them?"

Patrick was on a tight budget and insisted that when I took a shower, I should use as little water as possible. I was to wet myself, then turn off the water while I soaped up or I shampooed. Once I was all sudsy, I could turn the water back on and be done. It was hard to get used to bathing that way. One of the things I loved most about taking a shower was the luxury of being pampered with hot water running all over my body without interruptions. Most likely something to do with growing up poor and my parents not being able to afford a tub much less hot water from a shower.

Patrick was fanatical about everything being spotless, but when it came to having sex, he had no restraints. He asked me not to bathe before going to bed. "I love the natural smell of your body," he said.

He had a lot in common with Napoleon Bonaparte who, according to history, indicated in his romantic letters to Josephine that he was coming home soon from the battlefield and she was not to bathe. Men!

There were other odd things about Patrick. He collected his fingernail clippings in jars, which he kept in the medicine cabinet downstairs. Besides being strange, it was gross, but I didn't ask him why because I loved him and as such, I should accept his peculiarities. I did ask him about his last girlfriend.

"I'm more than happy to tell you," he said. "I was terribly in love with her, and when she threatened to leave me without a good reason, I showed her my gun and told her I was going to shoot myself in the garage. I was only pretending, but she called the cops and got a court-order against me. Can you believe it?"

"You poor thing. What you had to go through." I hugged him.

"Yeah, but now I realize it was for the best. You're my one-and-only and I love you with all my heart."

He was a bit weird, but so was everybody else in one way or another; besides, I loved him.

My friends from school, Donna and Cody planned a trip to Mexico with ten other students at the end of the quarter and invited me to go with them. We would be working as volunteer chiropractic doctors for a week at a hospital in a town called Delicias, in the state of Chihuahua. Two licensed chiropractors would be overseeing us. This trip was a great opportunity to practice my adjusting technique. The more I perfected the art and science of adjusting the spine, the better results I would have when I would be treating patients at the college's clinic in about six months. They also wanted to use me as their translator since I spoke Spanish.

I asked Patrick if he would like to go with me. He loved the idea so much that he invited his sister and her two children and his son to meet us in Delicias. After our week in Delicias, his family would join us and we would take the train to Mazatlán. The whole thing sounded like a very exciting adventure.

Because I had sold my portable adjusting table before leaving Georgia, I had to buy a new one to take to Mexico and it wasn't cheap. Donna and Cody warned me about the Mexican police at the border. If they asked me the value of my adjusting table, I should say, "This old piece of junk? Five bucks." Otherwise I would be "taxed" to death. I passed this bit of information to Patrick.

Patrick showed me two rolled up posters hidden behind his doubled sided antique desk in his bedroom. An artist named Thomas Kinkade had painted the originals, and the posters were worth thousands of dollars each. I couldn't see how a poster of any kind could be worth much. He was most likely trying to impress me.

"When I divorced Joan, my second wife, I worked out a deal with her. In exchange for my Nissan which we had bought together, and these two posters, I gave her two thousand dollars cash and let her keep the other two posters, which had little to no value."

"Why did you get divorced?"

"She knew every trick in the book when it came to pleasing a man. It wasn't until I married her that I figured out she couldn't be that good unless she had been a prostitute."

"She told you?"

"No, she never confessed, but I no longer trusted her. Even my family didn't like her."

Wow, how good could she be in bed? Maybe that's where he'd learned so much about pleasing a woman. I wondered why his family didn't like her but I wasn't going to ask him. They liked me and that's all that mattered.

Patrick asked me again, why I still live with Roberta and pay for rent and utilities when I spent most of my time at his apartment.

"You should move in with me now, before the end of the quarter. We're leaving for Mexico right after and when we get back we'll be busy starting a new quarter. How about you move in this weekend?"

"I don't feel right doing that while Roberta is away in New York. I should wait until she gets back from her seminar on Monday."

"I thought you loved me. Don't you want to be together?"

"I guess I could leave her a letter explaining."

"That's right. This calls for a special celebration." He put on the stereo and sang me one of his favorite cowboy songs while walking around bowl-legged with his thumbs in his pockets. I laughed so hard that I had tears rolling down my cheeks and could barely breathe. Then he laid me down on the couch and we made love. Later he told me he expected me to join his gym so he could be my trainer, and then we made love again.

I planned to move in with Patrick on Sunday afternoon. Between that and finals on Monday, I barely had time to eat. Luckily I had finished my written assignments, but it took most of Saturday to pack everything and dismantle the plastic crates. I had done a good job putting them together and had to work hard at pulling out the corners. My fingers were very sore when I finished. Patrick came by on Sunday morning with his pick-up. I left Roberta a letter saying that I had moved in with Patrick but had been in every day to take care of her pets while she was gone. I enclosed next month's rent.

In my heart, I knew I was wrong to leave while she was away.

On Tuesday morning, I drove to Roberta's house to apologize. Her car was outside but she wouldn't open her door.

When I got home I called her on the phone, but as soon as she heard my voice she said, "Remember what you promised me. Good luck. You're going to need it." She hung up.

Before we left for Mexico, Patrick taped two ping-pong balls behind our bedroom door.

"If these aren't in place when we return, I'll know *they* came into our bedroom."

"You mean your roommates?"

"Yes, them."

He probably got the idea from watching so many James Bond movies. Kind of sad though, that he didn't trust anyone.

~ *Chapter Thirteen* ~

VIVA MEXICO!

June 20

After flying to San Diego and crossing the Mexican border into Tijuana, Patrick and I met with the other chiropractic students for the ten-hour bus ride to Delicias. By volunteering our time to work in the hospital we all felt like we were doing something meaningful. Everyone was in good spirits. Donna and Cody came over to talk, but Patrick turned toward the window and ignored them.

"I hope you're more interested in being with me than with a bunch of phonies," he said after they left.

"I've known them since we attended college in Georgia and they are very nice people. You met them at my birthday party, remember?"

"I do and I also know they talk behind my back because they're friends with my ex-girlfriend. These are your friends not mine. I have nothing to say to them." I knew they weren't talking about him, but I decided to change the subject. "Have you noticed how many crosses with flowers are along the highway? The people in Mexico must be very religious."

"It has nothing to do with being religious. Those spots are markers where someone died in a car accident. Everybody knows Mexicans are lousy drivers. I'm surprised you didn't know that."

We arrived to Delicias at eleven at night. One of the students who had been to Delicias recommended a hotel he had liked, so most of the students opted to stay there. Patrick had made arrangements before we left California to stay at an inexpensive motel. When I asked the bus driver where it was, he recommended we take a taxi because it was five long blocks from the bus station. Patrick felt it was a waste of money. He hauled both portable adjusting tables, which were extremely heavy, and I carried both backpacks.

We immediately took notice that the sidewalks were as high as two feet and if we didn't watch our step we could easily break an ankle when stepping off. "Watch out for the potholes." Patrick pointed to the sidewalk in front of us. It was a broken down city in dying need of repairs. Except for two taverns, all the stores along the way were closed. All the housing and shops were one level and I had a feeling that we were on the western side of the city. "The weather is just like in Georgia, hot and muggy." I stopped to wipe my face.

Forty-five minutes later we saw our motel, lit by one light bulb over their office entrance. "I didn't know they had Motel 6, here in Mexico." I laughed.

The room was clean, had a queen size bed, bathroom and a sink in the room. According to Patrick we were only three blocks from the hospital. We were both happy.

Patrick and I arrived at the hospital at seven-thirty the next morning carrying our tables to meet with the other students and our two supervising chiropractic doctors. A hospital staff member and a nurse greeted us, and told us that it had been all over the radio and television, that American doctors were volunteering their services at the hospital. The huge lobby was filled to capacity. The white chalk walls, reminded me of the hospital my mother had taken me when I was five years old to have my tonsils out. The stagnant smell of iodine, sickness, heat and lack of oxygen, made my stomach tighten up. The only difference now was everyone spoke Spanish.

I asked the nurse, who to my surprise was also called Veronica, "How many people are here to see us?"

"Each person has a numbered ticket, and according to this list, one hundred and ninety-seven. I expect it will double after lunch."

Two other students joined us. The four of us, were shown to an empty room, just big enough to fit the adjusting tables and prepared ourselves to see patients until five o'clock. Patrick set our hand sanitizer and hand soap on top of the corner sink with a handwritten note next to them, "Do not use." It was meant for the other two students. I asked Veronica for paper towels to dry our hands and she brought us half a dozen white cloth towels. I told her I had never met someone with my name. She smiled and said, "Veronica was a saint. It is a very popular name in Mexico."

My first patient was an elderly man. "Please fix my husband's knees, I miss dancing with him." His wife handed me a homemade pineapple pie. I was ready to address all kinds of health issues except the stagnant hot air and body odors that within an hour saturated the room, making Patrick and the other two students sweat like open faucets. Unable to cool off because I don't sweat, I felt nauseous and dizzy. Mark, the tallest of us stood on his adjusting table and was able to open the window half way. It didn't help. What we needed was an air conditioner. Joyce, the other student, put away her table and left for the day. Patrick and I took several *breathing* breaks outside and when lunch time came we took our time walking to the motel and back.

On the second day, I nearly had a heat stroke walking from the hospital to the motel during our lunch break. I had a pounding headache and felt profoundly weak. I removed my clothes and laid like a star fish spread out on the bed. "Patrick, unless you get me some ice to cool off as soon as possible I believe that I'm gonna die." He ran out of the room and came back with a small bag of ice. He wrapped some ice cubes around my head and stroked my body gently with a wet towel. "I love you Veronica." He smiled before kissing me softly on the lips. As soon as I felt better, we went looking for a spray bottle. I found one at a hardware store. They sold only cheap plastic sprayers, but it was better than nothing. I used it daily when walking from the motel to the hospital and back. Occasionally people in the street would smile at me and point at themselves, encouraging me to spray them. When we left Delicias, I wondered if water spraying had become a trend among the population.

Patrick was afraid we would catch some intestinal bug. He had brought along a bag of limes to sanitize the raw food we bought in the market. He used the sink in our room to wash the fruit and veggies with soap and bottled water, and then he rubbed everything with half a lime to kill whatever might still be alive. Personally, I thought he was going overboard.

One day for lunch we checked out a small restaurant close to our motel. They served tacos and other Mexican dishes. Patrick was impressed with the prices and that everything seemed to be fresh. We liked it so much that we began having lunch there, every day.

Neither Patrick nor I came down with Montezuma's Revenge, like the other students did, but I got constipated. After three days of not moving my bowels, I decided not to leave the bathroom until I accomplished my mission. It felt like an eternity. I diligently massaged my belly around and around and then pressed in, on the left side, and then eased myself into a supine position with my legs straight out, but even that failed. I had a vision of myself in a Mexican hospital where they would have to cut me open to clear my impacted intestines.

Patrick pushed a small twig underneath the bathroom door.

"Try using the stick to pull the poop out." He laughed with gusto.

"That's funny, that's really funny."

On the way to the hospital I bought some prunes. I knew I would be fine by the evening.

Another hospital requested our services, but with only twelve of us and more than enough patients, we declined. Then a local television station sent three crewmembers to interview us. When they saw me translating for the other doctors, they assumed I spoke Spanish. I do speak Spanish, but with a Portuguese accent. They asked me questions about chiropractic, and I did my very best to answer them. I knew my Spanish was okay for small talk, but not for an actual interview. People watching television that evening would no doubt be wondering what in the world was I saying.

Our patients brought us homemade meals, fruit pies and handmade glass candleholders. Some tried to give me cash, but I told them our work was voluntary. I saw a lot of shoulder problems from carrying heavy weights and ankle injuries, most likely due to the potholes in the sidewalks. Good thing I had brought along my small handheld toggle piece. I used it to adjust knees and ankles. The mother of a young boy came by the hospital one morning to give me homemade bread as a thank-you for having fixed her son's shoulder. Some people I treated had never seen a doctor, and their fractures had healed incorrectly. Others had health issues like heart problems and diabetes.

Donna and Cody stopped by the room where we were seeing patients one morning and invited us to join them for dinner at their hotel. Patrick told them we already had plans of our own that evening.

At the end of the day we were walking back to the motel and I asked him what were the plans. "We don't need friends, we have each other. Don't you feel the same way?"

"I like having friends. C'amon let's join them. It will be fun, you'll see…"

"I don't want to go. You're not going to put me through that are you?" He was angry and stopped walking. "Well, do you love me or them?" He stared at me waiting for an answer.

My mind was racing. I was afraid to lose him. "Of course I love you. You know that you're more important to me than they are." I kissed him and he kissed me back. I could not resist him.

The medical doctors and staff would come in for adjustments first thing in the morning before they admitted the patients waiting in the hallways. The hospital was the perfect environment for learning. I counted my blessings for the opportunity to travel to Mexico and practice on so many people every day. I didn't do any manual adjustments. I stuck to the Activator Technique of adjusting the spine, which I felt it was a lot gentler and yet effective. Sometimes I had to smile when a patient that had just been manually adjusted by Patrick would get up and, upon seeing me using the Activator instrument, would ask to have the same treatment.

Patrick took care of disinfecting our food and I did the laundry by hand in the bathroom sink. We brushed our teeth with the bottled water we bought in a grocery store. I wondered if the water had come from a regular water faucet, like they do in the US, according to one of my teachers in Georgia.

In the last three days we were in Delicias, Patrick became obsessed with Lucia, the young daughter of Mr. Ramirez, one of his patients. Patrick felt she needed to have her teeth fixed because otherwise she was a knockout. He wanted to invite Lucia to come to the US and was willing to pay for her trip and dental bill. I already knew how frugal he was, and his willingness to spend money he didn't have meant he truly liked her. Given the opportunity, he would take her as his girlfriend, even though she was only fifteen years old.

"Veronica, you have some money. How about helping me out with Lucia's dental expenses?"

"I'm sorry, but I'm saving that money to open my practice after I graduate." Sometimes he was way out of his mind.

When his family arrived the next morning, Patrick made arrangements for Paul, his son who was fifteen, to go out that night with Lucia.

"Dad, I don't know the girl. I don't know what to say. I don't speak Spanish."

"You're such a looser. I wish I was your age. Let me give you some pointers on how to score tonight." He took Paul on the side to provide him with some man-to-man advice.

The next morning, we headed to the train station.

"I'm a bit nervous about the looks of this train." Nancy said. "My sister did a lot of traveling in Mexico and she warned me that they were far from safe."

The old wooden train reminded me of something out of a cowboy movie, but that didn't bother me. I was more scared about the railroad tracks and wooden bridges we would be crossing. Patrick picked a seat away from everyone. I divided my time between visiting his family and sitting next to him. He was upset because Paul had let him down. "Would you believe the fool didn't even kiss her? He's got no balls. He's not my son."

Paul heard him and said, "Dad, she was a nice girl. I couldn't just kiss her. I didn't even know her."

"I wasted my time talking to you last night. You're nothing but a disappointment to me."

How could he be so cruel to his own son? I looked at Paul worried about his feelings but he wasn't bothered by his father's remark. He went on, "I'm so excited, Veronica. Isn't this a great train ride? I can't wait to get to Mazatlan. Veronica, you're going to teach me to play guitar when we get back, right? Promise me."

"I promise."

"I can't wait to play as good as you. I want to play like Jimi Hendrix. Can you teach me, weh, weh, weh weh?" He voiced one of Jimi's riffs while acting like he was plucking the notes on a guitar. I laughed with him.

"Excuse me while I kiss the sky, weh, weh, weh, weh." He sang out of tune.

"I know that song." I said.

"Of course you do. You're the greatest."

"Thanks for the compliment, but you haven't heard me play yet."

"I'm sure you're great. Do you like Mexican food?"

"Yes."

"I love Mexican food. Beef burritos and enchiladas are my favorites. What's yours Veronica?"

I didn't have a chance to answer.

"Will you shut your big fat mouth?" Patrick yelled. "Get off my face and go sit somewhere else. You're driving me crazy with your gabbing. You sound like a girl." Patrick yelled.

Paul went to sit next to Nancy and stayed away from his father for the rest of the trip.

Nancy had made reservations at a nice hotel in Mazatlan. Upon entering the lobby, a well-dressed girl approached Patrick and me and offered us free tickets for dinner at a hotel, along with top entertainment and dancing. All we had to do was attend a one-hour meeting on time-shares that afternoon. I had never heard of such thing, but Patrick had and according to him, it was well worth the one hour of his time.

It wasn't easy to get out of the meeting without buying a time-share. But nothing they said or did bothered Patrick because he had no money. Before we left California he had showed me a stack of charge cards. Even though he was a tightwad, he still lived above his means. He had charged everything he owned. It was the American way.

Throughout the meeting, I kept quiet, like he had told me to, and I was glad when we finally made it out of the room. They'd kept us like prisoners trying to change our minds. When the hour was over, Patrick stood, gave the lead salesman a firm, deadly look, and said, "The two free tickets, now."

That night we dressed up to attend the free fiesta at a luxurious hotel where dinner and entertainment were being provided, compliments of the time-share enterprise. I drank two bottles of Mexican beer with dinner. It tasted like warm water. Thank God Nancy and the family were not with us because I felt a little tipsy. A young Mexican woman stood on the raised dance floor and announced that she was going to teach the Macarena to anyone that wanted to join her. I couldn't resist.

Wiggle the shoulders, wiggle the hips, bring your right hand out palm down, the same with the left, turn them over and keep shaking your booties. Cross your hands over to the shoulders, one at a time and then behind the ears one at a time, cross your hands to the opposite hips then one hand at a time to each bum, roll the hips all around and clap to the beat of belting out, *Hey Macarena*. Jump as high as you can and turn to the right to start all over again. What fun! Yahoo! I was ready to perform on my own. Afterwards, the live band continued to play and the dance floor opened to the general public. Patrick joined me for one dance and then sat at our table. I couldn't sit. I loved to dance, and the Mexican beer didn't make me sick. I could've sworn my feet didn't touch the ground as I danced and jumped up and down, feeling light as a feather, across the Universe, leaping from one star to another.

Patrick laughed as he helped me to walk back to our hotel.

The next day he wanted to go to another time-share session. The prize was a free boat trip to an island and included a buffet lunch and horseback riding. I had truly enjoyed going out the night before, but the thought of sitting through another drilling experience at the hands of several salesmen was not something I wanted to do again. "Hey Patrick, why don't we take a walk on the beach and enjoy the ocean view. What do you say?"

"Boring. We can do that anytime. I'd rather go horseback riding and enjoy a nice lunch on an island for free."

The timeshare salesmen were a lot tougher than the last ones. Three of them stood around us like thugs. It felt to me that we would have to fight our way out, when they began arguing with Patrick that he had to buy a timeshare, because he had just wasted their time when he knew he didn't have any money to spend. He stood up to them like a pro. "I lost an hour of my time listening to you. I want my two prizes now, if you know what's best for you." We did get the tickets, but I was relieved when he agreed not to attend any more time-share meetings.

The next morning, a large speedboat took us and other folks to an island not far from Mazatlan. Except for our hosts serving us a delicious lunch buffet on the beach, it seemed to be uninhabited. While we waited for them to bring the horses, they played the Macarena tune over the intercom. Five women, all tourists, stood side-by-side, but they weren't sure of the hand movements. I looked at Patrick. "What do you say? Should I help them?" And then to the women, "I just learned the Macarena last night. Would you like me to show you?"

Patrick snapped my picture while I taught the group. I felt a certain amount of pride for no longer being the shy person I used to be.

When it came time to go horseback riding, I asked for an old, beat-up horse with no spunk. Instead, they gave me a nervous stallion that was clearly in love with the mare ahead of us. When she took off, he dashed after her, galloping behind her on the beach and then into the woods. I held on for dear life. I didn't even see Patrick take off. He was gone before I blinked.

I yelled to the mare's rider "Hey, you on the horse, can you please slow down?" Either he couldn't hear me or he was ignoring me.

When I saw Patrick standing by his horse I knew I had arrived at the end of trail. He helped me off. "I was wondering how long it was going to take for you to get here. Where did you go?"

"You'll have to ask my horse. I was holding on to him like a leech."

"You were afraid to fall?"

"No, I was afraid to go flying before falling. I've never ridden a horse."

That evening he bragged to Nancy about me.

The next morning, we joined his family at the beach. Everyone went for a swim, except me. I can't swim, unless I'm in a pool and the water is about my waist height. I can do breast stroke for as long as the water doesn't get into my eyes. One large wave and I'd go under. It was a lot safer to stroll by the seashore. I barely wet my feet when I felt a sharp sting on the side of my left foot. I looked down and didn't see anything that could have bitten me. It had to be some kind of jellyfish. I ran into the closest hotel, yelling in Spanish, "Lemons, anyone have a lemon?" I jumped up and down, pointing to my swollen ankle. It hurt like a burning volcano.

"If you want a lemon, you need to go to the bar outside the hotel," said the hotel clerk.

I ran outside. The heat pounded on my head, but it was nothing compared to the hot throbbing pain on my foot. I hopped across the sand towards the bar. The bartender looked over the counter to look at my foot and said, "Didn't you read the warning signs?"

"For Pete's sake, I just need a slice of lemon."

"You have to buy a drink to get a slice of lemon."

"Can't you see? I'm wearing a bathing suit, I have no money."

"No money, no lemon."

I was forced to use my Aunt Heydee's survival protocol.

I yelled, "Mama mia, look. Look over there." I pointed behind him. When he turned, I grabbed a handful of sliced lemons, and ran as fast as I could. Patrick was just coming out of the water. I sat on the sand and rubbed my ankle with the lemons.

"What happened to you?"

I pointed at the jellyfish warning signs. "They got me."

"You must be kidding."

"I know. I didn't even go swimming."

Thank God, the next morning I didn't go on the inflatable banana ride with everybody else. From the shore, I watched in horror as they fell off the banana like dominos when the speedboat pulling the banana did a few inappropriate zigzags. Patrick and Nancy's daughter and son did fine. The people behind Nancy and Paul dragged them into the water, leaving them with a couple of good bruises.

I did go parasailing though, after I saw how easy it was for Patrick and the others to take off and land. I hadn't counted on my fear of heights kicking in so fiercely. I seized the harness, clenched my teeth, and squeezed my eyes shut. The crushing pressure in my chest prevented me from taking a deep breath, and I lacked enough air to scream. I was at the mercy of the boat's crew. I opened my eyes. It surprised me that I didn't see my whole life pass before me, as so many people had described when knocking at death's door. I knew only that dying wasn't going to be a pleasant experience. Either I'd fall into the deep ocean and drown, or I'd hit land and splatter like a raw egg. I cried, "Mama, Mama." Then I took a good look at my situation. If that was going to be my last day on earth, I might as well enjoy the view and stop acting like a scaredy-cat. With my life hanging by a string, I took turns between laughing hysterically and crying profusely.

To my surprise I landed fine. Patrick told me he admired my courage, but my legs shook like an epileptic, and my heart beat loudly and out of rhythm. I felt anything but brave. A British woman standing nearby said, "Only in Mexico can they get away with this. Parasailers are supposed to wear life jackets to prevent drowning and helmets to prevent head injuries. You wouldn't catch me dead in one of those. Look up there." She pointed to one parasailer taking off. "They're using canopies instead of parachutes."

Great information, but I had no intentions parasailing again, not even with the proper equipment.

Except for a few dinners with the family and the two days we spent at the beach, we barely saw them. Everybody was busy doing their own thing.

While in Mazatlan, Patrick insisted on making love to me after blindfolding me and tying my wrists and ankles to the bedposts. I wasn't sure I could trust him. I wanted him to believe I was a woman of the world and opened to out-of-the-ordinary sexual activities, but he seriously frightened me sometimes. Yet like a moth, I couldn't turn away from the brightness, even if it killed me.

There I lay on my back, blindfolded, wrists and ankles tied with rope to the bed frame, naked. I waited among the silence that surrounded me like a tomb. I waited and began wondering if he had left the room. His family was in the room next to ours. Maybe he had joined them and had forgotten all about me. I heard some footsteps and silence once again. This went on for a while and I was starting to get bored. Obviously he was walking around the room trying to scare me. It wasn't going to work, I knew it was him.

I offered to tie him up and blindfold him the next night so he wouldn't feel neglected, but he refused.

On our last afternoon, in Mazatlán, Patrick and I took a walk around the town. We didn't go into any of the shops, but there were lots of street vendors and I bought a beautiful silver bracelet in the shape of a dolphin, for five dollars. About an hour later the heat quickly caught up with me. My head pounded and I felt dizzy. I'd forgotten to take my spray bottle and hat and knew I'd be in trouble if I didn't do something soon to cool off.

I bought a small bottle of water at a grocery store and sat on the curb pouring it slowly over my head. It dripped down my back, shoulders and chest. It was like finding an oasis in the middle of the desert. I smiled with joy.

Patrick loomed over. "What are you doing? You just wasted a whole bottle of water. You have no right to do that." Patrick yelled, standing over me.

"Excuse me?" I looked up, still feeling weak to stand up.

"You heard me. You just wasted a bottle of drinking water."

"I didn't waste anything. I was getting sick from the heat and had to bring my temperature down."

He screamed, "You're pathetic, you know? You're worse than my first wife when it comes to spending carelessly. How can you be so unconcerned with your hard-earned money?" He kicked the curb.

"That's right. My money. The lousy dollar I spent on the water is my dollar. Matter of a fact, I'm going to really splurge and buy another one." I stood and stomped back into the grocery store and bought another bottle. Once outside, I took a mouthful and poured the rest over my head.

We walked back to the hotel in silence. Before entering the hotel lobby, he said, "I don't want my family to know about what happened. I just can't stand squandering money the way you do."

"My life is worth more than a buck."

"I'll be back." He left the hotel. I didn't have the key to our room. I wasn't sure what to do if his family was to walk in and ask for him. Half an hour later he showed up, all smiles, like the Patrick I loved. He handed me a flower with a little love note. "I didn't mean it. Will you forgive me? Yo te amo."

I forgave him.

~ Chapter Fourten ~

Patrick's Allure

Back at school, I had to divide my time between Patrick, my regular curriculum, and studying for the Chiropractic National Board Exams Part II.

Living with Patrick was a thrill of the senses. There was rarely a boring moment. I understood more than ever that life was too short. It made me sad every time I thought about how Mama had spent the last years of her life, confined to someone else's apartment with no way out except to go to the hospital. Her poor health had made her an invalid, dependent on other people to care for her needs. She had been a misunderstood woman, wishing in vain to have someone to love her for who she was. Mama represented everything I hoped never to become.

I promised myself never to look back with regrets. I would savor each day and seize life with all its radiance. For Mama and everyone stuck inside a self-made cage, I intended to climb as high as I could. I would climb the highest mountains, and then slide down to climb them once again.

Since Patrick and I returned from Mexico all he talked about was throwing out our roommates.

He had shown me *their* room a few days before we left. Except for the two single beds and a small dresser, the room was eerily sterile as if no one lived there. I wondered if he even had roommates.

I remember the day we came home from the gym, and he went directly to the kitchen opened the kitchen shades and pointed to the counter. "Over there, right over there, I can see water spots. Do you see them?"

I bent over. "I don't see anything. Maybe it's the shadows in the room tricking your eyes."

"You're not bending down enough. That's why you can't see it. If you look carefully, you'll notice they missed several water spots. I'm not going to stand for it if they don't clean up after themselves."

"Yeah, you should talk to them." At this point I still had not heard or seen any evidence that they existed.

Sunday morning we went to check out a garage sale. Patrick was driving his pickup truck. An old woman in a small sedan passed him on the left side of the road. He hit the horn long and hard and then kept smacking his fist into the dashboard while cursing the other driver. The small ivory skull that covered the stick-shift broke off and flew through the air. I looked at him horrified by his anger and pulled myself back into the seat crying. I was afraid of him. He saw me crying and pulled the truck into a parking lot.

"I'm sorry about losing my temper. I didn't mean to upset you. That woman had no business cutting me off to make a left turn."

That evening we were having dinner at home when he said, "I've something to share with you that's very personal, but since we're now living together you need to know about it."

I kept chewing my food and nodded.

"Once in a while something happens to me that I can't explain. I go into a phase of depression that makes me hide, usually inside a closet. I'll stay in there for three days or even a week." He looked at me waiting for my response.

"You don't come out at all?" I put down my fork and tried to look calm.

"That's right."

"What about going to the bathroom?" My mind was racing. I needed to get the heck out of there. He was crazier than I thought.

"I'm sorry to say but I won't be in shape to use the bathroom. I'll need you to be understanding. When that happens to me, you're not to call a medical doctor. They'll give me drugs that will affect my mind and make me sicker. It's important that you immediately call Dr. Wilson, our teacher at the college. He knows about my condition and he's the only one I trust. He'll know what to do. You must understand that during a time like that I'll be acting a bit strange and will remain inside the closet until I recover. I will not be washing myself or eating."

"What can I do to help when that happens, besides calling Dr. Wilson?"

"Come in the closet with me. Cuddle me. Make love to me. Hold me in your arms and be patient until I recover."

I told him that I would help him the best I could, but that I wouldn't be cuddling up to him after his description of days without bathing and living inside a closet. Then he quickly changed the subject. I didn't have the courage to ask any more questions.

I was in the kitchen mincing garlic—Patrick ate one clove of garlic every day as part of his healthy diet—when he came from behind me and whispered in my left ear, "I'd like to get a broomstick and stick it up your ass."

I wiggled out of his embrace without acknowledging what I had heard. My bad hearing could have caused me to hear something different than what he'd said. I turned around and said, "Here's your garlic, all ready for you." I kissed him lovingly.

After dinner he said, "I tested you earlier to see if you could hear me by whispering something nasty and you definitely can't hear in your left ear. You're definitely deaf."

My instinct told me not to share that I had heard him, but I also came to the conclusion that he was just very playful, and I shouldn't take everything he said and did seriously.

When the time came for me to take the National Boards, I felt confident that I was ready for it after taking a weekend seminar that provided lots of clues on how to do well with the tests. Patrick came with me and used the time to wash his car. After the stress of the exams, it was nice to come out of the building and have him waiting with a huge smile. I treated him to lunch as a thank you. I believed that I did well, but one never knows until the results come in the mail. I still had to take Chiropractic National Boards parts III and IV.

I was ready to drive off to school one morning when Patrick ran out of the house calling me. He knocked on my car window and handed me a cassette tape.

"Veronica, if you're truly my girl, you must learn to love country music. I made this tape with my favorite country songs, just for you. Put it in your cassette player and listen to it while you drive to school."

"Oh, that's so sweet of you." I threw him a kiss.

I didn't mind dancing to the beat of a good country *rock* song, but to listen to someone whining over love with a nasal sounding voice drove me crazy. It was worse than the *Fado,* the Portuguese blues.

I listened to a couple of songs and then realized I was alone in the car. I put the tape in the glove compartment and turned on my favorite music station. I would never force Patrick or anyone else to listen to music they don't like.

Patrick must have been blessed with an incredible IQ. He sat at his desk, reading his notes, while swirling his chair around two or three times. Then he turned towards me and said, "I'm ready to take my exams tomorrow. How about you?" He was able to absorb everything in class, and if he had any homework left, he did it while working at the computer lab. He couldn't understand that I needed more time to study. I stopped having lunch with him in the schoolyard and used that break and the time between classes to study. Once school was over, he wanted to do things together, but studying was not one of them. Instead, we went directly to his gym, a real man's gym, no frills or pretty girls. It was an old garage filled with sweaty men pushing, pulling and lifting weights. He kept a meticulous record of our workout. One day we worked on the upper body and upper extremities, the next day the lower body and lower extremities. "If you keep it up you might gain a few pounds. It would do you some good."

I had no intention of gaining weight.

Over the weekend, Ralph drove down from Oregon with Heather, his new girlfriend, a petite and pretty artist who seemed to be very nice.

It was wonderful to see Ralph again. I couldn't help but admire his new jeep, but he advised me not to get one. "The mileage sucks and they're very uncomfortable. I'm not looking forward to the ride back to Oregon."

Saturday morning we took them to Sacramento to meet Patrick's family. In the afternoon, the entire gang drove into the country and we stopped at Horsetail Falls Mountain. I don't know who came up with the idea, but it was decided that, except for Bonnie, Patrick's mom, we'd climb to the top of the granite mountain. I had never climbed a mountain. The huge boulders and striking cliffs petrified me, but I was more afraid to tell Patrick I didn't want to do it.

There was no trail to follow just large round boulders to climb. We followed Nancy, Patrick's sister. She reminded me of a mountain goat as she guided us without an ounce of fear. Halfway up, Heather complained about the steepness and refused to climb any further. So did Paul, Patrick's son. Ralph remained with them. I wanted to stay too but Patrick insisted that I was doing fine. All I had to do was hold his hand. I concluded that everybody was an expert cliff climber except Heather and me. I should have remained seated in the shade next to Patrick's mom. Nearing the falls, the canyon narrowed over larger boulders which felt slippery upon stepping on one of them. "Are there any trails?" I asked Patrick.

"Of course there are, but this is a lot more fun. Look over there, have you ever seen more impressive waterfall?"

"Oh, wow." I went back to keeping track of where I put my feet. Every once in a while Josh, Patrick's brother, or Sean, Nancy's husband, would give me a hand by pulling me up. Patrick didn't hold my hand like he promised. If it wasn't for them I would have never made it.

I expected to be standing on the tip of the mountain when we reached the top. Instead, we found a stream bordered by flat land. On the other side sat a middle-aged man seated on one of the rocks. He faced us naked with his legs open as if oblivious of our presence. We tried to control our laughter and not stare in his direction, but it was hard not to.

I appreciated breathing in the crispy unquestionably clean, fresh air and the awe-inspiring view that surrounded us but the euphoria only lasted a few minutes before one important question took over my psyche. How would I get down the mountain without breaking my neck? Going up had been challenging enough and most of the time I didn't dare to look down. To descend, one had to look, and there was no way to ignore the steep drop beneath my feet.

We followed Nancy as she took another path from the one we had climbed. She confirmed my fears when she stood at the tip of a large and very round boulder put her hands up, and announced, "There's no way down from here. We need to go back up and see if we can find a better route."

Patrick took over as our guide. As we began to descend I did my best not to look towards the rushing water cascades now on my left. I followed everyone as if I had blinders on. When we came up to a straight cliff Patrick found his way down by holding on to a rope that both Sean and Josh held onto and he slipped down a narrow path. We took turns at being lowered that way. Even after we reached a lower plateau, we were still high up on the mountain, and the granite rocks had multiplied by lots of smaller pieces all the way down. My weak, shaky legs made it harder to keep my balance. Sean and Josh took pity on me. They each grabbed an arm and carried me like a child, in the air, until we reached flat ground. Patrick, who already waited at the bottom, snapped a picture of what later would show the look of a pitiful wide-eyed woman between two wonderful and caring guys. Ralph, Heather and Paul applauded my arrival.

After we left the park Bonnie, Patrick's mom said, "While I was waiting for you guys I talked to a ranger who told me that even professional climbers sometimes get hurt climbing to the top of this mountain. I was worried about some of you."

Patrick held my hand and said, "I'm very proud of Veronica. She has a lot more courage than my son and all the other sissies that stayed behind."

No one had been hurt, and that was all that mattered. I had always wanted to climb a really tall mountain, and my wish had come true. I would just have to be more careful with wishes.

Ralph, Heather, Patrick and I headed back to the Bay Area that evening. The next morning we took them to Berkeley. It was ten in the morning when we got there. Heather wanted to go shopping and that wasn't one of Patrick's favorite things to do. We decided to split up and then meet them at noon at a corner street by a bagel shop.

Patrick and I stood by the bagel shop promptly at noon.

"He knew we were to meet here at noon. Where is he?" Patrick yelled.

"I don't know where he is. But it's only five minutes past twelve. Maybe he's waiting to cross a street? You know… the lights?"

"I'm not going to stay here waiting for him. It's his problem." He walked to the corner and waited for the light to change.

I remained on the corner by the bagel shop acting as though I was looking over the crowd.

"C'mon, Veronica, let's go."

Just then, Ralph and Heather appeared. I waved at them as they walked towards me. Patrick joined us but he wouldn't talk to Ralph.

Ralph whispered. "What's wrong with him?"

I pointed to my wristwatch.

"It's ten after twelve. Big deal. We're only ten minutes late." He shook his head in disbelief.

From Berkley, we drove to Chinatown in San Francisco. While walking around, Ralph suggested we have lunch since it was two o'clock.

"Ralph is nothing but a spoiled brat. We shouldn't be forced to eat with him. We have food at home."

"Three-ninety-nine for a meal is far from being extravagant. I want to eat with my son and his girlfriend. If you can't afford it I'll pay for your lunch."

When we came home, Ralph told us that he had decided to head back to Oregon that afternoon. I knew Ralph well enough to know that he wasn't comfortable with Patrick's overall attitude and that was the reason he was leaving so soon. I felt embarrassed that he was my boyfriend and decided to let him know. I asked him to sit on the couch next to me. "Patrick, things aren't working out between us, I can't handle your fits of anger. I'm sorry, but I'm going to make arrangements to move out."

He began to cry. Then, without saying a word, he leapt to his feet and stormed out of the apartment. I remained seated, not knowing what to do next. For some stupid reason I had expected him to react differently, like, begging me not to leave and that he would promise never to lose his patience again and, he would stop being so cheap. My goodness, what had I done? All my stuff was storage in his garage. How was I going to move and where would I go? I would have to call Dexter. I knew he would help me. How humiliating.

Someone knocked at the door. It was Patrick. He handed me a daisy and a note. *Will you give me a second chance? I'm so happy and proud that we are sharing our lives together in the same home. It is as it should be. I love you more than mere words can reveal.*

My gut feeling told me that I should have remained focused and moved out, but I didn't have the courage to go through with it.

On Friday, during dinner, Patrick suggested we go to Sacramento early the next day. "We'll stay in my parents' house and on Saturday evening I'll take you to a casino in Lake Tahoe where they serve a very expensive, but incredibly delicious dinner buffet. What do you think?"

"I'd love it, but why are you doing that when you always say that spending money on food is a waste?"

"It's my way of making up for the way I acted when Ralph came to visit us last week. Matter of a fact, let's leave tonight."

It was nice spending the next morning with his Mom and Dad. After breakfast we drove over to the cemetery where his grandfather was buried. It reminded me of an old prairie cemetery with old worn-out headstones. It possessed a mysterious quiet beauty, the way it sat peacefully on a hill by itself. Patrick looked at the surrounding trees and the mountains across from the cemetery and said, "I like the way it feels here, being surrounded by nature. When I die, this is where I want to be." Then we left for Lake Tahoe.

The casino was nice but didn't have the splendor of the casinos in Atlantic City, New Jersey. We played the nickel slots for a couple of hours. Then he took me to their buffet dinner on the fourth floor. The buffet was a wall-to-wall array of sea food, including sushi, salads, soups, and desserts. He had just finished a small dish of rice pudding when he looked at me and said, "I must have overeaten, because I can't quite breathe." He put his hands to his chest and bent over slightly. Our waitress came by our table and asked him what was wrong. "It feels as if something is stuck in my chest." The waitress called the restaurant manager.

"Patrick don't scare me now. What's the matter?"

"You can sit down. I'm okay, honey. This has happened to me before. It will soon go away." He smiled.

The restaurant manager didn't charge us for dinner. I wondered if Patrick put on an act to get a free meal.

The next morning, in Sacramento Patrick asked Lauren to lend me her bike.

"I've never learned to ride as a kid," I said, "and the idea of starting at my age is a bit intimidating."

"Don't worry, I'll teach you. You'll learn in no time."

Back in the Bay Area, on Monday, when we came home from school, he put the bike in his pick-up and drove me to a middle school parking lot in Castro Valley.

"Get on the bike and I'll push you."

"How about if I get on the bike and try to learn to balance myself first?"

"No, you get on the bike and start pedaling when I push you. That's the only way you can learn."

He pushed and I pedaled. I yelled out, "How do I stop the bike?"

I couldn't make out what he said and I crashed into the school wall, bruising my arms and legs. Patrick grabbed the bike and threw it in the air. Then he picked it up again and threw it into the pickup bed, cursing. I cowered against the wall, scared he would beat me up.

While driving home he kept cursing and yelling that I was nothing but a disappointment in his life because we would never be able to go riding together. I felt terrible that I had led him down and remained silent. When I got home I ran into the bathroom to cry and locked the door. I felt emotionally abused yet I understood his frustration towards my inadequacy. In his eyes I was a failure and I couldn't bear that thought. I needed to prove myself. Not much time passed before he knocked. He must have gone outside to pick up a flower from one of our neighbors' yard, because when I opened the door he was standing against the wall holding a daisy and smiling. He apologized for losing his temper and I promised to learn to ride the bike so we could start going on outings together.

According to Patrick, that's how his daughter Lauren had learned to ride her bike. He would push her down the hill, over and over until she finally stopped falling. That was how she caught on to the idea of peddling.

Thank God, Lauren arrived the next weekend and stayed with us for a week. After school, Lauren held the bike in one spot until I was able to balance it on my own on flat ground. After a few times of doing just that, I began peddling around our parking lot. When Patrick came home, I made the big announcement, "Lauren taught me this afternoon how to ride a bike and I'm now confident enough to ride on my own."

"All right, let's see how good you really are. Let's go to the high school nearby and ride our bikes around the track. If you can do that without falling then I know you can do it."

Patrick lent one of his bikes to Lauren and the three rode to the high school and then around the track field a few times before going home for dinner. I was overjoyed with my accomplishment, but without Lauren's help I would have never been able to do it.

Later, when I was setting the kitchen table for dinner, she said, "I love you. When you and my dad get married, I want to call you mom and come live with you. You're so much fun." She hugged me.

I loved Lauren and Patrick, but marriage was out of the question. I would have to be out of my mind to lose the freedom to leave anytime I wanted.

The next day I asked Lauren if she would keep an eye open for Patrick's roommates. She didn't know anything about her dad having anyone living there. I wanted to know what they looked like. I showed her their room. Perhaps they were home while I was in school.

The next day, Patrick took us on a hike through the countryside. It was high noon, with no shade in sight. We walked for an hour. I was surprised I had lasted that long. It felt hotter than in Mexico, and without a water bottle to drink from or spray myself with, I feared the end was near. Lauren wasn't doing much better. It was difficult for her to keep a steady pace, she was breathing shallow and her face was flushed. I could see that she was also overheating.

"Veronica, I don't feel good in this heat."

"I don't either. We can rest under one of those trees ahead. Patrick, we need to take a break to cool off."

"Dad, I need to take a break."

He walked ahead, ignoring our pleas.

"Patrick, she's not feeling well, and I'm overheated too. Please let's stop for a few minutes under this tree." Lauren and I sat on the grass by the tree.

"I don't know why I brought you girls along. You make a pitiful pair. If you can't keep up with me, that's too bad." He disappeared up the trail.

"I hate him," Lauren said. "I wish he would die. I hate him. I'm having my period, and I just don't feel good with this heat. I hate him."

"I'll stay with you, and we'll walk together. Don't worry, we'll find our way out of here on our own."

I had a nasty, pounding headache, so we remained seated under the tree until we both felt better. We found him standing against a tree, on the side of the road. He smiled when he saw us and began telling us jokes as if everything was back to normal. Lauren was not ready to forgive him and remained silent for the rest of the day. It really bothered me that he was so inconsiderate about our needs, but instead of saying how I felt, I acted as if nothing had happened by laughing at all his jokes.

After leaving Lauren at her Mom's house, in Sacramento, Patrick and I drove once again to the old cemetery on the hill. He liked standing between the trees and scanning the surrounding area, taking in the overall feeling of nature. Patrick loved nature as much as he loved his grandfather who was buried there. "When I die I can't think of any other place on earth I'd rather be than next to my grandfather."

While driving back to the Bay Area he asked, "Do you have my parents' address written down?"

"No."

"Why not? Get a piece of paper and write it down."

I pulled a notebook out my backpack and wrote the address he gave me.

"Write the directions to their house too," he ordered.

"What for? We're always gonna go together."

"I said write it down. "He pounded his fist on the wheel and glared at me. "You'll need the directions when you go by yourself."

"Okay then." I didn't want to argue and wrote the directions. He really could piss me off. It was like he had multiple personalities, and at that moment he had the one that made no sense. Why would I ever go see his family without him? And there were his roommates. Lauren never saw them while she stayed with us. I was starting to believe that the roommates were a figment of his imagination, but when I asked him, he said they were on vacation.

Patrick's family was the epitome of what a family should be. Bonnie, held the family together. She cooked for everyone and made her house a warm, welcoming place for all to gather. They played games together, sat around talking and laughing, and love could be felt all around. Once I treated Bonnie for sinus headache by working on pressure points, which helped her feel better, now every time we visited, that was the first thing she asked me to do. I loved touching Bonnie's face.

I'm a grandmother again! Steve and Diane are the proud parents of a baby girl. Shayna was born on July 9, and they tell me that she looks like a mini me. My goodness, I'm so lucky to have two grandchildren. I wonder when Ralph is going to have a family.

Patrick asked me again to marry him. He said, "It's not right for us to live this way, we're living in sin." I'd rather live in sin than be stuck. Like Ralph said on the phone, Patrick and

I had no kids, and it wasn't likely we would, so what was the purpose to getting married?

Every weekend, and sometimes after school or the gym, Patrick taught me a different sport. Once he made up his mind, there was no stopping him. I hoped that sooner or later he would realize that I lacked any aptitude for any sports. He taught me—I should say he tried teaching me—to play volleyball, basketball, tennis, and ping-pong, and I failed miserably at every one. I simply didn't have what it took to be physically sporty. He insisted I run with him but I would quickly get out of breath and couldn't keep up. I hated running, but I did it to impress him.

Patrick was magical. I felt alive when I was with him. That was the kind of feeling I had never experienced while married to Al.

One afternoon I was driving behind Patrick after we had finished working out at the gym. When he stopped for a light I saw him looking at me in his rear-view mirror.

I blew him a kiss.

When we entered the apartment, he closed the door and grabbed me from behind and kissed the nape of my neck, one of my most erogenous zones. We had sex on the steps to the bedroom. Afterwards he said, "When you blew me a kiss I got so excited, I could barely wait to have you in my arms."

That was the kind of passion that twirled me around his fingers making me forget his bursts of temper and rudeness.

After finishing classes on Friday, Patrick took me to play golf for the first time. He drove his pickup. When we arrived he parked under a tree, backing up to a ten feet chain link fence.

He jumped over the fence from the back of the truck, and asked me to hand him the clubs, the golf bag and a container of golf balls he called range balls.

"Why are we jumping over the fence? Don't they have an entrance?"

"Yes, of course, but it's more fun this way. Let's go. It's getting late and it's your turn to jump over."

"Oh my God, I can't jump a fence this high, and even if I could, how in the world are we going to get back?

"Look, I expect you to jump over the fence after you climb on the side of the truck. It's no big deal. Now do it!"

"I don't want to." I clutched at the fence with both hands. "The whole thing is stupid. I don't mind paying to get in."

"Are you going to disappoint me?" He glared at me with a severe look.

I climbed on the side of the truck, and pulled myself half way stretched across the fence. He opened his arms encouragingly. "C'mon, jump. I'll catch you."

And he did.

Many years ago when I lived in New Jersey I had seen a professional golf course from a hot air balloon and a few times in my life I enjoyed playing mini golf, but this was a driving range to practice the golf swing. Patrick swung his golf balls high and far and all in the intended direction. The only thing I did well was chopping out chunks of grass. I swore never to make fun of golfers. I used to think it was a joke for grown men to hit a little ball around, but playing golf was a serious sport.

The sun slid behind the hills and covered us in shadow. When we were ready to leave, I stood on his shoulders and grasped the top of the fence. Like a circus performer, I pulled myself over the fence and dropped into the truck's bed. He passed the equipment over the fence and, in one clean sweep, climbed over. I admired his physical prowess and how brave he was. He asked me to wait because he had a surprise for me. He turned on the engine and put in a cassette tape with his favorite country tune. We made love under the stars in the open bed of his pick-up parked next to the golf-course fence.

I woke the next morning with pinkeye. Patrick gave me some of his Johnson's baby shampoo and said it would get rid of the infection.

By evening the pinkeye was gone.

I learned a lot with Patrick, like using baby shampoo to clean contacts. He said it was better than the commercial lens cleaners and it was a lot cheaper. As a student, I spend as little as possible so I could save for the future. I prided myself on being a smart shopper, but Patrick was even more frugal. He literally accounted for every penny he spent.

One afternoon, after I arrived home from school, Patrick said, "I threw our roommates out. They're gone for good. I get sick of having to clean up the kitchen every time they make a mess."

It surprised me he was willing to lose income because of the water spots on the kitchen counters. Later, I peeked into the extra room. It was empty of furnishings. I smiled. I wouldn't have to go downstairs to use the bathroom in the middle of the night.

I called Papa to see how he was doing. We talked to each other once a month, but this time he sounded very sad.

"Veronica, my daughter, I'm a very lonely man ever since your mother died. I'm still living with Luisa and her family, but my life in her house is not good. I need to move out. I wish you were here."

I told Patrick what my father had said.

"Let's go to Portugal and take care of him."

"Are you kidding? What about school?"

"It's more important we go see your father. When we get back, school will still be here. It's only right that you do this for him. Call him back and tell him we're coming."

One thing about me was that I could be talked too easily into doing things that made no sense. Maybe it was because they were so senseless. They had a certain appeal. On top of that, Patrick had a power over me that I'd been aware of since before I moved in, what some people called charisma. Yes, I would stop school and take care of my dad. It was my duty as his daughter.

I called Papa and he blessed me over the phone and cried with joy. I promised to call him back when I had the date.

All week long, after getting home from school, Patrick and I planned our trip. It was all we talked about. He wanted to stay in Portugal for at least six months. I agreed, but we needed to figure out where we'd get the money to buy the airline tickets and rent a two-bedroom apartment in Lisbon. Patrick recommended that we take my portable adjusting table so we could generate some income. "This trip will also provide the opportunity to see if we want to practice in Europe after we graduate. Your father can live with us, but we need to get married before we go to Europe. Your family won't accept me if I'm not your husband. I'll be an outcast."

"I don't care what they think. We are adults. We can do whatever we want."

"How do you think your father will feel when you introduce me as your boyfriend?"

"We are not living in the middle Ages. I'm sure he will understand."

"If you really loved me you would say yes to marriage." He sat on the couch pouting.

"I do love you."

"Then prove it." He stood and looked demandingly at me.

"I don't see why we have to get married."

"That's because you don't value my feelings toward you. I love you enough to leave school, my friends and family." He put his arms around me and his eyes softened. "Let's get married. I want to make our relationship legal."

"I don't know what to say."

"It's easy. Call your father and tell him that I'm asking him for your hand in marriage, and if he says yes, then that's what it is."

I called Papa and told him that Patrick, my boyfriend, wanted to ask him for my hand in marriage. I thought that the idea of asking my father was very nice, but at my age I felt it was ridiculous, and I should be the one to decide if I wanted to marry.

"Is he a good man?" asked Papa.

"Yes, he is."

"What's his name?"

"Patrick."

"Is he willing to provide for and take care of you?"

"Yes."

"Do you love each other?"

"Yes, we do."

"Then you have my blessing, Veronica. Tell him that it makes me happy to know he will be my son. What's the name of my son again?"

We set our wedding for November 3. Three days later we would leave for Portugal. I told Patrick that besides taking care of my father, I had another mission to accomplish in Portugal. I had promised my mother to buy a pink marble stone for her grave. He was all for it.

Autumn of 1995

Patrick told me I would have to sell my car if we were going to have money to travel. He had no money.

"What am I going to do for transportation when we get back? You have a car and a truck. Why don't you sell one of them?"

"It makes more sense to sell your car. Because it's like new, we can get a lot more cash. Don't worry about transportation when we get back. You can borrow my pickup if you need to do errands on your own. I'm going to leave it with my brother and have him work on it while we're in Europe. We don't need three vehicles when we return."

"I don't know why I have to drive your old pickup to do errands. I'd like to have equal rights to driving your car."

"Before I allow you to drive my car again, you'll have to prove to me that you've developed better driving skills. When I let you drive my car a month ago, you drove over the median line without regard for the wear-and-tear on my tires."

"I did it once, but that doesn't mean I'm a bad driver. You keep saying that everything we have is ours to share. Your car is also mine to drive when I want to." I stared at him the way he does when he is angry.

He grabbed me gently and laid me down on the couch next to him. "That's right, we belong to each other, and when we die I only hope to be cuddled up to you this way. I want us to be connected forever, through the end of time. That's how much I love you."

I put the car up for sale for twelve thousand dollars and told Patrick I would go as low as eleven thousand. When I came home from school, he waved a mass of money in his hands and said, "I sold the car. When you left for school someone called, I told them ten thousand cash and they came by and picked it up."

May God forgive me, but I had a gut feeling he had sold the car for twelve thousand and wasn't telling me. I couldn't accuse him without proof. I argued, "Why would you do that without speaking to me first? You know that my car was worth twelve thousand. I was willing to go down to eleven, but that was it. This is not right what you did."

"What are you complaining about? I got cash for it."

"I didn't ask you to sell it for me. The car was only in the paper for one day, I could have gotten at least eleven thousand."

"That's the thanks I get for taking care of the sale. Next time you do it yourself."

"I'm sorry. Thanks for selling the car for me."

"We still need to raise more money."

"We have ten thousand that should be enough."

"Are you serious or not about us taking care of your father?"

"I am...."

"Well, then, how much money do you have saved in the bank?"

"Twelve thousand."

"Let's take the money we made selling the car with us, and put the twelve thousand in a joint account to pay our bills while we're gone."

I felt a tight feeling in the pit of my stomach. He was *taking over* my savings to cover *his* bills. I had no bills to speak of and I had suddenly become responsible for his debts. He must have read my mind.

"What I have in personal assets, like furniture, and so on, is worth a lot more than what you're putting in *our* joint account. Just the stereo alone with the speakers and the television are worth at least five thousand dollars. You're basically investing nothing into our marriage when it comes to finances. The least you can do is help me to pay for all this stuff that we're both using. Now give me the money we made on the car, so I can keep it in my money belt while we are traveling."

"It's *our* money, so half is mine to carry."

"I can't take that chance. You're more likely to be robbed because you're easy prey."

"It's *our* money. I'm entitled to half by the law of common sense."

"Okay, you win. You take four and I'll take six, because I'm the man."

"No, you take four and I'll take six, since I'm the woman that's putting out all the money."

"Alright, we'll go half and half."

I put the five thousand in my money belt and then said, "By the way, when we get married I'm keeping my last name."

"As my wife your last name should be my name. That's how it is in marriage."

"I like my last name and I will not change it."

"Are you ashamed of my name? This isn't right what you're doing. You know that, don't you?"

"If this is no good for you, let's not get married then."

"You're being unreasonable. But I love you, so go ahead and keep your name."

I had made a promise to Roberta, and a promise was a promise. Once in a while I could be assertive, but it took a lot out of me to do that.

October 12

We picked up our International Student Identification cards. Patrick said that was an essential card to have while traveling. It gave us free entry and discounts to museums and also some health insurance coverage if one of us got sick.

My father must have told our family in England about the wedding plans, because I received a letter from my cousin Max, in London, congratulating us. The wedding present: two airline tickets from Portugal to England. Once in Portugal, all we had to do was call him, and he would make the arrangements.

That evening, I heard Patrick talking on the phone to Katie, a friend from school who had graduated a year prior. She had gotten married and was living in Hoorn, Holland.

"That's great, we'll be glad to visit you and meet your husband. Yes, I'll let you know when. Thank you for the invitation."

"We have a free place to stay in Holland," he announced.

"I thought we were going to Portugal to take care of my father."

"I've always wanted to go to Holland. It's only fair that if we're going to spend a lot of time with him that I spend just a few days visiting a friend."

We planned to have a garage sale after our school finals, but when it came time to do it, Patrick changed his mind and decided to put all his stuff into storage. I went ahead anyway and sold everything except for old family heirlooms that I just couldn't part. I even sold my acoustic guitar and both my old wine barrels. We made thirteen hundred dollars over the weekend, which was pretty good, because it helped me pay for most of our airline tickets.

Our special student airline tickets were good up to one year to return to the US and as long as there was space we could use them any time we wanted. We would fly from California to New Jersey and then to Holland, before going to Portugal.

We were done with our finals at school. The next two days we made several trips in his pickup to the storage facility. We had fun racing through the long hallways and up to the second floor of the storage facility. Everything had to be a game, a challenge. Of course he always won, but for me it was more about the enjoyment of doing something together.

He taught me how to balance the refrigerator on the hand-truck. It was fun to move such a large appliance and not get hurt doing it. Then he showed off his collection of guns, which included two long rifles, before hiding them between the couch cushions in back of the storage unit. I didn't share with him that I also had a gun, hidden in a safety deposit box along with five thousand dollars that I had put away when I first moved to California. I didn't feel comfortable telling him about it, probably because I knew he would find a way to take it from me.

He also showed me a small container with Native American beads he had taken from their burial grounds. I couldn't touch them. I believed that it was acceptable to have historical artifacts in a museum to help preserve history, but plain wicked to keep them hidden in a closed container just for one's own pleasure. I imagined *their* souls crying out for revenge.

I hadn't realized how much stuff he owned until he tried to fit everything into the rental space. He had furniture and boxes packed all the way into the ceiling, and even though it was the largest unit available, he could barely close the door. I imagined that when we returned from Portugal and opened the unit door, everything would pour out, like when I used regular dish soap in my dishwasher instead of dishwasher soap.

When we were done putting everything away we headed back to our empty apartment. We were supposed to leave for Sacramento that afternoon, get married two days later and then fly to New Jersey. "I don't know about you, but I'm tired," he said. "Let's have a romantic evening in our empty apartment and leave tomorrow morning instead. I'll be right back. Don't move." He winked at me as he went into the kitchen and brought out his lunch box with cheese and crackers and a small cartoon of orange juice. It was just like him to have everything pre-planned. He took a blanket from the coat closet and laid it on the floor.

"It's a picnic!" I clapped my hands delighted.

His face glowed with happiness. "Yes. It's a picnic of love. You and me, having tasty snacks, sharing our thoughts, holding each other lovingly and making love for the last time in this old apartment."

Before leaving for Sacramento the next morning, he took a bag of birdseed and his three bird feeders to Mrs. Krum, the maintenance lady at our apartment complex.

"I know how much you love birds so I'm leaving these feeders for you to use until we get back from Europe. If you want you can use this bag of seeds, but if you do I expect you to replace it."

I couldn't believe that she agreed with him.

Patrick drove the pick-up truck to Sacramento, because he was the only one that could handle the bad brakes and other mechanical problems. The horn in the truck was also not working since he had smashed it with his fist. He was very strong. Sometimes I thought about the two guys that attacked him when he was running one morning. He told me that he punched them to death. I believed him.

I drove the ZX and had to admit that I enjoyed being by myself, without a back-seat-driver telling me what to do, but my mind was not at peace. Why am I marrying a man that goes nuts at least once a week? Go ahead, Veronica, answer that.

I love him!

Why am I leaving school and spending all my savings?

Like Patrick said, I owe my father and school can wait.

Maybe so, but why am I paying his bills?

Because being married means sharing everything.

Then why am I getting married?

None of my answers made sense, and beneath those answers, one line kept hammering in my head like a woodpecker. *You're making a big mistake. Don't do it!*

I turned on the radio to muffle my thoughts.

The day after arriving into Sacramento, Patrick woke with a toothache. He decided to wait until the next day, our wedding day, and see if it would go away. The next morning we signed the documents at the courthouse and we became officially man and wife. He wore a suit and tie and I burrowed a simple cream-colored dress from Nancy, his sister. Bonnie gave me a small bouquet of pink roses. After we signed the papers, Nancy took our picture. It was a very simple wedding. Patrick's children and his parents came to the occasion. Ralph couldn't make it. I believe he didn't approve and preferred to remain out of it. I didn't invite any of my friends from school. Patrick would be upset if I did.

Patrick's toothache grew worse, and the idea of flying with a possible abscess was not a pretty picture. Bonnie called the dentist as soon as we got home. They were closed for the weekend, but Bonnie knew Dr. Bergsten's home number. When Patrick found out the tooth would most likely have to be pulled, but that there was no dental assistant available over that weekend, he told Dr. Bergsten that I would assist with the tooth removal. So on our wedding day I became a dental assistant. The tooth broke in half as it was being pulled. There was a lot of blood loss, and the dentist had to dig around quite a bit to pull the rest of the tooth and root. I felt like a Florence Nightingale, as I held the vacuum-like tool to suck up blood and spit from his mouth, but I didn't have what it takes to be a dental assistant. Several times during the procedure I got queasy at the sight of the dentist digging into his gum while pulling the root piece by piece.

Afterwards, Patrick could barely stand because of the painkillers and went to bed as soon as we got home.

That evening his mom ordered Hawaiian Pizza from Papa Murphy's (the best pizza I had ever had), and the whole family joined into the festivity. We had ice cream and Bonnie's homemade apple pie for dessert and stayed up late playing

Monopoly. When Patrick's ex-wife came to pick up her children she hugged me. "I wish you my very best," she said. Bonnie and Nancy shared some funny stories about Patrick, when he was a child. I felt loved.

Patrick put his mom's name as part of our new bank account. He kept one charge card for our travels and gave all his other cards to his mom with specific instructions for paying his monthly charges and the other bills he owed that would be arriving to her address.

When she asked him where he got so much money he said, "It's Veronica's money. But now that we're married, it's ours."

~ *Chapter Fifteen* ~

The Honeymoon

Patrick put a lot of effort into building a cardboard box to carry my adjusting table. He reinforced the corners with duct tape and attached a rope handle. Then he wrapped the table with a wool blanket, inserted it into the box, and threw in four large chiropractic books to keep it from wobbling. I couldn't lift the box off the floor.

"Don't worry. I'll carry it." He lifted it with one hand.

I kissed him. "You're my hero."

Patrick packed his suitcase full of winter and summer clothes, vitamins, and toiletries. Although I had packed clothes and personal stuff, I had filled my suitcase mostly with chiropractic books—so we could stay up on our studies. In addition to the suitcases and portable adjusting table, we would each carry a large backpack for our most personal items.

The next morning Nancy offered to drive us to the San Francisco airport. I carried my share of money, driver license and Student ID in my money belt. Patrick did the same, but he also insisted on carrying both our passports and airline tickets.

When we landed in New York, my son, Steve, was waiting for us outside the terminal with his store van. Patrick enjoyed watching Steve and I go through our traditional Kung Fu greeting where Steve allows me to defeat him when I throw my leg up in the air and touch his shoulder. He was, however, freaked out when Steve drove on to the shoulder to get around the slow traffic and sped through a few extreme turns before arriving safely home. I told Patrick that was how I drove while living in New Jersey.

Diane had not changed much. If anything she looked younger. Jacob was now two-and-a-half and liked being hugged. Shayna looked like a beautiful porcelain doll. She smiled every time I held her. No one had told Al I was in New Jersey, and I was glad we had kept that way.

Patrick and I slept in Jacob's twin bed, but because we always slept as if glued together, it was quite comfortable.

The next day Steve lent us his car. Patrick and I drove to Philadelphia. We visited Independence Hall and I took his picture standing by Liberty Bell. With so much to see in Philadelphia I was shocked when he said, "I was only interested in seeing the Liberty Bell. Let's go back to New Jersey."

The following morning Steve slipped a hundred dollar bill playfully into my hand. "You're going to New York. Spend it as you like it, and have fun with your young husband. I'm proud of you Mom." He winked at me and gave me a hug.

I parked the car at the Port Authority Bus Terminal in New York City and we walked from there to the famous 42nd Street, or as we call it in New Jersey, Sin Street. Having lived in New Jersey for almost thirty years and only an hour from New York City, I was very familiar with all the sights, but no matter how many times I had been to New York City I was still in awe of its majestic architecture and took my time along with him to look up at the skyscrapers. We stopped at the Empire State Building, but because I had been up several times, we agreed that he should go alone. I stood at the street corner, watching people go by.

By the time he returned it was one o'clock and I was ready for lunch.

"You can't go to New York and not eat a hot dog from a street vendor. It's the best in the world," I told him. "I'll treat you."

I paid for the hotdogs with Steve's one hundred dollar bill.

"Let's save the rest of the money Steve gave you. I'll take half of it," he said.

"Steve gave it to me to spend as I like it. It's my money."

"You keep forgetting that we are married and as such, everything you have is also mine! Now give it to me!" He extended his hand waiting. I took my time counting the change before I gave him half.

My mother would be proud of me. I was a good obedient wife, just the way she had trained me to be, before she pre-arranged my marriage to Al.

In Chinatown we shared a plate of Chicken Chow Mein and had fun hopping from one Asian shop to another. When we walked across Greenwich Village I suggested we attend a show at my favorite comedy club, but he said he was tired and rather start walking back to the bus terminal. It was already growing dark by the time we reached Broadway and Times Square but the city had just awakened to the celebration of the senses. We were surrounded by a multitude of lights, multicultural restaurants and food carts emitting exotic aromas. The surrounding sound of cars honking, hitting the brakes, and people yapping as they walked pushing to pass us, played like a well-rehearsed orchestra. We stared in amazement at the flickering and ever-changing façade of huge billboards. Their vibrant colors were as abundant as the prostitutes, their pimps, and the drug dealers that offered us their services unrestrained along 42nd Street.

"We need to get out of here. I'm done with New York." He held my arm with a strong grip and pushed his way through the crowded street.

But then we passed a live peepshow and he stopped. I was glad when he said, "Only twenty-five cents. Let's go in." I had always wondered what it was like inside those places.

Inside, a short, obese man sat in a recliner and watched a cowboy movie on a small black-and-white television. He collected fifty cents from Patrick and led us down a dark narrow hallway. He opened the door to a room the size of a phone booth. "Stand by the glass window." He turned off the light and closed the door behind him. I felt like Patrick was as nervous as me, we both giggled. A light came on the other side of the one-foot window, revealing what seemed to be a dressing room. Two out-of-shape women in their mid-forties sat in their underwear, talking to each other. One began pulling on silk stockings, and the other took off her bra exposing large flat breasts. The light went out and the man opened our door.

Outside, I asked Patrick, "How can women so out-of-shape be part of a peep show. I thought they would have to be beautiful."

"Some men like their women that way. They find them sexy." Patrick smiled.

I wondered if he was one of those men. It was nice to know that one didn't have to be young or have a model's figure to be considered attractive.

The next day we drove an hour-and-a-half to Atlantic City, but as soon as we started walking on the boardwalk he said, "I don't like it here. I'm more interested in seeing the famous Stone Pony Club in Asbury Park." So we drove back north to Asbury Park, but we didn't stop. He only wanted to see it from the outside. I was very disappointed that we didn't go in. I would have liked to check it out.

From there, we headed west to Freehold. I took him to my old neighborhood and showed him the house where my family and I had lived for fifteen years. The neighborhood still looked the same, except that the house that Al and I had paid eighteen thousand dollars in 1963 was now worth two hundred and fifty thousand. I wanted to show him The Simy Dinner Theater at the Kobe Japanese Restaurant, where I had produced theatre for over nine years, but he didn't want to go in and waited outside while I said a quick hello to Mr. and Mrs. Ounuma and Jerry the bartender.

Steve paid for all our meals when we went out for dinner, and before going to work in the morning, he treated us for breakfast at his favorite diner.

The morning before leaving New Jersey, I paid for breakfast, but after we dropped Steve at work, Patrick threw a fit. I wasn't to spend anything unless I asked him first.

"If I want to treat my son to breakfast that's my prerogative."

"Yes, but it's *our* money and, as such, we don't do anything without consulting each other first."

I wanted to tell him that I had never met anyone so cheap, but didn't want to get into an argument.

Neither Steve nor Diane could drive us to the airport the next day because they had to work.

"I promised to take you to the airport," Steve said. "I hope you don't mind that I've arranged for a limousine to pick you's up. It's all paid for."

While waiting for our plane I told Patrick, "It was really nice that Steve paid for our meals when we went out and gave us money to spend. He didn't have to do that."

"Steve has a lot of money. It's only right that he paid."

How pathetic. Steve didn't owe us anything, he and Diane worked hard for what they had and they were far from rich. It bothered me that Patrick lacked any appreciation for the richness of their hearts.

~ Chapter Sixteen ~

Holland

On the plane to Holland, I thanked God for being able to have seen Diane, Steve and the grandchildren one more time.

Katie picked us up with her car, at the Amsterdam Airport. She practiced chiropractic in the town of Hoorn, about an hour, north of Amsterdam, where she lived with her husband Gavin. She had beautiful brown eyes and long brown hair. Patrick and she talked mostly about their days at chiropractic college while I gazed at the green flat fields intertwined with an overly abundance of streams and canals. I imagined with a bit of rain, the region we crossed was susceptible to major flooding.

I had expected the people in Holland walked around in wood clogs and Dutch bonnets to match their typical costumes, but they looked no different from people in the US. They wore sneakers and winter coats over jeans. A few wore accessories like wool scarves and hats. She stopped at a mall composed of three shops. "You're probably hungry, so I thought you might want to pick up a sandwich or something at one of the deli's here."

"We had lunch on the plane." Patrick responded. "We're going to wait for dinner."

I guessed he considered two mini bags of peanuts, as being lunch. I had given him my bag because it had a smoked flavor.

Their home reminded me of the miniature wood-block row houses I used to play with as a child. Their simple but contemporary style furniture fitted perfectly. Gavin was a tall, tough looking guy. He worked as a cop in Amsterdam and owned two big exceptionally mean dogs that he kept in separate metal cages in their backyard. He used them to sniff out drugs and had trained them to go for the throat if necessary. According to Gavin, the Turks brought in most of the hard drugs into the country.

For dinner, Katie served us small pieces of toast, thin slices of cheese, and cold cuts.

Patrick whispered to me, "They call this dinner?"

Shortly after we finished eating, she said, "As you can see our home is very small and there's not enough space for you to stay with us. I'm going to drive you to a very nice hotel not far from here where you both will be very comfortable."

Patrick's love for Katie flew out of the window when she dropped us at the hotel. The cost for each night was ninety-five US dollars and included breakfast. Patrick called it robbery, and, at that price; we couldn't afford to buy dinner that night.

Katie and her husband worked the next day and couldn't come by the hotel until that evening. We spent the day walking around town, window shopping, and cringing at the price of shoes. Given the number of affluent shoe stores Hoorn must have been the Mecca of shoes. We also noticed that there were a lack of automobiles and a lot of bicycles, probably because of the narrow cobblestone streets. Like so many old towns in Europe, when they built them, cars didn't exist.

We agreed that there wasn't much to do in Hoorn since he didn't want to spend any money to look at museums. We planned to leave the next day for Portugal.

That evening, Katie and Gavin took us to a restaurant for dinner called the same as the harbor's name, The Hoofdtoren. Patrick looked at the menu and then said to our hosts. "Do you mind ordering the food for us? We don't read Dutch." I had fun reading the Dutch menu, because I could actually understand what was written if I read it slowly. I also noticed that the average price for a three-course meal was about thirty dollars and was surprised that Patrick was so relaxed about it. During dinner Patrick talked about crime in the U.S. and Gavin informed us that robberies in Holland were going up because people didn't put curtains on their windows. When crooks walked by they could see the valuables inside and whether anyone was home. When they offered to pay for dinner, Patrick smiled and said politely, thank you.

~ *Chapter Seventeen* ~

Portugal

We arrived to Lisbon's airport at eleven-thirty in the morning. Patrick followed me through customs and then outside to the street. The typical cool breeze I associated with Lisbon in the winter greeted me by messing up my hair and spitting a piece of dirt into my left eye and lodged under my eyelid. I blinked a few times to wash it away. I felt comfortable in my turf, surrounded by the familiar sounds of traffic and slightly polluted air.

Patrick set the box with the table on the sidewalk. "Are you sure you know where the bus stop is? I don't want to carry this all over the forsaken place."

"I lived here the first eighteen years. I know this city like the palm of my hand."

The bus driver opened the door, but as soon as he saw the box and luggage he yelled, "Oh no, you're not bringing those on my bus. This is a public bus. Take a taxi."

"Hey, I'm Portuguese. You're not going to deny a fellow citizen and her husband the use of your bus are you? Besides, this bus is half empty."

"Alright, c'mon in. It's just that I'm sick of foreigners coming in from the airport with a load of bags and taking over the space we need for our own folks."

Within three stops, riders jammed the bus and soon Patrick couldn't breathe. The driver was glad to let us out when I told him my husband was having a panic attack. We exited the bus and waited for one less crowded. But it was lunchtime, rush hour, and I knew we'd be waiting forever. He refused to take a taxi. We walked two hours before reaching the same pensão where I had stayed with my school friends over a year ago.

We left everything in our room except for our backpacks and headed over to Luisa's apartment to see my father. Luisa's cousin answered the door. "Your father no longer lives here," she said. "He left two weeks ago and is renting a bedroom in someone's apartment." My heart speeded up. My poor father, he was all alone and he really needed me. I thanked Patrick for making me take this trip. She gave me his address—a block from where my Grandmother Rica used to live, on the other side of the city.

On our walk there, Patrick said, "I don't like Lisbon. Let's get out of Portugal and go to a different country."

"What? For goodness sake, we haven't even seen my father. It was your idea to come and take care of him, and that's what I'm going to do." I kept walking. He was as unstable as nitroglycerine.

Papa was thrilled to see us; we hugged each other over and over again. Patrick said he wished he looked that good when he reached ninety-three. Papa insisted on taking us out for lunch and ordered a large seafood platter for us to share. Patrick wouldn't touch the food. "It's disgusting how much money your father is spending on lunch," he whispered to me. "Don't you pay for any of it."

"Don't worry. He would be offended if I even offered."

Papa spoke in Portuguese. "What's the matter with your husband? Doesn't he like seafood?"

"He only likes bread and cheese."

Papa turned towards Patrick and said in English, "Son, you better eat something other than bread and cheese or you'll get sick."

Patrick didn't answer. With his arms crossed, he sat erect and stared into space. I felt like someone had just dropped a bucket of ice over my head. I was worried that Papa was going to ask me why I had married a man with such an attitude problem. I said in Portuguese, "Please don't pay attention to him. When he is tired he can't eat, and he is sitting with his arms crossed because his back hurts from flying and… he isn't feeling well." I finished the shrimps and smacked my lips to show him how much I appreciated lunch.

Papa called a taxi and took us to meet Carina, his girlfriend at a coffee shop. She looked a lot like Mama and that gave me the creeps—especially, when she showed me the ring Papa had given her. I was upset because I had wanted it. It had no monetary value. It wasn't even a real stone, but it had belonged to my mother. Papa must have given Carina the ring because it was pretty. What else was he going to do with it? Wear it? The reality of the situation is that once we're gone, our material things mean nothing to others. I was still angry with him.

Throughout the next two days, Papa talked and talked. No matter how hard Patrick or I wanted to respond, it was mostly a monologue.

What he had meant on the phone was that he was lonely without Mama and could use some company. He had no intentions of leaving Portugal and laughed when I told him that we were in Lisbon to take care of him. "Thank you, my daughter, but Luisa's daughter-in-law comes by once a week to pick up my dirty laundry and who knows, if things get better between Luisa and me, I may move back to her place, but for now I like being on my own."

That same afternoon Patrick wanted to go to the post office to pick up postcard stamps. Papa offered to walk us there. When we arrived, he sat down and Patrick and I got in line. Papa yelled, "You, stupid. Can't you see that you don't have to be in line to buy the stamps? Stupid woman!" Then he mumbled and shook his head.

Patrick said, "Did I hear your father calling you stupid?"

"Yes, because we don't have to be in this line. I didn't know." I flashed back to my childhood, when Papa would speak in that same tone. "I'm fifty-one years old and my father still reprimands me like a child." But as soon as I said that I knew I shouldn't have voiced my feelings.

"I don't care if he's your father. Nobody talks to my wife in that manner."

He walked over to Papa, pointed a finger in his face, and yelled, "You, old man! How dare you talk to my wife in that manner? It's disrespectful, and even worse in public. For your information, your daughter is a lot smarter than you. We're leaving you for good."

A woman standing nearby said in Portuguese, "How dare he talk like that to an elderly man. I've never seen anything like that. It's despicable!"

Everybody looked in our direction. Patrick grabbed my arm. "Let's get out of here."

That woman might have been right but Patrick had defended me. Yes, it was wrong, but of all of Patrick's outbursts of temper, that one my father had it coming.

The next morning Patrick woke me at five and said, "According to this map there's a stadium not too far. I'm going to walk there and run the track."

We planned to meet at noon, back at the pensão. I was going to use my morning to call my cousin Max in England so he could make arrangements for our airline tickets to England. Max encouraged me to buy a phone card so I could call him without having to keep putting coins into the phone box and then getting disconnected anyway.

I bought a twenty-five dollar phone card at the post office. I liked the idea that I could use it to call anyone I wanted without fumbling for change or asking Patrick for permission. But the card wouldn't work on the street phone and, thinking that I was doing something wrong, I asked for help from a passerby.

He tried it and when it didn't work he remarked, "All these phone cards are a piece of shit."

I asked someone else for help who basically made the same observation and then added, "You'll have to buy a card that works."

"Not me. I just bought this card. I'm going back to the post office and get it exchanged for one that works."

"Good luck with that."

The post office worker who had sold me the card was still behind the counter. I felt lucky.

"Hi, remember me? This card you sold me ten minutes ago doesn't work. I need to change it for one that works."

"That will be twenty-five dollars."

"I need to change this one, not buy another one."

"It's twenty-five dollars if you want another card."

"No, you don't understand. I just bought this card a few minutes ago from you, and it doesn't work. You sold me a defective card and I want it changed for one that works."

"Next!"

I wasn't going to move. I asked to speak to his boss.

"Madam," said the polite postmaster, "you need to go to our central post office to get the card changed. There's nothing we can do at this branch."

"And where's the central post office?"

He wrote the address down and gave me the directions. I had to take a bus to the other side of the city.

At the central post office, the postmaster, a short middle-aged man, laughed at my request and told me to get out of his post office.

I jumped on the counter and, facing the customers, yelled, "Someone call the police. I've just been robbed by the post office and I want justice!"

Two employees helped me off the counter and took me to see their so-called branch manager. She was pissed off at my attitude, so I told her I felt the same way towards everyone working there, including her.

"Give me your address and I'll mail you the refund."

"I live in the United States, and I don't want a refund. I want another card to replace the one I bought but doesn't work."

"Here, you can have my card. Have a good day."

"I'm going outside and use it on the street phone by your door and if it doesn't work I'm coming right back." I walked out feeling like Clint Eastwood in the movie *Dirty Harry*.

Five minutes later I dropped the card on her desk. "Your card doesn't work either."

"You're lying. It's impossible."

Both my hands went flat on her desk as I moved my torso forward. My eyes opened wide and then narrowed down as my lips tightened over my teeth just like Clint Eastwood would have done if in my shoes. "How dare you call me a liar? If you don't believe me, you get off your fat ass and go outside and try the phone card yourself."

My words were as bad as I could make them given that I hate being called a liar unless it's true. She signaled me to follow her.

She put a card in the phone outside, but it didn't work.

"Now, apologize." I looked straight at her without blinking.

"So many people use their cards and then bring them back and say they don't work that we don't trust anyone anymore."

"What happened to my people? I'm ashamed to say I'm Portuguese. What a way to live where you don't trust anyone. What happened to customer service? I've wasted my whole morning between the other post office and this one. I can't wait to go back to the US where you can return anything you want without being treated like a criminal."

"I'm so sorry. Please wait here and I'll be right back with another card."

Neither one the three cards she tried worked. It was her turn to curse at the cards. She went back into the post office and upon returning she handed me a phone card saying, "This one should be fine."

I grabbed her arm firmly. "I need to call my father. You're staying right here until the phone call goes through." She did, and then she left when the call went through.

"Papa, I'm calling to apologize for what happened yesterday."

"I'm the one who needs to ask your forgiveness for being so rude. Patrick was right to get upset with me."

"Thank you for telling me that, Papa. I accept your apology. I also want you to know that Patrick and I are leaving for London. When we get back I want to see you again, but I don't know if that's going to happen. He's angry at you. He has a very bad temper and wants everything his way and…"

"Veronica, my daughter, you're not going to like this, but your husband Patrick uses women to get what he wants. He's nothing but a user, a *chulo!* Please be careful. Meanwhile I'm going to pray to God to protect you from him. So don't worry. We'll see each other again."

I called Max-Leão, my brother, who lives in the south of Portugal. He said he couldn't wait to see me again and meet Patrick. I told him that Patrick and I were heading to England for a week but when we returned to Portugal we would come to visit him. We were to call him when we arrive to Ourique, the town where he lived.

Back at the pensão, I told Patrick what I had gone through that morning to get the phone card so I could talk to my cousin Max. He laughed and said he was proud of me for not giving up to a bunch of nitwits. I made sure that he knew my cousin was going to give me the money for the card.

I had told Patrick the first day we used the Metro in Lisbon that those who didn't purchase a regular ticket most likely had a pass. "I don't believe it, he said. "I've been watching and I don't see any subway cops."

"They're everywhere and when they catch you, you go to prison."

"I take full responsibility." And so we used the subway to go everywhere in the city free of charge. I was a nervous wreck worrying about getting caught.

While Patrick was in a bakery's restroom I bought my favorite Portuguese pastry, a *Pastel de Nata,* a small round flaky pastry filled with cream. I swallowed it in two bites. I knew he would have a fit if he saw me spending money without talking to him first. To him food was a waste of money. Two things in life he wished he could get rid of: food and sleep.

For lunch we had water and a *Papo Seco* a small Portuguese bread roll very much like a French roll, crusty on the outside and soft on the inside. It included two thin slices of cheese. To my surprise he also bought two fruitcake pastries. They looked like supersized scones. I took a bite of mine and then gave it to him. I hated fruitcake, especially these. They were big and cheap, most likely the reason he bought them. They filled his belly for a quarter each. The pastry I wanted was seventy-five cents, so I bought one. If I was going have a dessert it should be a dessert I enjoyed, not something that he had to approve of.

I still had a mission to accomplish that afternoon. I was told at the synagogue's office that the pink marble tombstone Mama had asked me to buy would cost three thousand dollars. Patrick only stared. I knew better than to buy it. Outside, our talk was short.

"We're not in a position to spend that kind of money. Wait until you start working, and then you can buy your mother's stone. We need all the money we have for traveling. After we return from England, I want to go to Spain since we're so close."

"I thought we were going home after we returned."

"Don't you want to see Spain with me?"

I would have to return to Portugal another time to buy my mother's tombstone. But knowing how tight he was with money, I was fooling myself even to consider that would ever happen.

I called my cousin Max in England. Our airline tickets were waiting for us at the airport. We would be leaving Portugal in two days.

For dinner we stopped at a fast food restaurant close to our pensão and each had a cup of soup and a *Papo Seco* again with two thin slices of cheese. For dessert he bought two fruitcakes for himself. I decided to skip my favorite dessert and avoid being called a spendthrift.

The next morning, while riding the trolley to the train station in downtown Lisbon, we ate a breakfast of bread and cheese. The old Rossio Railway station still looked exactly the way as I remembered when, as children my brothers and I would wonder around, before taking the train to the beach. The building was a magnificent example of the romantic period connected with the Neo-Manueline architecture, showing off two intertwined horseshoe entrances, and a soaring clock tower with lots of crafted wall sculptures. "Are you sure this is a train station?" said Patrick. "It looks more like a palace."

Inside it was just like any other busy train station, except that the platforms were covered by cast iron. Our destination was Sintra, a picturesque, nineteenth-century town north of Lisbon. It had been the summer residence of the kings of Portugal. It was our intent to head directly to its famous palace, *Palácio da Pena* and then the castle, *Castelo dos Mouros* that belonged to the Moors during the eighth or ninth century. Patrick was very excited about the excursion since he had never been to a palace or a castle.

When we arrived at Sintra's train station, I could not remember which road lead up the mountain to the palace. I asked several people for walking directions, but they had no idea. One man pointed to a bus stop across from us and said that was the best way to get there.

Patrick crossed his arms and shouted, "You lied to me when you said you knew the way. You're nothing but a liar!"

"I'm sorry, but it's been over thirty-five years ago when I walked to the palace with my brothers and my Aunt Heydee. I realize now that things have changed since then. I just don't know the way by foot anymore." Tears filled my eyes.

A man standing on the platform next to us grabbed a pigeon flying past him and snapped its neck with both his hands. He walked away holding the dead pigeon in one hand.

"My God, Patrick, did you see what that guy did to that pigeon? He broke his neck!"

"I didn't see anything, so don't go making more lies. I'm not going to trust you anymore."

"Patrick, I drove my parents up there about a year ago when I was visiting them but I followed the road signs. Let's take the bus over there."

"No, we're not taking the bus."

A teenage boy walked by, and I asked him for directions.

His answer was very Portuguese. "Follow me and I'll take you."

Raul was his name, bless his young soul. Of course Patrick didn't believe this kid would take us to the palace. He thought Raul was just a punk who would try to rob us. Patrick relented and we followed Raul up the hills. I could tell he was taking shortcuts that only someone who lived locally could know.

"We're not paying him a dime." Patrick insisted. "It's his choice if he wants to be our guide. Tell him that."

I said in Portuguese to Raul, "Thank you for taking us all the way up to the palace. I'll be glad to give you five dollars for your work."

"I'm not doing this to get paid. I'm on my way up there to join some friends."

"Did you tell him?"

"I didn't have to. He doesn't want any money from us."

When we reached the town surrounding the palace, Raul waved goodbye. Patrick was content. I was happy to see him smile and be back to his old self again. We sat on a bench and ate the bread and cheese sandwiches we had brought along.

After eating, we headed to the palace, but there was an entry fee, and he didn't want go in. I felt Patrick was missing a very important part of Portuguese history but nothing I said was going change his mind. I'd been inside the palace several times and didn't need to see it again. I resigned to the thought that he could do whatever he wanted from then on and I would just enjoy his company, which was the greatest when he was normal. I told him about the Moorish castle nearby and how it was free to the public. The walk to the castle turned into a bit of a hike but we both enjoyed the forest scenery and I thanked God for everything.

We explored the castle for an hour and then began walking down the road toward the valley below, but we got only a couple two hundred feet. Patrick dropped his backpack on the ground and announced, "I'm not walking any more."

I tried to emanate a relaxed tone to my words. "Okay and how are we going to get into town if you're not walking?"

He stood against one of the large boulders with his arms crossed over his chest and staring into nowhere.

"Patrick, it's getting late. I've noticed that there haven't been any buses going by, only families in their cars. We need to start walking before it gets dark."

He turned his back on me and faced the wall. He had never acted this crazy before.

I ran back up the hill toward the castle looking for help. In the parking lot I saw a small black car with an old couple inside. The driver had just turned on the engine. I went up to their window. "My husband doesn't feel good and is standing down the road. Would you be so kind to give us a ride down to the town? Please?"

"Of course. Get in." They stopped to pick up Patrick. He had not moved from where he had been standing.

He was in a spiteful mood and sat silently in the back seat. Mr. João Sousa and his wife, Maria, were animated and keyed up about Patrick being an American, especially João, who spoke better English than his wife. Portuguese music blasted from the radio and João began singing along.

"Tell the old man to shut up."

"Patrick, it's his car and his radio. I'm sorry, but I can't tell him to stop singing."

João stopped singing and said, "Look, my friends, just look at the beautiful mountains that surround us. Have you ever seen a more beautiful place in the world?" Our happy-go-lucky chauffeur waved his arm out of the window.

"Big freakin' deal!" Patrick said to our driver, "If you saw our mountains in California you would crap in your pants."

João turned off the radio. No doubt he had understood what Patrick had just said. I saw his wife holding his hand in hers. If Patrick were to get into a fistfight with João, I knew who would die. I did the same as the woman; I held Patrick's hand and begged him with my eyes to calm down.

After a long silence, I said in Portuguese, "Please forgive my husband, he gets cranky when he is hungry." One could see that Mr. Sousa was a jolly, kind person who couldn't hold a grudge. "I'm going to take another road even though it's a little further. You must see one of Portugal's natural attractions, *O Buraco do Inferno* which means *Hell's Hole.*" You can't leave Portugal without seeing it. Don't worry there are lots of restaurants close by."

Again I answered him in Portuguese. As long as Patrick didn't understand what we were saying, he wouldn't have anything to pick on. It worked because Patrick remained quiet the rest of the trip.

They dropped us off by the shore, and I waved goodbye. Patrick looked at the site, crowded with tourists, and said, "It sucks just like the old man."

We found a tavern and I ordered two codfish sandwiches and two *Pastel de Nata.* After he had finished the sandwich, all hell broke loose. "You're still doing whatever it pleases you. Without regard for my wishes, you keep going on a constant spending frenzy. You just blew a dollar and a half on two desserts that can't even fill up a cavity."

I had to laugh at his description.

"It's nothing to laugh about. I can buy a lot of desserts here for half of what you just spent. Once again, let me remind you that before we started this trip, we agreed that you were not to buy anything without first talking to me. But you insist on doing it anyway."

"Okay, I promise not to buy anything without asking you first. Are you eating your dessert?" He walked away without answering me.

I picked up his *Pastel de Nata* and, before reaching the door, I stuffed it into my mouth. He was right, they were small.

Papa must have thought that I was nothing but a helpless pitiful woman under Patrick's spell, but I concluded I was purposely punishing myself for leaving Al. I had married Patrick because I didn't deserve anything better. Maybe I was addicted to Patrick the way I was with chocolate—deadly allergic to it but I still ate it. Like with any other addiction I couldn't stop, even if it killed me. Or maybe it was just like my father said, I was stupid. Either way, it didn't matter anymore. I had to keep going. Whatever he wanted us to eat, that's what it would be. Besides, I didn't mind bread and cheese. It was actually very fulfilling when I was hungry.

Back in Lisbon, the manager at the pensão offered to put all our belongings in storage until we returned from England. We left with our bare necessities inside our backpacks.

~ *Chapter Eighteen* ~

England

Max was waiting for us at the airport. I hadn't met him before. He looked to be in his mid-sixties, over six feet tall and very handsome. But his blue eyes impressed me the most. They radiated kindheartedness. He wore an impeccable gray business suit and had very distinguished manners. I told Patrick, "I bet he works out."

On the way to his home in the country, he drove through London, taking his time to point at the most important attractions, like Buckingham Palace, Big Ben, the Palace of Westminster and some historical parks.

"I'd like to be your personal guide, but I can't take time off from work. I apologize for neglecting you. When we get home, I'll give you train passes to London and some phone cards. In case you get lost or something, you can call me. I'll be home at the end of the day and look forward to having dinner with both of you. You'll find that my wife, Hilde, is the best cook in the world."

Just like Max, Hilde greeted us warmly and her smile brightened my spirits. Although she seemed to be about Max's age, she was the most youthful person I had ever met. I couldn't help hugging her constantly. She was like a love magnet. One afternoon she asked if I had any advice, as a future chiropractor, for making her legs stronger.

"I enjoy skiing, but my legs aren't working as well as they used to." She pointed to one of her legs. "You'll notice that this leg doesn't go as high as the right." She raised one leg way up to her chin height and then did the same with the other. She had me laughing hard.

Hilde was pure joy to be with, and she had plenty of stories to share with us—most to do with Max and when they were young. After a half century together, he was still the love of her life. She told us that Max was a chemical engineer and had used his skills in the manufacture of pigments before starting up his own adhesives company in 1960. He also ran a Research and Development laboratory at Cambridge Science Park and was involved in the work of the British Adhesives and Sealants Association and the British Standards Institute. I was impressed.

Their bathroom had heated towel holders. It was absolutely divine to get out of the shower and wrap my hair in a warm fluffy towel while I dried myself. I had never experienced anything so luxurious. Their old house was just the way I imagined a typical English home, with a quaint herb garden and fruit trees in the backyard. She was the gardener and very proud of it.

Patrick and I left early every morning, to explore the London's sites. I invited Hilde to go with us but she insisted that as honeymooners we should be by ourselves.

A few times I asked Patrick if I could borrow his camera, but he wouldn't let me use it. He said he had to save on film, and besides, I might drop it. He did let me take his picture when a bunch of pigeons surrounded him, some sitting on his head and others on his arms as he stood still like a statue.

Patrick thought the announcement over the train intercom, was annoying. Every time the train stopped to let people in and out a voice announced, "Mind the gap." I agreed with him but one had to admire such an effective and inexpensive solution to warn train passengers to take caution while crossing the gap between the train door and the station platform.

In America that would never work. Someone for sure would get hurt and sue for neglect and lack of safety.

When Patrick and I came home at the end of the day, Hilde would be in the kitchen making dinner. Patrick sat in the living room and looked at his map of London, marking the places he wanted to see the next day, while I helped to set the table. Soon Max would arrive home and we would have dinner. He always brought out a bottle of wine and before serving it would tell us the history behind it. He was very entertaining and so was Hilde. Afterward, Max would follow Hilde to the kitchen and help clean up. Though they wouldn't allow me to do anything, I remained in the kitchen talking to them. They were the portrait of love, acting like teenagers on a first date, kissing and making jokes and laughing. Patrick would remain in the living room, looking at his map.

One afternoon prior to Max getting home, Patrick and I sat on the couch in the living room waiting for Hilde to join us. Suddenly, he said, "I can't stand the sight of Max. Let's get our backpacks and leave now."

"Are you serious? You want to leave, just like that? Why don't you like Max?" My heart dropped out of my chest. I wasn't sure how to handle the situation. Good thing Hilde was upstairs getting dressed for dinner.

"He thinks he's better than me because he's rich. I don't like the way he talks down at me as if he knows it all. He has no right to look down on me."

"My goodness," I said smiling. "Of course he has to look down. He's so tall." Knowing he was jealous of his sister for being taller than him, I thought my joke would lighten up his spirits. Had I just goofed!

"So now I'm too short. You don't show any respect for my feelings."

"I'm sorry. I didn't mean it that way. You make me nervous, talking about Max the way you do and wanting to leave for no good reason. Hilde and Max have been nothing but nice to us. Patrick, please don't act this way. They are my family."

"Either you're with me or against me. When he walks through that door I'm telling him that he's nothing but a rich snob and I'm sick of listening to his observations when we're having dinner. I'm not staying here another minute. Do you hear?"

I cringed at the thought of what might happen. I put my arms around his neck and kissed him. "Of course I'm with you, but have you thought what it would cost for a London hotel and for food until we leave? C'mon, honey, at least we have a free place to stay. Just think of all the money we'll save."

"Okay then, but I'm not going to speak to him for the reminder of the time that we have to live in his house."

That evening, Patrick sat at the dining table eating but stared in the air as if no one else was present. I did my best to remain calm and act as if everything was normal. I knew that drinking wine would make me sick. I knew too it would make me act silly, so I drank some. I made jokes and so did Hilde and Max and dinner would have been great if Patrick hadn't remained speechless and distant.

When dinner was over, he stood and said, "Veronica, I'm going upstairs. Are you coming with me?"

"I'm going to help Hilde with the dishes and then I'll come up."

I took my time clearing the table and then stood in the kitchen talking to Hilde and Max. When Hilde said, "That's okay Veronica, Max and I can take care of the rest."

I said, "I really don't want to go upstairs."

"We understand," said Max. "When you get back to the US, you need to take him to see a psychologist. I'm no expert but I can tell you he needs help."

That night I couldn't fall asleep. Knowing that Max had noted something abnormal about Patrick confirmed my suspicions. What if Patrick started hating me for no reason? Would he just leave me stranded somewhere or get rid of me like I had seen in movies where the Mafia tied cement blocks around the neck of people they didn't like and then threw them into a lake.

I turned in bed and he did too, putting his arm around me. He loved me too much to ever hurt me. I fell asleep.

The next evening when Max got home he hugged us, kissed his wife and said, "Hilde, my darling, Patrick has told me that he used to work with his brother-in-law in landscaping and he knows a lot about trees. Why don't you show Patrick the fruit tree you've been having problems with." Then he turned to Patrick, "I'd be very grateful if you could provide some of your expertise to my wife. The tree is not doing well and she could use your professional opinion. Can you do that?"

When they left, Max took me to the side. "Veronica, I have been thinking about your husband and I feel it's better if you both stay with my sister Meta, instead. I already spoke to her and her husband this morning, and they said they would love to have you both over for the few days you have left in England. I feel it would be a good idea considering your husband behavior towards my wife and me. What do you think?"

I appreciated Max's kindness for not throwing us in the street. I told him that I too didn't know what was wrong with Patrick. I hugged him and said thank you for being understanding.

The next morning, Meta, Max's sister came by Hilde's house to pick us up. Shortly after talking to Meta, Patrick said to me, "I've never met such a beautiful older woman in my life. So much energy and in such great shape, I could easily fall in love with her."

Instead of feeling jealous, I was relieved. When he met her husband, who walked with a limp and used a cane, Patrick liked him immediately. "He's genuine," he said.

Max and Meta had been the ones who had paid for our plane tickets to England as our wedding gift. They also provided my parents with financial support with a monthly check to cover their living expenses. They didn't have to do that. They did it out of the goodness of their hearts.

Meta drove us all over the countryside and treated us to lunch every day at different village pubs, providing us a true flavor of the country and the English people. Patrick's favorite was fish and chips and would order them every time we went out.

One night, Meta made dinner of roast beef, roasted potatoes, vegetables, and Yorkshire pudding. Patrick begged that she do it again the next night.

Meta made dinner every night, and I helped her with the cooking and cleaning. Patrick sat in the study talking to Meta's husband. He would gladly have remained longer in England, but the invitation was not extended.

Before we left for Portugal, Meta gave me a bluish wool scarf and a handmade wool shawl that used to belong to my grandmother, Mutter, my father's mother.

"This winter is going to be a cold one. Her shawl will keep you extra warm while traveling. My mother would have liked you to have it."

God bless my family in England!

~ Chapter Nineteen ~

Back to Portugal

We arrived in Lisbon late in the afternoon. We were about to go down the metro steps when two transit cops came from behind and asked for our tickets. Patrick acted as though he didn't know anything about it, and I did the same by acting like a foreigner. They let us go after calling us ignorant Americans.

The next morning we carried our belongings from the pensão to the bus station, we would be heading south to Ourique, where my brother Max-Leão lived. While waiting for the bus, we sat on one of the wood benches in the terminal and watched an inebriated man seated on the bench across from us. He tried to sit upright, but kept falling sideways. Patrick laughed heartily, his camera on hand, ready to take the shot if the man fell on his face. We had no right to watch somebody's misery. I closed my eyes and made believe I was resting.

We arrived at Ourique, at six o'clock that evening. The bus stopped in front of a tavern. It was a small town. The waitress knew my brother and so did her boss and everybody else in the tavern. He was an architect and builder, so a lot of the men in Ourique relied on him for their work.

The waitress called my brother, and in less than twenty minutes, he and his wife, Patricia, arrived at the tavern. We hugged each other joyfully. I had met Patricia only once, fifteen years ago, the last time I had seen my brother. We had a lot to catch up on.

They lived on an old farm, and their house was a typical Portuguese country home made of stones. Their son, Leo and daughter, Tara, were traveling and we wouldn't be able to meet them. My brother and Patricia, who was British, both spoke English, but her accent was typically British. She served us a homemade Portuguese dinner, which I savored with gusto—fresh codfish cooked with potatoes and steamed vegetables and delicious olives on the side. For dessert she had made flan! Wow, I was with my brother, his wife, and eating the kind of food I had grown up with. I couldn't ask for more. Patrick was behaving quite well. He liked the food and the idea that everyone spoke English.

After dinner my brother drove us in his 1940's black Mercedes, about thirty-five minutes from his house, to a farmhouse he was restoring in what felt like a nowhere-land of darkness. "You guys are on your honeymoon, so have the place all to yourselves. The house is still under construction, but the bedroom and bathroom are ready to use. Enjoy it!" He opened the front door to a small unfinished foyer still covered with dirt and then a double unpainted double door to a large fully furnished bedroom. As he was about to drive off, he put his head out the window and yelled out, "I almost forgot. If any of the horses comes trotting into your bedroom, don't worry, they're friendly. I'll come by in the morning to pick you up for breakfast."

It was a simple bedroom with naked white walls and a new matching set of modern French style furniture, with a queen size bed, tall armoire and a long dresser. There was plenty of space for us to storage our goods and we agreed that our bedroom was very luxurious. What got to me was the bathroom. It was like something out of a James Bond movie, with thick block glass walls surrounding an open shower. I had never seen anything so sexy in my life. The counter tops went all around the room, with wall-to-wall mirrors. The counters had two large sinks that looked like they had been brought from Arabia due to the exquisite ceramic pattern and the Portuguese soap and shampoo emanated a delicious clean smell. After the shower, I wrapped myself in one of the towels, the size of a blanket.

Patrick was busy in the bedroom unpacking. When he went to take a shower he commented, "Some farmhouse with three shower heads. I can't wait to see the rest of the place tomorrow morning." While he showered I took a better look at the bedroom with its tall windows and old-fashioned wood shutters, no glass or screens. In the south of Portugal, the winter rarely became rigorous.

I could hear the shower running in the bathroom. I smiled because he didn't turn off the water once. When he came out, he was wearing only a smile. I dropped my towel and slipped under the warmth of the four inch thick goose-feather bedcover. Patrick crawled in. He kissed my feet, one toe at a time, and then slowly made his way up to my lips. He was a great lover and knew how to bring out the best in me. Until I met him, I had always worn pajamas to bed. He liked the idea of us sleeping naked. That way we could feel each other's bodies and be ready to make love any time of the night. I was all for it, besides it felt good to be held all night, even while sleeping. In California, he had his clothes on his side of the bed in case he had to run outside because of an earthquake. I had learned to do the same. Being in Portugal was no different. We were prepared in case of an earthquake.

The next morning, Patrick shook me awake. "Veronica, you ain't gonna believe this house. Come and check it out. This is truly an amazing place."

As we opened our bedroom door to the unfinished vestibule, we walked carefully not to trip over the demolition debris as the hallway opened into an open area where the only thing standing was one of its original stone walls with a fireplace that ran the full twelve feet length of that wall surreally facing one of the stables. The wind blew briskly across our faces. The possibilities of what that room would look like in the near future left a lot to the imagination. Obviously my brother had yet to work on that part of the house.

Max-Leão soon showed up, and he gave us a tour of his property. We stopped first at the stables. He had a pregnant mare, a black stallion, and two ordinary horses. Patrick was enthralled by the novelty of everything and worked hard along with my brother cleaning the stables. "If I could bottle all this manure and find a way of selling it as a cure for all diseases I would be a millionaire." They were both laughing.

Then he showed us the man-made lake he and some of his employees had dug. I could hear the pride in his voice. Then he took us to the other side of the house, where he was ready to install an in-ground swimming pool.

"Max-Leão, remember when we were children our parents wouldn't allow you to excavate a pool in our backyard?"

"Yes I remember." He laughed. "Now I can make lakes and pools to my heart's contentment."

Turkeys, ducks, and chickens ran freely in the property. Patrick and I agreed that when my brother finished building the house, it was going to be a remarkable ranch.

Max-Leão drove us to his home where Patricia served us delicious homemade bread, hot-from-the-oven, goat cheese, homemade peach jam and soft-boiled eggs. They drank coffee and Patrick and I had tea. We sat in their kitchen talking until lunchtime and then Patricia served us ham sandwiches and a salad.

"It's time to show you our ponderosa mountains. Are you ready to go hiking?" Max-Leão proudly showed us his property, which was humongous, and definitely a hunting and nature paradise. Some of the mountains produced slate, which brought in some income. By the time we finished hiking, we were famished.

They treated us to dinner at a restaurant and we talked about our experiences as children and our parents. "Papa had no right to sell his house and all his possessions without conferring first with me, his only son. I'll never forgive him for not calling me. I could have helped him and Mama to get out of the situation they were in."

He confessed to being jealous of me when he was sent to England at fifteen and I stayed home. I told him that I wished I could have gone with him. At least he was free to marry whomever he loved. We talked a lot about the past and I knew the cobwebs between us had been cleared when he began telling jokes. He had me laughing so hard that tears ran down my face. Patrick was also good at telling jokes and joined right in, and we all laughed heartily. The midnight hour soon arrived and he dropped off Patricia at home and drove us back to the farmhouse, but fifteen minutes into our drive, his car stopped dead. He turned the key several times, but the engine wouldn't kick in. It was pitch black all around us and not a single car was going by.

He sat back and crossed his hands in back of his neck. "You might as well make yourselves comfortable back there. So, how did you two meet?"

"We attend the same college," I said. "Max-Leão, does this mean that we're stuck?"

"The engine will turn over when it's ready to. There's no rush. Life is too short to worry about stuff like this."

"How can you just sit there when we're stranded in the middle of nowhere?" Patrick asked quite calmly.

"Do you see any gas station? What good will it do to get upset?" My brother wore a serene smile.

"Are we going to spend the night in the car?" Patrick continued to remain calm, which surprised me a lot.

"I hope not, but if it's meant to be, it will be. Take off your shoes if you like. Get comfortable." Max-Leão took off his shoes and stretched between the two front seats.

We talked about all kinds of mundane stuff, such as the weather and how life was a lot more stressful in the US. A half-hour later, Max-Leão turned the key and the engine kicked in. "This car definitely has a mind of its own." His smile grew joyful.

When he dropped us off at the farm, I encouraged him to call Patricia to come and get him.

"Don't worry, Sis. My car will get me home." He hugged me and drove off.

We turned out the lights inside the house, took our blanket outside, and laid it on the ground. Patrick and I held hands while looking at the sky lit up by the Universe above us. I felt as though we were the only two people on the planet. We lay out there for an hour, just staring at the starry heavens.

"When we're doing well financially, we should come back and buy this property from your brother. Do you think he would give us a good deal? I'd be happy living here."

"Possibly." I lacked enthusiasm. I preferred to live where my sons and grandchildren lived, in the US. Even though we were having a good time visiting my brother I wasn't very sure that I was happily married. If anything, I couldn't wait to go home and back to school.

"I admire your brother, the way he remained so calm and relaxed when the car broke down. I'm gonna try being more like him and control my temper."

The next morning Max-Leão came by promptly at eight and took us to work with him. He wanted us to see what he did for a living. He bought properties with century-old, beat-up homes. He then renovated the houses to fit today's modern standards, but made sure the exteriors didn't lose their typical Portuguese look. Inside the house he created what his clients wanted—modern bathrooms, huge fireplaces, and stone floors made to order.

Patricia worked in real estate, and together they made a great team, along with their son, Leo, who followed in his father's footsteps. We also learned why Max-Leão was so successful. He worked very hard. He wasn't just an architect who drew plans. He climbed on top of houses and helped his workers lay tile, and when he couldn't find someone skilled to put in floors, he did it himself. He complained that a lot of the old carpenters and artisans had become a thing of the past, and sometimes he didn't have the skilled labor he needed to do the work. His knees suffered from the hours spent putting down floor slates, not to mention other tasks that required him to lift heavy equipment.

He took us to visit a grapefruit farm that left us with our mouths open. The workmanship and detail my brother had put into the construction of the farmhouse was astounding. I wondered how he had designed the kitchen sink, with such beautiful intricate patterns on the inside. The entryway floor was in itself a work of art, and any artist would be proud to say they had designed it. Everything had been done professionally, with attention to the smallest detail. He kept us busy all day, looking at properties and ranch houses he had built into small palaces that even a king would be proud to own.

After five days Patrick decided he no longer liked my brother because he owned too many properties. He was a know-it-all architect who made money from the sweat of the village people.

That night in bed, he said, "Have you noticed the guy installing the slate floor in the entry? How would you like to have sex with him?"

"Why in the world would I want to have sex with him?"

"My fantasy is to watch you with another man."

"If that's your fantasy, you're wasting your time. I'm not interested."

"Don't you have fantasies?"

"Of course I do. Everybody has fantasies."

"If you love me, you'll stand naked by the window tomorrow morning and invite him into the bedroom."

"So you want me to have sex with someone else to prove that I love you? That doesn't make any sense."

"I'm giving you the freedom to enjoy yourself. That's how much I love you."

I tried to appeal to his common sense. Fantasies can't be turned into reality or they stop being fantasies. That didn't work. He had one track mind. I remained silent and waited for him to fall asleep.

I woke the next morning very concerned. How I was going to fight for my rights as a human being and not do what he wanted me to?

Patrick rushed into the bedroom. "Damn it! I've been looking for the worker all over the place. It looks like he isn't showing up today."

When having lunch at my brother's house, Patrick had the nerve to ask my brother if his worker was coming back to finish the floor. My brother said he had given him a few days off because his wife was in the hospital. That night, he continued to push his warped sense of sexual dysfunction. "When we get home, I want to put an ad in the paper for another couple to have sex with. Won't that be exciting? It will be great for both of us."

"Not for me. I already told you I'm not interested in having sex with other people."

"Things will have to change when we get back. You need to get with it. I also want to get a dog. I get very aroused about having sex with animals."

"Stop it. I'm going to get sick. I'm not having sex with other couples, much less with a dog."

"You can watch me then."

Once he was obsessed with something, nothing I said would stop him. Once again I let him talk while I remained silent, waiting for him to fall asleep.

I offered to make dinner before we left, so Patricia took us to the town farmer's market. Patrick had a fit. According to him, they could afford feeding us and we shouldn't spend any money on them. I wanted to cook at least once to thank them for their hospitality. Once Patrick decided that he didn't like my brother, he had stopped talking and began giving Max-Leão dirty looks.

"What's the matter with Patrick?" my brother asked. "Did we say something to offend him?"

"He has a hormonal imbalance and suffers from mood swings."

"Like a woman, hum?" Patricia laughed and so did my brother. I was glad that we were leaving the next morning, while things were still good.

The plan was to travel just with our backpacks and leave all our possessions with my brother and his wife. I packed my backpack with underwear and socks, leg warmers, long johns, two tee shirts, a sweater, Meta's bluish wool scarf, and my favorite Pittsburgh Steelers wool hat. I don't know what Patrick was carrying, but his backpack was filled tight to the top and so heavy I had to help him to put it over his shoulders.

I also carried my goose-feather winter-coat. It was a bit worn out, with most of the goose feathers gone, but I figured that could work to my advantage. It would still keep me warm, but it would be easy to squeeze it into my backpack on warmer days.

The next morning we took the bus to Faro, a city in the south of Portugal. From there we would pick up another bus to Spain.

On the ride to Faro, Patrick said he wanted to go to Tangier, Morocco. Sometime ago I had made the mistake of telling him about my trip there with Ralph where we had been kidnapped by an Arab posing as a government official, luckily we were able to escape from the Kasbah in the middle of the night.

"Have you forgotten what I told you happened in Tangier? I don't feel it's any safer now. Honey, let's go home after we visit Spain."

"If an Arab even comes close to me, I'll beat the crap out of him." He had made up his mind. From Spain we would go to Morocco.

We arrived in Faro at ten in the morning. Patrick wanted to spend the night there. I told him about the hotel where Ralph and I had stayed a few years back that was very economical. "You and Ralph have expensive tastes. Let's check out the other places."

We found nothing cheaper than ten dollars per night, and all we did was waste the whole morning. By the time we arrived at the bus station to buy tickets to Spain, there was a sign on the window that read, "All tickets sold out. We'll open again on Monday." We would have to stay in Faro for two more days.

We finally found a fast food place to eat that he felt was economical enough. Several people stood in line before us, waiting to place their orders with the two employees behind the counter. We had stood there less than a minute when Patrick yelled, "This place sucks when it comes to service."

"Patrick, there are only six people in front of us."

"This type of service would never make it in the US." The couple in front of us turned and stared at him. "What are you looking at, you creeps!" Then, he turned his anger on everyone else on line. "In America you would be considered morons. You're nothing but morons, do you hear me?"

If I was a man and stronger than him I would have slapped him, instead I asked him to sit at a table while I stayed in line.

He sat holding his head between his hands, staring at the table top. I brought him two cheeseburgers and fries.

"I'm going to step out. I'll be back."

His face softened. "Where are you going?"

"I'll be by the front door. Take your time eating, I need some fresh air."

I stood outside with my back against the building. I didn't care that people could see me bawling. I didn't want to travel any more, and most of all I didn't want to be married to Patrick. The man I loved was impossible to live with. I wanted to go home, get a divorce, and get back to school. I was beginning to fear for my life. He had too much violence inside of him.

I took a deep breath. It was my fault for being in this situation. Mama had warned me many times, "The bed you make is the one you sleep in." I had even written in my diary that it would be a big mistake if I married him, but I did it anyway. What a pathetic fool! I deserved everything I got. I would continue with the trip and do the best I could, because even though I was starting to hate him, I also felt sorry for him. I asked God to give me strength before I entered the restaurant.

When he saw me, he stood and hugged me. "Sorry about the way I behaved. Will you forgive me?"

We began walking towards what we thought was the road to the shore. Two hours later we were still walking. Finally we put our thumbs up. A disheveled young man riding a beat-up Fiat with no back seats gave us a ride. Patrick sat upfront and I kneeled over the metal base of the trunk-like space, feeling much like a hula dance doll on a car's dash, every bump shaking my bones. Still, I was happy I didn't have to carry my backpack another mile.

By the time we reached the beach, the sun was rapidly disappearing behind the horizon. We filled a small plastic bag with a handful of sand. I had proposed we collect sand from each beach we visited. I'd told him about Dr. Morphinot, one of the teachers at school, who had an assortment of small colorful spice jars in her office. I had asked her why she had so many spices when there was no place in her office to cook. It was a sand collection from all the beaches that she had visited. Patrick loved the idea.

Patrick agreed to take the bus back to Faro, rather than walking back, in the dark and possibly getting lost. Even so, once on the bus, he announced, "We have just wasted a dollar in bus fare." We would be eating bread and cheese that night.

The next day we took our time exploring the city. We stopped in a church that had been built in 1713. Inside, we found a small chapel built with human bones. The inscription over the chapel door read, "Stop here and think of the fate that will befall you—1876." He felt cheery about the chapel, but I thought it was gruesome to be surrounded by the remains of over a thousand monks. When I asked him if he wanted his picture taken next to the altar covered with skulls, he posed for me with a big smile.

After we left the chapel, we walked for hours, looking for a place for lunch with food he liked and that fitted our budget. We finally found a restaurant at two o'clock. When the waitress took our order, Patrick asked for the fried chicken advertised on the menu board outside.

"I'm sorry but we ran out of that. Lunch stopped being served an hour ago. I can still get you a salad if you like."

He jumped to his feet and threw his chair backwards, then with both hands he turned the table over and walked out. I sat as if paralyzed and then said in Portuguese, "I'm really sorry."

"Is he your husband?"

"Yes. Please excuse his manners."

"He is an American, right?"

"Yes." I helped her to pick up the table.

"That's what I figured. Americans are rude people. I feel sorry for you."

I had to run to catch up with him. He walked fast and wouldn't talk. I led him into the same quick food service shop we had been to the day before. He sat at the same table with his head between his hands. I ordered fries and two-cheese sandwiches for him, and one for me.

"What can we do to prevent you losing your temper?"

"When I get hungry, that's what happens. I have no control over it."

"What if you carry snacks in your backpack for in-between meals?"

"I like that. We'll look for a supermarket every morning and buy our daily food and carry that in our backpacks. That way we don't have to eat at restaurants."

"Fine, but we need to add some vegetables to our diet, besides bread and cheese. You take vitamins every day but I don't."

"The money we have is for traveling and for postcards to send to the family, but I can see us sharing a tomato or a green pepper once in a while. I'm trying to manage our finances so we don't have to dig into our bank account."

I agreed that we should spend as little as possible.

~ Chapter Twenty~

Spain and North Africa

The bus ride to Spain was very comfortable. Patrick stayed busy chatting with a young Australian woman. Once the bus driver began stopping at every town tavern to talk to friends, Patrick became irritated, and I had to pull all my resources to keep him distracted. When I ran out of funny stories, I asked him to sing his favorite country song to me.

The blissful ambience soon ended when a guy sitting up front lit a cigarette. Patrick cursed at the smoker. The man cursed back. The bus driver stopped the bus and told Patrick and me to get off. We were in Seville.

We waited less than ten minutes but the next bus was jammed packed. Patrick started to shake, his eyes opened wide, and grabbed his chest as if grasping for air. "I can't breathe, get me out of here." He repeatedly pressed the bell for the bus to stop.

"I'm going to kill that asshole driver." He pushed passengers out of his way to get to the front. The driver must have seen him in the mirror and slammed on the brakes. The side door opened and the bus driver called out, "Hey, crazy man, get out!"

Patrick kneeled on the sidewalk and yelled, "I hate Seville. I hate Spain. I hate Europe. Let's go to Mexico instead."

"Mexico? Patrick, do you even realize what you're saying? Do you know where we are?"

"Let's take a plane to Mexico. Let's go back to Mazatlán."

"How about we take a plane home instead?"

"No. I want to go to Mazatlán, I like it better there." He began to cry.

I didn't have to be a psychologist to realize he was out of his mind. I dropped onto on my knees put my arms around him and rocked him gently.

He smiled and I told him he had a beautiful smile. We kissed.

"Let's find out where we can take the boat to Morocco." He spoke as if nothing had happened.

We would have to take a bus to Tarifa. We had a three-hour wait for the bus to Tarifa. We left our heavy backpacks in one of the secured storage compartments at the bus station and walked through the city. We saw an old church with a very tall tower that appeared to offer a good view. And it was free with a student ID.

"Patrick, please don't get upset, but I left my card in my backpack after using it the last time. But it's only fifty cents."

"You're such an airhead, a total idiot. I can't depend on you for anything. A lousy ID card and instead of keeping it where it belongs in your money belt, you put it in your backpack. Where are your brains? Did you leave them there too?"

"I'm sorry, Patrick. I'm very sorry. It won't happen again. I'll put the card on my money belt as soon as we get back to the bus station."

I sat on the cold stone floor with my legs crossed and put my head between my hands. He returned with my ticket. "Next time you forget your ID, I'm going without you."

I climbed the worn-out stone steps without stopping. My breath grew short and my heart beat faster. Nothing would stop me until I dropped dead from a heart attack. I asked God to have pity on me and put me out of my misery since I was too much of a coward to leave him. I cried all the way to the top of the tower.

On the way back to the bus station Patrick asked me to forgive him. I said okay, but after a daily dosage of excuses from Patrick, his apologies, had lost their meaning.

On the bus to Tarifa he put his head on my shoulder and fell asleep. Once in Tarifa we walked all over the city looking for economical accommodations for the night. Looking for accommodations had become an expected but exhausting part of our journey where we would spend hours walking with our heavy backpacks until all possible motels and hostels had been evaluated for the best rates.

When we walked by the dock, I thought about pushing him into the ocean. He would drown, and I would be free to go home. That was never going to happen. He knew how to swim and would probably kill me with his bare hands after he reached the shore.

The sun was going down when a man in his mid-twenties tried to sell us hashish. Patrick told him to get lost, but he kept following us. It didn't bother Patrick, though. In fact, he enjoyed it. Even after we checked into a hotel room, Patrick went directly to the window to look outside. The young man stood on the street corner, smoking a cigarette and looking as if he were waiting for us to come out.

"I'll be right back," Patrick said. "I'll take care of that bastard." He left.

With luck, he wouldn't come back.

I checked out the bathroom down the hallway. It had a shower, only cold water, but still, it was a shower!

Patrick's face glowed when he returned. "When he saw me coming, he walked away, but I followed him, then he ran, and I ran after him. I scared the crap out of him. I've never been this content in my life. It's only ten o'clock. Let's celebrate with a good dinner."

A block from our hotel we found a restaurant with a sign on the window, "Dinner Special, four dollars." It was the worst chicken with rice I had ever eaten. No wonder it was so cheap. They had burned it and were trying to get rid of it. I gave Patrick my plate.

"You're too picky about food," he said. "Don't blame me if you get hungry. Hey, it's still early, let's go to a bar and enjoy the night life." Usually we were in our room by ten, playing cards.

We walked into a tavern and sat on the bar stools. The bartender asked what we would like. Patrick said, "Tell him we're waiting for a friend."

We talked and held hands and looked into each other's eyes, smiling. A young woman sat next to him and in very poor English began chatting to him. She was dressed to attract and Patrick *was* attracted.

I knew what he was thinking before he even said it. "This is an opportunity for us to have a *ménage à trois,"* he whispered in my ear.

"What if she has syphilis or something worse?" I whispered back. "Are you ready to lose your penis?"

"You're right." He turned to her and said with a friendly smile, "Excuse me, but I'm with my wife." And he turned to me all lovey-dovey.

The next morning we picked up some nuts and other items for him to snack, plus our ration of food for the day. Breakfast was no longer part of our diet, unless it was included with our lodgings. We caught a local bus to the port of Tarifa, where we boarded the ferry to Tangier. The ferry carried a load of cars and the passengers were mostly men. The smell, a blend of fumes and gasoline, made me feel like I was in a cargo ship. As we neared Tangier, about an hour later, I realized there was a good possibility he would get murdered in there and I would be going home.

When the ferry arrived at the pier, Patrick reminded me of Pavlov's dog. Tangier offered him the once-in-a-life-time opportunity to practice his karate, and get away with it. After going rapidly through customs, since they didn't even check our backpacks, a well-dressed man approached us, just like what had happened when Ralph and I had visited Morocco. The man asked Patrick and me to follow him. Patrick was expecting it, since I had described to him how *they* worked.

Patrick shoved the man out of his way. "Get out of my face, you mother fucker."

"You're a very nasty person," said the man. "I'm just trying to make a few dollars by offering my services."

"Read my lips, go fuck yourself!"

The man backed away a few steps and then followed us out of the terminal. I led Patrick toward the main avenue that led into town. Patrick and I were in control of where we wanted to go. We planned to have lunch on the beach before heading into the Kasbah.

The man that followed Patrick and me had two more buddies working with him. Each took his turn walking with us and trying to make conversation.

We were still walking along the shore when Patrick told me to stay put. He walked to the street corner and put his backpack on the ground. Then he took off his leather jacket, pulled his sleeves up, and said, "You fucking vultures. Get off our backs or I'll break your necks."

I admired his courage. Two of the men fled. The other followed us at a respectable distance from across the street. We walked to the beach, sat on the sand, and ate the cheese sandwiches while enjoying the Mediterranean air. I laughed along with him about our adventure in Tangier. The guy who had been following us had given up and was gone.

We filled a small plastic bag with a handful of sand and then headed up the hill towards the old part of the city, called the Kasbah.

I had warned Patrick about the Kasbah and how easy it was to get lost in its narrow labyrinth-like streets, but he had it all planned out. He pulled out his notebook and, using his special astronaut pen that could write upside down, he drew each street as we moved deeper into the Kasbah. He wrote right, left, left, right. We didn't go very far before his claustrophobia kicked in and we had to leave.

While we rode the ferry back to Spain, Patrick showed me the map where he had marked our travel itinerary. After Spain, he wanted to go to Nice, France, and Monaco. He no doubt knew where we would go after Monaco, but he wasn't sharing his plans with me.

At this point I was juggling mixed feelings towards him. His outbursts of anger scared me and when they were directed at me, I hated him. Yet, he could make me feel very special and loved. Just about every day I found a little love note under my pillow or inside my backpack, and when we walked by a garden he would pick a flower for me. We held hands whenever possible and kissed passionately every night no matter how tired we felt. Most of the hotels and hostels where we stayed offered only a small bed, but if we had two twin size beds he would move them next to each other. He couldn't sleep unless he was holding me. I liked that. It felt good to be held lovingly at the end of the day. It made me forget how unhappy I was.

We took the train to Valencia, just because he'd read that it had a nude beach. It was a long walk to the beach, but a small price to pay, for a bag of Valencia sand. A boardwalk resembling the one in Asbury Park, New Jersey, extended along the shore with no one in sight except for five men who stood together staring at the beach below. The beach was empty except for a naked, out-of-shape middle-aged woman sunbathing.

"This is supposed to be the Spanish Riviera where beautiful women lay naked on the beach," Patrick said. "She looks more like a whale marooned on the sand!"

She kept changing positions without modesty. Then she smiled at a good-looking young man wearing an out-of-place business suit. He walked over and lovingly kissed her on the mouth, then handed her a glass of red wine. It was a spectacle worse still, I was the only woman standing among those men, while Patrick kept repeating, "I can't believe it. I just can't believe it. It's disgusting."

I wanted to say, nobody is forcing you to look, but instead I laughed along with him. When he was happy, so was I.

He couldn't find anything else he liked in Valencia, so we walked back to the train station and took a train to Barcelona, where we spent the rest of the day looking for a budget motel before retiring for the night.

The next morning, we had been walking under a misty rain for about an hour when for no apparent reason he began picking on me, despite having enough snacks to eat anytime he wanted. "There's something I've been meaning to tell you. It bothers me that you never thanked me for going with you the morning you took the National Boards."

"I always say thank you for everything you do for me."

"Not that time, you didn't."

"What are you talking about?"

"I took the morning off from school just to be with you and you didn't thank me for it. Don't expect me to forgive you for that."

What this was all about, I would never know. The best I could do was to stop defending myself and let him complain until he ran out of steam. Later he would apologize.

Considering that it was winter, the weather in Barcelona was quite warm even when it rained. I thanked God for the rain, a gift from the heavens concealing my tears.

We walked into a large plaza where several musicians stood under a small canopy playing a sort of flute like instruments. I hadn't heard that style of music before. I continued to cry silently but didn't last too long as the haunting sound of the Andes music had such a joyful beat that I began tapping my feet, and I was happy again. Since he prohibited me from wasting any money on one of their cassette tapes I promised myself to get one when I got back to the US.

Later that day we came across a Christmas craft fair. I was surprised when he said, "Let's buy a small trinket to give each other at Christmas."

"Really?"

"Yeah, as long as it's under a dollar, I'm fine with that."

We gave each other an hour to shop. Then we would meet by the exceptionally tall Christmas tree in the center of the square.

Oh my gosh, this was my chance. A whole hour to catch a bus to the airport. By the time he realized that I ran away, I would be on my way home. The fantasy lasted only a few seconds. He carried both our passports and return airline tickets.

~Chapter Twenty-One~

France

We spent the night on a bus to Nice, France. Patrick made small talk with Gisele, a German girl sitting next to him. It was four in the morning when the bus driver dropped the three of us off at a large plaza. When she asked us where we were staying the night, Patrick said we had slept enough.

"Patrick, we spent the night on a bus. I need to take a bath, stretch on a bed and get some real sleep."

"We rested, and that's good enough for me. Besides, the night is already gone. Why pay for another day at a hotel?"

He offered to escort Gisele to the hostel where she would be staying, since it was still dark. I expected racecars passing me by and movie stars walking the streets. Nice seemed to be a gloomy city. At least it had stopped raining. We walked until she saw two young guys with backpacks, standing by a doorway talking to each other. She asked them for directions.

"For a good fuck, I'll give you the directions," one said. Then he and his buddy laughed.

Patrick marched up to the doorway and yelled at the guy who had insulted her. "Apologize to this young lady, or I'll beat the shit out of you."

"Sorry, man. I was just playing around. I didn't mean anything by it."

I was proud of Patrick for defending the girl. Despite his violent temper and screwed-up thinking process, he had a lot of good qualities.

The two young men were either English or Australian. I couldn't tell the difference in their accents. Most likely Aussies, as Patrick called them, given that the only English-speaking people we met during our travels were from Australia.

The three of us walked to the hostel. When we arrived, we said our goodbyes, and then Patrick and I went looking for the train station. Once we found it, we waited for it to open, under pouring rain. My coat was not leather like Patrick's, and the rain soaked through the thin layer of goose-down feathers. The cold wetness seeped through my coat deep into my skin and my bones. It was daylight when someone told us that the railroad workers were on strike. We would have to stay in Nice.

We spent the rest of the morning looking for a hostel, but finding lodgings in Nice that fit our budget was like panning for gold. We finally found a hostel for a decent price, but the bathroom was one floor below our room and had to be shared with the other guests. Nice had a refined look, its manicured gardens and boulevards reminded me of Estoril, an elite Portuguese city that was famous for welcoming the rich and famous.

After we got settled, we located a market place that sold bread and cheese, but then we discovered that the street cart vendors sold pre-made sandwiches for a lot less.

We spent the day walking, first along the beach, as far as we could go, and then through the city. As we walked back to our hostel, I saw a clothing store named Toledano. I pointed to the sign and said, "Look, that's my grandmother's middle name. Maybe the owners are my cousins." I entered the store.

A young girl worked behind the counter. When I told her that my grandmother's middle name was Toledano, she quickly welcomed me.

"My first name is Simy," she said.

"Oh dear, Simy was my mother's name."

"How exciting, perhaps we are family." She hugged me. "My parents and I own this store." She waived to her parents who were talking to customers. I waited and when they came over to meet me they were just as friendly as Simy.

"This is absolutely incredible." I said, unable to contain my joy. "My husband is waiting outside. But I would love to stay and talk to you."

"We close in a hour." said Mrs. Toledano. "Would you and your husband like to join us for dinner at our house?"

"Let me tell my husband. I'll be right back." I ran out to get him.

He was pacing on the sidewalk in front of the store.

I told him what happened and how excited I was and that we had been invited to their home for dinner.

"I'm hungry now and I refuse to wait another hour. Besides, I've no interest in socializing with a bunch of French snobs."

"They are not snobs. You haven't even talked to them. What's with you and meeting people? There's more to traveling than just keep going and going. This is a wonderful chance to possibly meet family from my grandmother's side."

He wasn't listening and I knew better than to agitate him. He wouldn't socialize with anyone, unless it was an attractive woman who paid attention to him. They were disappointed when I told them that, my husband wasn't feeling well and we had to go back to the hotel.

On the way to the hostel, we passed a restaurant where whole chickens were being grilled outside on a rotisserie. Patrick said we should buy one and share it. I couldn't conceive eating just a chunk of meat. My body was begging for fresh green vegetables. I had to settle for a lettuce salad, the closest thing they had to raw vegetables. Patrick ate the chicken and I satisfied myself with salad. We agreed to do the same thing for dinner the next day.

Before going to sleep, he said, "Tomorrow let's find out about taking a train to Sarnen, Switzerland. That's where my mother's family, the Jaquois, originally comes from."

"And then we go home, right?"

He laughed so much that it got contagious.

The next morning, when we were walking to the train station, I saw a car rental place. Traveling by car sounded a lot better to me. No sitting on buses and trains, listening to Patrick complain about people smoking or other conditions beyond his control. And no more panic attacks.

"Let's see what it costs," I encouraged him. "It doesn't hurt to ask."

After hearing the price, Patrick concluded that if we slept in the car, the money we would save in accommodations and other forms of transportation would more than make up for the cost of the ten-day rental fee. The next day we would drive east and then north across France, through Italy and into Switzerland. We would use the car to carry our belongings and when tired we could just park and rest.

"I'll drive and you'll be my navigator," he said.

As we were leaving the car rental, a man dressed in a black tuxedo was walking toward the building. Just then, a flock of pigeons bombarded him with white poop, covering the poor man from head to toe. Patrick couldn't stop laughing, and used his handheld tape recorder to record the incident. He recorded everything that struck him as funny. He was a great storyteller.

~ *Chapter Twenty-Two* ~

Switzerland

Our car was a dark blue Fiat 500, stick shift, sparkly clean inside and out. I knew Patrick liked it when he stroked his hand over the hood and smiled at me. I held the opened map on my lap, ready to give directions. On the way out of Nice my French came in handy when I read the sign toll ahead. He repeatedly hit the horn, and then pulled an abrupt U-turn, to avoid going through the toll, but there was no way off the highway without paying. I felt as though we were on the New Jersey Turnpike. No one drove in or out without paying.

Of course Patrick called me a useless good-for-nothing navigator. I blocked him out of my mind and concentrated on the scenery. Soon I forgot he was there. I was traveling in a world of magical wonders. Surely, God must have spent a little extra time creating France. The farmlands were a rich pallet of multicolored pastels, a carefully planned collage of rolling hills and streams cutting through lavish shades of green and gold fields.

When we crossed into Italy, it was time for dinner. Patrick drove into a parking lot in front of a large office building, where three cars were parked inside the fence. We had our bread and cheese and the rest of our tomato and green pepper leftover from lunch.

"Must be a government building to have such a tall metal fence around it," I said.

"Yeah, a perfectly safe place to spend the night."

Two cars started leaving through the main gate. When I saw the last car in the lot driving off I had a premonition.

"Patrick, don't ask me any questions. Start the engine now and follow that car."

As we drove out of the parking lot we saw the driver of the car in front of us, getting out of his car and locking the gate entrance. He waved at us smiling.

"Bastard," Patrick said. "He knew he was locking us in."

The next day was Saturday. If we had not acted, we would have been stuck behind that fence until Monday morning. We needed to pay more attention to where we parked for the night.

Not too far from there we parked behind a church and fell asleep, but I woke within an hour. My blood felt as though it had turned into ice. It was snowing.

Patrick turned the engine on for a few minutes. "The longer we run the engine," he said, "the more gas we'll use. Let's wait until we're both shivering."

"Patrick, we need to find a warm place to sleep. I'm scared we'll freeze to death."

He laughed.

"This is no joke. It happens to a lot of people, even in America. You know that, right?"

After driving for two hours, we found a hotel, but it was for rich foreigners. Even I cringed at the prices. We decided to rough it. We found a dirt road that led to a farmhouse, and parked under a tree. Every hour or so Patrick turned the engine on to heat up the car.

Once in Switzerland, the weather worsened. A blinding snowstorm stopped us cold. Snow covered our windshield like a thick mat, and the road had grown invisible. We had no choice but to look for the nearest lodging. The price didn't even matter.

It was a real hotel. And what a hotel it was! We made love inside our own private hot shower and then took turns washing our jeans, shirts, underwear and socks. The wall heater became our clothes' dryer. The extra thick goose down duvet was like a mound of hot whipped cream over our bodies. We laughed and hugged and made love again. I don't recall how long we stayed awake but it was late in the morning when we woke. Our clothes had dried and we were ready to move on. A thick blanket of snow covered the roads, but it was no longer snowing.

Switzerland's landscape of mountains topped with castles was like traveling inside a fairytale book. I thanked God for having given me eyesight and allowing me to see so much beauty. It also helped that Patrick was in a great mood. I believe that Switzerland's scenery had a calming effect on him.

According to the map, the town of Sarmen lay next to a lake by the same name in the mountains ahead of us. We knew it was south of Lucerne but we just couldn't figure out how to get there due to a lack of road signs. Patrick turned at the first left we found going up a steep road that was also very narrow, with no way to turn back. We drove through a small village covered in snow, but found no signs or people to give us directions. He continued to drive until we reached a road that took us out of town.

A blizzard now blew off the mountain. Suddenly, we saw a man walking on the road ahead of us.

Patrick slowed down and I opened the car window and called out in my best French, "Psst, pssst, could you please tell me the way to Sarnen?"

"Sorry, but I don't speak French."

Talk about miracles. After three days on the road and getting lost in the middle of nowhere, we found a British man who was visiting Lauren, his daughter in Sarnen. Lauren was married to a Francois Jaquois, Patrick's family name. We offered him a ride and he took us to his daughter's house. I was impressed with the wall-to-wall white carpets and that the front porch was about ten feet from a cliff. Lauren served us hot chocolate and gave us directions to the cemetery where

Patrick's ancestors were buried. When I told Mr. Warden about my cousins in England, he knew them. They were neighbors and acquaintances!

We spent about thirty minutes at the cemetery looking at gravestones. Patrick wrote the birth and death dates of his family ancestors in his journal. He planned to show that list to his mom when we returned to the US.

Patrick had no interest in meeting Francois Jaquois. I was looking forward to socializing with anyone, besides Patrick, and tried to convince him to stay and at least say hello, but Patrick wanted to get back to Nice.

On the way back, he was opened to see Geneva but we couldn't find a free parking spot. The traffic was no different from New York City except for the lack of skyscrapers. Outside Geneva we found a spot off the highway, to spend the night. I woke a few hours later and couldn't move my eyes, my breath poured from my nostrils like smoke and I used it to warm my fingertips before touching Patrick. "Patrick, I'm very, very cold." I couldn't stop shattering.

"I'm freezing too. I'll turn the engine on."

I believe that the newspaper was what saved us from turning into human ice cubes. That morning, the wind had blown it along the road like tumbleweed and all I could see was a blanket. I got out of the car and ran after it. Patrick had said it was a stupid idea, but that night he gladly wrapped a few pages around his legs. I stuffed the rest of the newspaper up my legs and around my torso, with plenty of space left to also insert a half a plastic garbage bag that I shared with him. The next morning, he saw the water in our bottles had frozen and said that using the newspaper and plastic bag, was the best idea I had come up with since we had begun our trip.

We drove most of the following day, except for stopping for gas, going to the bathroom and getting some groceries. As soon as it grew dark, Patrick parked under a grove of trees. I didn't know where we were, except for being in Italy and in the mountains. It wasn't as cold as Switzerland, but I still shivered all night, and my lower back kept cramping up into spasms.

He agreed that once we returned to the South of France there was no more sleeping in the car, but we would use the rental days we had left to take day trips along the Riviera coast.

We found an inexpensive hostel in Saint Maxine. It was Christmas Eve and he wanted to do something special. After searching several grocery stores, he splurged on an inexpensive bottle of champagne, two cookies, and a handful of almonds and dried fruit. We walked to the beach. He dug a hole in the sand and buried the champagne bottle so it would be cold when we returned later.

We borrowed two glasses at the hostel, and at 11:30 that night, we headed back to the beach and sat on the sand, talking while waiting for midnight.

"You're the best thing that has ever happened to me." He kissed me on cheek. "Neither one of my ex-wives would have stood for sleeping in a car like you did. You're a real trooper." He put his arm around my shoulders and held me close.

"Thank you." I kissed him back and stared at the calm ocean. Home was far beyond my reach.

"No, I mean it. I also want you to know that I'm aware of my behavior but can't help myself. It's the way I am."

"I understand." There was no sound of ocean waves beating against the shore, no wind, no moon, no one except us sitting in an empty world of sand and darkness. What was I doing on the other side of the world, seated on an empty beach, in the middle of the night with a mad man? There could only be one answer, I was having a nightmare.

"You're my angel and my salvation," He kissed me again and then got up and walked to the spot where he had buried the champagne bottle.

He carefully poured the bubbly into my glass but it spilled over. His laughter was contagious. We toasted to love and happiness and remained seated while we drank the cold champagne and ate the almonds and apricots.

"You're the only one who understands me." He kissed me in the lips and then reached into his pocket. "And now it's time to exchange the Christmas gifts we bought in Spain."

He handed me a little tree ornament wood circle with the date 1994. Mine had the words Feliz Navidad.

We kissed and then he put his arm over my shoulders.

"It's because of you that I'm less angry and learning to deal with problems as they come along. You've been a great influence in my life."

"Thank you. You have been a great influence in my life too." Being Portuguese I had been taught to always act polite, even if I didn't meant it.

He filled his glass again. "Go ahead and drink up. We can't waste French Champagne."

I don't like champagne but guzzled it anyway. I knew his euphoria would not last. The next day he would be annoyed at me for one thing or another. I smiled besides my sadness.

On the way back to the hostel, I tapped danced on the side-walk and we both sang Christmas songs obnoxiously loud. We were kind of drunk and definitely in high spirits.

As always, one of his love notes waited for me under my pillow. Earlier on I had drawn on a piece of paper a heart with our names on it and hid it inside his coat pocket.

He looked under his pillow. "It's Christmas and you didn't write me anything special." He pouted.

"Take a look in your jacket."

"I wondered all day if you would forget." He grabbed me and wouldn't stop kissing me.

~ *Chapter Twenty-Three* ~

Monaco

The next day we drove along the coast as far as Narbonne, passing through Cannes, St. Tropez, La Seyne, and Marseille. While Patrick was driving through the winding roads of Côte d'Azur, I thought about Princess Grace Kelly and the car accident that had taken her life. We sat in the car at all the lookouts along the road. We particularly enjoyed the one overlooking the Monte Carlo bay while having our lunch or dinner sandwiches. It was full of luxurious yachts and sailboats with the Alps rising in the far distance. I was very happy, but I knew that if I was happy one day, Patrick would do something the next day to make me cry. I accepted the happy days with gratitude.

We were delighted to find a parking spot not far from the Monte-Carlo Casino. Patrick was open to exploring Monaco. While walking up a garden path, we stumbled upon Monaco Cathedral where Princess Grace Kelly had been buried. There was no admission fee.

I had always admired Grace Kelly's angel like beauty and felt very privileged to be visiting her burial spot. Finding her grave like this seemed an omen that somehow I would survive my honeymoon. I stood as long as possible by her flat tombstone, only adorned by a bouquet of fresh flowers. I couldn't explain exactly what I was experiencing, but I felt calmer than I had since we left the states.

We sat on a wood bench in the old part of the city and had our sandwiches. "Can you believe that we are in the second smallest country in the world?" said Patrick.

"It could fool me. Which is the first?"

"The Vatican. That's where Satan lives."

"Really? The devil himself, that's impressive." I was having a hot flash.

"Don't make fun of me. Everybody knows that the Pope serves Satan, he hates Jesus Christ and… "

I stood and then sat on his right side, that way I wouldn't hear as much of his jabbering. I thanked God for being deaf on my left side.

As we walked back to where we had parked the car, the sun was strikingly hot. We passed a woman with two children eating ice cream cones. I would have given anything to have a French ice cream cone. I didn't dare suggest it.

When I proposed we check out the Casino Monte-Carlo, his answer was, "Good idea. I could use a bathroom."

I took a deep breath and smiled, as we entered the Casino's lobby leading to a white marble stairway. I pointed at the tall golden glass doors at the top of the steps. "What do you think? Maybe there's a bathroom in there that you can use."

Patrick didn't respond. He just followed me up the steps. When the concierge opened the door, we entered the casino's main lobby. My mouth fell open. I was in the set of *Casino Royale,* James Bond's famous movie. We were surrounded by glimmering gold ornaments and hanging crystal chandeliers. "Patrick, have you ever seen anything more magnificent in your whole life?" He did not answer. He turned his back on me and crossed his arms. He wore the "gray" look, I had come to dread when he was ready to have a fit of anger. I asked him what was wrong, but he continued to ignore me. Ahead of us men in tuxedos and women wearing beautiful long dresses, were entering a large gold-encrusted doorway. Upon seeing how refine the people were dressed I took a step back feeling like a beggar in my worn-out clothes. Still, I wanted to enjoy the moment. I took off my coat but immediately realized that

I looked better covered up. After wearing the same clothes for over a month, they had taken on an extraordinary hobo look.

I put the coat back on.

"C'mon Patrick, let's go see where those beautiful people are going."

He continued to stare at nothing in particular, with his arms across his chest.

"I'll be right back." I said, not willing to lose the opportunity of a lifetime. "I'm just going to take a peek."

On the wall by the gold encrusted doorway, a small gold plaque read, "Grand Theatre de Monte Carlo."

I stood at the doorway flabbergasted. Not in a million years could I've imagined the inside of a theatre to be so magnificent. It was even more spectacular and luxurious than the São Carlos Opera House in Lisbon, Portugal. The audience was dressed as if attending a king's wedding. Several crystal chandeliers shined from above amid the gold intricate designs that matched the walls and balconies. The seats were covered with red velvet, and there was a feeling of grandeur that had to be seen to be appreciated. The name said it all, the Grand Theatre de Monte Carlo! I ran back to get him. He had not moved an inch from the spot I had left him.

"Patrick, please come with me. I can't even describe what I just saw. You need to take a look for yourself." I clapped my hands briskly, several times like a child to show that what I had found was worth taking a look at.

"I have no interest. I'm going to find a bathroom and then we're leaving." He walked away.

"Okay," I said loud enough for him to hear me. "I'll wait for you here."

I didn't dare move from where I was standing, but like an owl, my head was turning in every direction watching the beautiful people go by chatting and laughing.

When he returned, he couldn't stop talking about the men's bathroom and the amazing toilet technology he had just experienced. "After I peed, the toilet cleaned itself. Go downstairs and check out the women's bathroom, I bet they have the same procedure with their toilets."

He was right. It was a masterpiece of plumbing. Its sensitive mechanism knew when I was done, and after flushing on its own, scrubbed the inside of the bowl and changed the toilet seat for the next customer. All it needed was for someone's hand to come up from inside the toilet and wipe one's butt. I sat down again and then watched the whole procedure once again.

We left the casino in a good mood, talking about the toilets and what we would be doing the next day. A block from the car he became quiet, and I noticed that his "gray" look was back.

"We need to talk," he said, stopping by the long stone wall overlooking the beautiful Monaco harbor.

Based on his look, this wasn't going to be pleasant. I felt hopeless wondering what I could have said or done.

"You've met my first wife, and you've seen how fat she is. Once I decided to go to college to become a doctor, she was no match for me. My second wife was a whore, so I had to get rid of her. I don't know what I'm going to do with you. You're definitely not the kind of wife I'm going to keep. You're no better than either one of them."

"I see. One was fat, the other a tramp. So, what am I to you?"

"You have been nothing but a big disappointment. You need to start acting more like a lady, a doctor's wife, and what you did to me at the casino was unforgivable."

I put both my hands on the wall overlooking the harbor. I wanted to slap him across the face, but I was afraid he would knock me out with a punch.

"What did I do?"

"When the porter at the casino opened the door for you, you walked ahead of me and left me behind. That's not what a lady would do."

"He opened the door and I entered." I laughed over the absurdity of his comment. "You were right next to me. We both entered together!" I yelled as loud as I could.

"Yes, we entered together, but a real lady would have taken her husband's arm."

"I am a lady, and you are not taking that away from me! I can't take it anymore. I want to go home and I want a divorce." I ran towards the car.

He ran after me crying. "I'm sorry, please forgive me. I love you. You know that I love you. I'll die if you leave me. I'll change I promise."

I told him that I forgave him. I didn't mean it.

We took the car back the next morning. It meant once again traveling by bus or train and watching Patrick throw fits when someone lit up a cigarette. The whole of Europe was like a smoke stack.

We'd be heading to Rome next, but first we had to stop in Florence. The German girl in Nice had told him that one couldn't go to Italy and miss Florence.

~ Chapter Twenty-Four ~

Italy

Our train arrived in Florence at six in the evening. I rarely have headaches, but that evening I had a sinus headache that even affected my vision. When I was married to Al, he would call me weird and make fun of me when I'd ask him not to bathe in cologne because it gave me a sinus headache. The smell of tobacco in the train was worse than Al's cologne. It not only gave me a headache but also made me nauseous and lightheaded.

We were getting out of the train when he said; "It's strange, but the tobacco smell makes me dizzy."

Once he told me that, I felt at ease sharing that I had the same problem. There was definitely some kind of chemical in the smoke from European cigarettes that was more powerful and nastier than American cigarettes. We had something in common, but I still couldn't go up to smokers and tell them they better get rid of their cigarette or I would kill them.

In Florence we began looking for accommodations. Nothing was cheap enough for our budget. To give myself time away from Patrick, I offered to check every hostel and hotel we came across, while he waited outside. It was ten in the evening when I finally found a hostel that met his financial requirements. The room was on the fifth floor. There was no elevator. Bath towels were available if we paid extra. The twin beds had springs, but no mattress to speak of. It was bitter cold because there was no heat and the wood floors had no carpet, not even a small rug. There were no curtains, on the tall windows, only broken shutters that barely closed. Besides the beds, a small table with two wooden chairs sat in the corner of the large room. A single low voltage light bulb hung from the center of the ceiling, creating monster shadows against the light gray dirty color of the walls.

The bathroom was at the end of the hallway, and we had to use our own toilet paper. After traveling through Spain we had learned how vitally important it was to always carry a few toilet rolls.

We moved the table and chairs in front of one of the windows so we had light to play Uno and Yahtzee. Both games had become a ritual every night. I didn't know which one I hated more, probably Yahtzee.

The first night in our new quarters I was introduced to the true meaning of fibromyalgia. Every hour I had to climb out of bed to relieve the hips and back pain. I would stand until I was shivering and then get back into bed and grab on to Patrick for body heat. I was amazed that the metal springs protruding through the thin pad didn't bother Patrick. At times like that I wished I had fatter hips. I imagine that the more tissue one had the less painful it was.

The next day, we headed to the Galleria dell'Accademia. Patrick was upset that our student IDs didn't cover the entrance fee. "I'm not paying to see a stupid statue."

"What are you going to tell your friends at home when they find out you were in Florence but didn't see one of Michelangelo's most famous works?"

That did the trick. He was quite thrilled when he saw the statue of David, and like everyone else, he walked around it several times. By then we had seen a lot of sculptures, but none touched me as much as that one. It looked like real skin covered the sculpture, and at any moment it would return to life.

He wanted to leave the next day for Rome. I talked him into staying in Florence. It made more sense not to go into a city like Rome just before the New Year. I was sure it was going to be impossible to find accommodations, and I wasn't looking forward to spending hours looking for a place to stay.

It poured every day. Patrick bought a cheap undersized umbrella, and even though we walked real close, I got soaked because he wanted the umbrella over his head. If it deviated even slightly towards my side he would get upset.

"I need my hands free if I'm going to fight a mugger. The least you can do is to make sure the umbrella covers my face."

While walking in the outskirts of Florence, we saw what looked like an old castle on a hill and hiked toward it. An hour later, we made it to the village surrounding the castle, and as we were walking up the steep cobblestone street, I asked two travelers if we were getting closer to the castle.

"Oh, yeah, you don't have far to walk. As you came up this street did you by any chance see Galileo's house?"

"Galileo? Where, please tell me where?"

"Right over there, on the left." The young man pointed to a stone wall.

I grabbed Patrick's hand. "Oh, my God, Patrick, I can't believe that we almost missed Galileo's house. I always admired him as a child. He was the inventor of the telescope!" I ran down the hill towards the wall.

We couldn't see Galileo's house because of the tall wall surrounding it, but just the idea that my feet stood on the same ground where he had walked and the idea that I was possibly breathing the same air he had breathed made me hum with joy. I was ecstatic and thanked God for giving me such opportunity. It was worth everything I had been through just to be there.

The castle ruins were no big deal, but the view of the villages below and the wide stretch of countryside were outstanding. I imagined those who had lived there fighting the invaders that most likely wanted to take over their castle.

On the way back to the hostel we crossed the Tiber River, and Patrick offered to climb under the bridge to collect some of its mud for our sand collection. I stood by the bridge with his backpack in between my feet. If someone was to try to steal it from me I was to yell as loud as possible and he would be back to fight the thief. He returned with a half cup of dirt wrapped in a plastic bag. "The river bank was gross beyond your imagination. Good thing I'm wearing boots. The ground was covered with syringes, condoms, and broken glass bottles, along with the vagrants' piss and shit. They live down there, if you can even believe it."

He put the contents into a second plastic bag and tied it tightly. "We need to be extra careful when we put this dirt into a container. Who knows what deadly virus or bacteria, is growing in it."

We explored every piazza and church in Florence, except Duomo-Santa Maria del Fiore, and the Baptistry, because there was a charge to get in, even with our student ID.

No matter how much we walked around Florence, we always wound up by the Ponte Vecchio, where several street vendors sold tourist trinkets.

On the way to Rome we stepped off the train at the town of Pisa. But the Leaning Tower of Pisa, where Galileo had conducted his famous experiments on the velocity of falling objects was surrounded by a fence and closed due to restoration and underpinning. We ran back to the station to catch the next train.

The train contained sections for smokers and non-smokers. We sat in the non-smoking section. When a woman lit up a cigarette, Patrick shouted, "You, better stop smoking or move to the smoking compartment."

She flipped him the Italian gesture for drop dead, and turned her back on him.

He stood and walked towards her. "You bitch. How dare you do that to me."

She didn't budge. He pointed a finger in her face and said, "I'm getting the conductor, and if he doesn't throw you off the train, I'll do it myself."

She gave him the finger and puffed away.

While he was gone, I said in a low voice "My husband and I are doctors, and we're sick of treating patients who are dying from lung cancer. It's not fair that you smoke in this compartment and put us all at risk." The other non-smokers nodded in agreement.

The train stopped at the next station, and the woman got off just as Patrick returned. "There's no conductor on the train, and we wasted our money buying train tickets. Where's the bitch?" I pointed her to him standing on the platform. She looked up to our window and gave us the middle finger. We returned the gesture.

In Rome we found a hotel that was even cheaper than the hostel in Florence. Sofia, the cranky hotel owner, handed us each two-bath towels and said, "No more than one shower per day, and don't use the heater in your room unless you want to pay extra." Even so, we felt like we had hit the jackpot. Our queen size bed had a thick straw mattress and on the wall above it hung a hefty black cross with a bleeding Jesus. Everything in the room, including the dark wooden dresser, was impressive in its bulkiness.

The four days we spent in Rome, we walked from morning until night. I loved walking and I enjoyed learning about the history behind every place we visited. It took me by surprise when a narrow cobblestone street suddenly opened up to a larger-than-life cathedral, like Saint Peter's. I was stunned by its architecture and Patrick commented on how much money had been wasted building it. We walked straight through Plaza Venezia, with the largest equestrian statue in the world.

There was no time to stop and admire anything in particular, as Patrick reminded me, we had a lot more places to visit.

When I was 11 years old and still living in Portugal I had seen the famous Trevi Fountain in the romantic American movie, *Three Coins in the Fountain,* with Portuguese subtitles. I stood staring at it until Patrick pulled me by the arm. "C'mon let's go, it's just a water fountain."

While walking an open field, on the way to the Basilica Santa Maria in Cosmedin, Patrick mentioned that field had been one of Rome's largest stadiums where chariots most likely used to race. "If we had more time, I would run it." He sighed looking at the empty field.

"Go ahead and run. I'll wait right here for you."

"There's too much to do yet. Time is of the essence, we need to keep traveling. We can't stop right now." We held hands as we crossed the street.

At Santa Maria in Cosmedin, there was a beautiful long porch with seven arches and seven windows but its main attraction was a grotesque, round, marble face, built into the wall, supposedly two thousand years old. Audrey Hepburn, my favorite movie star, when I was growing up, and Gregory Peck in the film *Roman Holiday*, had made it famous. The marble face was called La Bocca della Verita, meaning the mouth of truth. Tradition had it that, its jaw would snap shut on liars. I put my finger into its mouth and then asked Patrick to try it. He wouldn't do it.

We spent most of the next morning at the Colosseum admiring its magnificent structure of concrete and stone. It used to seat 50,000 spectators, who came to watch gladiators fight and lions eating Christians, hundreds of years ago, something like 70AD. The stone walls felt cold to my touch, and I knew that's the way they had felt to those who touched it before entering the arena with their families, to be mauled by wild animals. When no one was looking, Patrick took a small handful of stones for our stone and sand collection.

On the way back to our hostel we stopped at the Vatican wall.

"Patrick I would love to see what's behind this stone wall."

"I'm not supporting the Pope in any way, shape, or form. He is the anti-Christ and a devil worshipper. I'm taking some of the wall stones for our sand and stone collection. Keep an eye for anyone who might see us and call the police."

I did.

Before leaving Rome we bought postcards to send home. My cards all had the same picture. Michelangelo's famous painting of a girl's face under distress, looking as though she was running away from danger. Patrick read everything I wrote. I mailed the postcards to Papa, my sons, Ralph and Steve, and my best friends, Diane in California, Francis and Tracey in New Jersey, and Leila in Georgia. I hoped they would get the message from the picture, that I was in trouble, and one of them would come to my rescue. Just how, I didn't know.

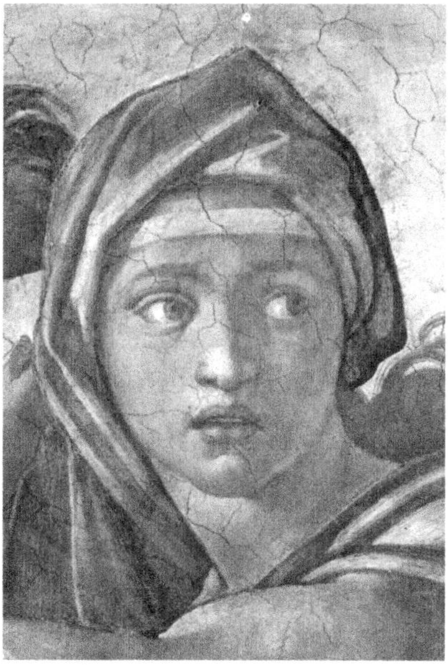

The Postcard

~ *Chapter Twenty-Five* ~

Greece

Greece was next on his agenda. We took the train south to Brindisi, in Southern Italy. On the train we met a young couple, Mark and Joyce. Patrick thought they looked like Barbie and Ken dolls. He hated Ken, but liked Barbie. Mark suggested we stay together since we all spoke English. We arrived to Brindisi at midnight. Mark and Joyce knew of a hostel, and at that hour we decided it was best to follow them. The next morning the four of us walked to the dock to buy boat tickets to Athens.

The more expensive tickets offered private rooms. The cheap tickets put us outside. Mark and Joyce were seasoned travelers and felt that for one night sleeping on the deck wasn't that bad. We did fine sitting on the deck's wooden benches having our sandwiches and talking until night came upon us. We asked for a blanket, but the crewmen told us that our tickets didn't include them. We each took a bench and lay down, but didn't matter how much I curled up. The cold wind off the Ionian Sea blew right through my bones.

Within an hour I had to pee and was forced to go inside to look for a toilet. All the doors in the ship's narrow hallway were closed and there was no one to give me directions. I took a chance and opened one door with a Greek signage, it was the bathroom. On the way back to the deck I saw a small narrow door flapping back and forth. Someone had forgotten to close the linen closet. I grabbed four heavy brown wool blankets and gave one to each of the others. They were impressed. Patrick said, "This is why I married you. You are the greatest." He hugged me and kissed me, before going back to his bench.

I felt warm as a puppy and was smiling when I fell asleep.

The new morning I woke to the voice of two crewmen yelling at us for using the blankets.

Joyce flashed them an angelic look. "The blankets were on top of one of the benches and we thought they were for us to use."

"Yeah," we all said, almost in unison. "It made sense to us."

They took the blankets and told us that we were in trouble. We didn't know how they were going to punish us, but as soon as the ship docked we ran off as fast as we could.

After we got a safe distance from the dock, the kids informed us that we were still a few miles from the city of Athens and needed to take a local bus. That's when we came to fully appreciate the full meaning of *it's all Greek to me.* After many failed attempts, we finally found someone who spoke enough English to give us directions to a bus stop.

While seated on the bus Patrick whispered, "Mark pisses me off. How dare he tell me what to do next? We don't need them. They're a couple of spoiled brats using up their parents' money to travel."

I didn't answer. We finished eating our lunch of bread and cheese just as we arrived at the bus center station in Athens.

When we got off the bus, Patrick turned briskly to them, and said, "We want to be on our own from now on." He walked away.

I said, "Goodbye, guys," and ran after him.

Considering that we couldn't read or understand Greek, it wasn't easy finding our way around. There was nothing in the price range we were looking for. Patrick hated Athens as much as Lisbon. I would have to agree that the pollution was pretty high, even I was coughing. Still, we spent the whole afternoon going from one place to another. In some, the bed sheets looked dirty, in others, the rooms smelled, and in one, the elevator had no bottom just two planks of wood. There was one with a private bathroom, but the toilet didn't flush and the water coming out of the faucet was brownish red. When we finally found a hostel for the right price, we were too tired and hungry to check out the room and just took it. We had made the right choice, the bed had a mattress, the sheets were clean, there was a bidet in the room, and that meant to Patrick we didn't have to use the bathroom down the hallway. Our hostel had another added benefit; there was a quick-service food restaurant right next door. It was 7:30pm, past our dinnertime and Patrick had just discovered there was more to life than bread and cheese. There were gyros! For seventy five cents one could get thinly sliced fatty pieces of what looked like compressed meat served inside greasy flat bread covered with sliced onions, lettuce, tomatoes, and a white creamy sour sauce. That night I barely slept, moaning with stomach cramps. Grease didn't agree with me.

The next morning we were walking up a steep street. I followed him slightly behind, doing my best to keep up with him, as my backpack, had become like a heavy appendage. He turned and said, "I'm going to cross the street and see if I can make heads or tails of the sign on the street corner."

I stopped walking to catch my breath. He ran across the street, but had to wait to cross back because of ongoing traffic. I began walking slowly up the hill. After a bit, I turned to see what was taking him so long. He had crossed the street but stood motionless on the sidewalk. I waved at him, but he didn't respond. "Are you okay?" I called out.

He put his backpack on the ground, crossed his arms and then turned his back on me. Obviously he wanted me to walk down to where he stood.

When I reached him, he threw the map at me. "Since you want to walk ahead of me, you go ahead and lead the way from now on."

It didn't matter how many times I apologized for not waiting for him. He wouldn't let go of it, and over the next few days he kept bringing it up. By then, I had begun humming inside my head when he went on and on about whatever.

Patrick ate gyros for breakfast, lunch and dinner, and because I refused to eat them, he grew upset.

I told him, "I'm sorry, but even as a child I could never eat fried food. I simply can't digest grease. It makes me sick of my stomach. I'll have a green salad instead."

"A salad costs dollar-and-a half American money. For that much I can buy two gyros. You're wasting our money!" He walked away.

I ran after him. "Patrick, I'll skip breakfast and have a salad for lunch and dinner, please don't get angry."

"Fine then, but when you buy a salad, it's only right that I get to eat two gyros."

I agreed. It was my fault that I couldn't digest grease, and needed more expensive type of food. It was one of those days where I felt I had no right to complain. He was more than kind to put up with my flaws. I had wished for a man that was the opposite of Al, a man that could make decisions, and be in charge, but now I realized there was a price to pay. Patrick was in charge of everything including my life. I had no say. This was his trip, and it no longer mattered to me where we went. For the most part, I just followed along quietly.

The next day, we stood at the top of a steep hill. Patrick ran-straight down the slope. I followed the sidewalk that curved down gently. I didn't see the need to take the steeper, slipperier route and risk being hurt. As soon as I reached the bottom, Patrick started with the insults, telling me I was nothing but a scared little mouse. I ignored him. *Hum, hum, hum.* I felt proud of myself for being strong.

That morning, on the way up to see the Acropolis, we bumped into Mark and Joyce. They told us not to miss the Greek island of Santorini, which, they thought was the best part of Greece. Patrick cut it short. As always he was not interested in connecting with anyone. In his world, it was just him and lucky me.

Patrick ran in the Panathenaic Stadium, not that it was open to mere mortals like us. We found it closed for maintenance and a tall wire fence with several signs in Greek, French, German and English, "Warning under penalty of the law. Stay off property. Under repairs." When Patrick said we were jumping over the fence, I knew better than to say I couldn't do it.

I ran less than a quarter of the track and then sat among some fifty thousand empty seats of white marble. He ran twice around the field.

He had run in a stadium he found in the outskirts of Lisbon as well as two other stadiums in Spain, but, like he said, none could compare to running on the first stadium to host the first modern Olympic Games in 1896 and built over a 330BC Greek arena. He was absolutely stoked.

On January 9, we boarded a ferry for the Island of Santorini. Before boarding the ferry I ate a gyro for lunch just to avoid his nagging. I paid dearly. The diarrhea and stomach pain were so severe that I remained seated close to the bathroom on the lower deck. I was very surprised when Patrick returned to tell me he had met a nice Greek couple in the upper deck. They were medical doctors on the Island of Santorini and wanted to meet me.

I dropped my backpack on the floor next to where he sat and said while running off. "I have to throw up." I made it to the bathroom just in time.

When I got back to my seat he said, "Are you feeling better now? Do you think you can make it to the upper deck to meet the Greek couple?"

Dio and Lydia Papadopoulos spoke a bit of English. "It would give us great pleasure if you became our guests," Dio said. "We have an extra home in Fira, Santorini where we live and practice. You're welcome to stay there for as long as you like."

"That is most kind of you," I said. "Thank you."

"Hopefully you'll fall in love with our island and when you graduate from school you return to Santorini to practice," Lydia said, and she handed me her business card. "Our island needs more doctors."

Before we left the ship, Patrick told me that no way were we going to stay in their home. He had changed his mind about them. It was our trip and he was not out to make friends with them or anybody else.

"Why?" I asked him. "You said they were nice."

"They will expect us to pay them and who knows what more they might want from us."

"If they wanted to charge us they would have said it. When they offered their place, I believe they were doing it out of kindness."

"You can believe what you want, but they are not my friends. They'll probably want us to adjust their spine."

"So what, I feel very confident about adjusting. Goodness, we both adjusted hundreds of patients in Mexico. What's the difference?"

"I don't trust those Greeks. Who knows if they're even doctors, and if they are, that's one more reason not to trust them."

I began my internal humming. Hum, hum, hum. And then I prayed, *Please dear God don't let me go crazy like him.* I went back to humming. *Hum, hum, hum.*

We docked in Santorini, in the middle of the night. It was raining heavily with a gusty cold wind. Dio and Lydia asked us if we would like to go with them in their car. They would be happy to take us to one of their homes for the night, but Patrick told them we already had a place to stay. They left.

We would have to take a bus to Fira, the closest village and the capital of Santorini. It was our only option. Once that bus left, we would be stranded in complete isolation without any refuge from the weather.

We diligently followed the other passengers to the bus. It left quickly and followed a long steep road into Fari. Once we arrived, we had no choice but to follow an old guy with a British accent who was renting rooms for the night. Santorini was far from an ideal place to look for a hostel, especially in the middle of the night. Whatever the guy's price was going to be, it was going to be. He led us down one dark street after another, until we came upon what seemed to be a small white hut. It was an exceptional dark night, and the strong wind made the rain intolerably cold. Luckily, the price turned out to be quite reasonable.

Patrick wore his leather jacket to bed and even though he wore two long-sleeved T-shirts underneath his two sweatshirts, he was still cold. I had to take my dripping jacket and shirts off. I had nothing dry to wear. I wrapped one towel around my chest and another around my bottom. Even though we slept glued to each other, there was little heat between us. If anything his leather jacket felt cold against my back. The sheets were cold and damp, and the two thin blankets were a joke for keeping anyone warm. That night, I held my jaw with both hands. I was afraid my front teeth were going to break from chattering so hard. The bathroom was outside our hut in another building. Out of necessity I quickly learned to urinate in an empty water bottle. Of course, Patrick had no problem peeing into the bottle.

I didn't sleep much. I was angry about my situation and felt that I had enough. I wasn't going to take it anymore. I spent the morning trying to convince him that we needed better accommodations, and we should at least visit Dio and Lydia and see what they had in mind. He finally relented.

Everyone knew them by name. They were the island doctors. They lived on the other side of the island. The British guy that rented us the room offered to take us there and he spoke very highly of the Papadopoulos. We had to walk through very narrow streets. An old rusted pick-up was turned over and we had to climb over to get to the other side of the street. Patrick complained about getting his pants dirty, and how much he hated the Greeks and Greece. I hummed, *This land is your land.*

Dio and Lydia's home was so warm I had to take my coat off while sipping hot tea and munching on butter cookies. Their house was just like the other small white houses with flat roofs we had seen as we crossed the island. Except for the occasional blue dome here and there, white was the predominant color, giving the whole island a bridal look of innocence.

Their house was overcrowded with antique French furnishings, Persian rugs and lots of porcelain figurines. I assumed they had lived in that house all their lives. They wanted to be our friends. That's all they wanted. It was winter, and the island was basically sleeping because of the profound lack of tourists. They enjoyed company. Patrick accepted their offer, and Lydia took us to see our home. Before opening the gate to our front porch, a beat up looking dog with a crusty eye approached us in a friendly manner.

"Shoo," Lydia said, pushing him off with the heel of her shoe.

Patrick bent over to pat him.

"That dog looks sick. You shouldn't touch him. I'll have to call the dog pound society to pick him up."

"This dog is not sick. You would look terrible too if I smashed your face in."

I bent my head down and then looked away. I hoped that Lydia had grown quiet because she wasn't quite sure if what Patrick said was what she had heard. Still, she was no dummy, and I saw her go from a happy pleasant hostess to not-so-sure-I-want-these-people-here. But she did give us the key to the house and showed us inside. There was a kitchen, bedroom, living room, and a bathroom. It wasn't only furnished, but it also had a portable electric heater that could be moved from one room to another.

Not once did she or her husband come by to visit us in the following days we lived there.

One morning while exploring the island, we found a long, steep zigzag stairway carved into a thousand foot rocky cliff to a caldera that opened to the ocean and we could see two large ships in the distance below. When we reached the bottom, Patrick wanted to walk over some slimy green rocks to see what was on the other side of the rocks around the caldera.

"I can't walk on top of those rocks." I said. "I'm afraid to fall."

"What are you afraid of? You're pathetic! Let's go, and don't make me wait!"

"I'm sorry, but when I was ten years old, I fell on a slippery rock like these covered with algae and broke my tail bone. Now I'm afraid to walk on them. Please, don't make me do it. I'm scared." Tears filled my eyes.

"I'm sorry to hear that," he said. "I understand what it's like to have fears. I don't like bees." He crossed back and carried me to the other side. I didn't tell him that I was also afraid of bees, heights, snakes, and him.

The other side of the caldera was no different from the side we had come from, just loose rocks by the water and the steep cliff to our right, made it a narrow path to nowhere. We didn't stay long and I was happy when he carried me back, over the algae rocks.

As we hiked up the steps, he began picking on me again, saying that I walked too slowly and was dragging him down. Instead of lashing back at him, I considered running up the stairs as fast as I could to see if I could kill myself. It hadn't worked when I climbed the tower in Spain, but with five hundred more steps perhaps I would drop dead. Or better still, he would drop dead from trying to keep up with me, given his asthma.

I began running. So did him of course. Who cared that I couldn't breathe and my heart was pounding hard. Nothing was going to stop me.

"Stop, you're going too fast. Let me catch a breath." He called to me several times.

I looked back, but didn't stop. Fall you miserable bastard.

A day rarely passed that I didn't feel emotionally abused. He would say he was sorry, surprise me with love notes, cuddling, and at night we always had sex. I would forgive him and then feel terrible for my sinful killer thoughts through the day.

Patrick did have a good heart. He just didn't know how to balance his anger with his kindness. He decided to save all the dogs on the island. He carried stones in both pockets and threw them at dogs running after cars. I had mixed feelings about seeing them cry out in pain, but it was better than getting hit by a car.

The gyros in Santorini were even cheaper than in Athens. Patrick ate several for lunch and for dinner. I could eat them if I skipped the meat and the white sauce. I had just discovered Gyro vegetarian style, pita bread stuffed with lettuce, onions, and a slice of tomato, but after five days of this, my whole system cried out for something else. One afternoon, we walked by a small restaurant with a sign on the window, "Today only. Vegetable soup special $2.00."

"I'm going to have some hot soup. Are you coming?" I swiftly made my way in. He sat across from me, but wouldn't order any food. He stared into the air and said nothing. At first, I ate like a glutton but quickly realized that if I kept that up, the gastronomical experience would soon be over. I stopped and tasted each spoonful, like a miser counting pennies. I lingered over the aroma, savored each bit of potatoes, carrots, zucchini, cabbage, tomatoes and asparagus. I called the waitress. "This is delicious, what do you call this soup?"

"Hortosoupa."

"I can't believe it! Soupa also means soup in Portuguese, but what about Horto?"

"Horto is a very beautiful Greek fishing village."

Afterwards we walked to the gyro stand and he bought two gyros and an order of large fries. We sat at a table inside. Now that he had food, I assumed he was himself again.

"Patrick," I said, "You know I can cook, right? Imagine how much money we could save if we used our kitchen to make meals?"

We began shopping at the local market. The butcher, who spoke fairly good English, told us that if we came to live in Santorini and work as chiropractors, and treated him and his family, the meat would be free. I kept his card.

According to Paul, the owner of the gyro stand, Santorini was a jungle of tourists in the summer. We were lucky that it was winter. The island was practically ours. He encouraged us to rent a motorcycle from him and *really* see the island.

The next morning Patrick would drive and I'd sit blissfully with my arms around him. It took me back being a kid in Portugal. I would hold onto my father while he drove his motorcycle. My feelings towards Patrick had become as unstable as him. When he was mean, I hated him. When he was kind, loving and fun, I loved him.

Having a motorcycle to explore the island, took us to parts we would have otherwise missed. We followed the coast and stopped to explore beaches of different colored sand. I especially loved Kamari, the black sandy beach, where even the water looked black, and the Red Beach, smartly named after its red sand. At every chance, Patrick would take off and race up and down the sandy hills and smaller cliffs along the shore. Sometimes he would disappear and then yell down from one of the sandy hills, "Hey look up here! I'm on top of the world!"

It was midafternoon when we reached Akrotiri, an excavation site discovered in 1967 by archeologists. The town had been buried in 1450 BC when a volcano had erupted and destroyed most of the island, leaving it less than half of the size it used to be. We were lucky the site was opened to the public.

A metal dome covered the site. White ash covered what was left of the buildings and streets of what was once a beautiful and prolific town. It even covered some tall clay jars and a few frescos.

When we left the site, Patrick asked me to follow him across the street. He pulled two metal spoons out of his backpack. "Start digging," he said and pointed to the sandy hill in front of us. "This whole area was probably part of the town. We might find our own archeological site."

We dug for ten minutes before we gave up.

After returning the motorcycle we went home for dinner, my own concoction of Hortosoupa, and meatloaf with mashed potatoes. After dinner, we left the dishes soaking in the sink and rushed out to watch the sunset like we did every evening, by standing on one of the several overlooking walls along the cliffs. To miss such magnificent display of colors against the ocean could only be excused if we were blind. Most of the time we were by ourselves but once in a while one or two young couples would join us to watch the spectacle. We all stood in silence until the last ray in the sky disappeared.

The next morning, after breakfast, Patrick announced, "We have been in Santorini for eight days and I'm ready to move on."

"Me too, let's go home. I'm so tired of traveling. I miss school. Don't you miss school?"

He opened a map. "I'll let you know when we're done with traveling. I'm not sure if we should go to Turkey or the northern Europeans countries. What do you say?"

I could only visualize my future when we returned to the US and asked him for a divorce. I would have no money and no car. I would be on the breadline. I wasn't looking forward to that part of my future. Suddenly the idea of going to Turkey was like someone throwing me a lifesaver. Turkey was going to be my salvation, I was sure that the Turks wouldn't take any abuse from him, and they would kill him. That thought gave me the hope I needed to speak up.

"Turkey is closer to us. We can always go to the northern countries afterwards."

"We'll leave tomorrow morning." We kissed.

The next morning an ocean storm prevented ships from coming to the island. All the stores were closed, including the gyro shop. Though the wind was mild and the rain was insignificant, the ocean was off limits to traffic. There was a feeling of doom all around us. We both agreed that being on an island sucked. We were stuck.

It took some work but I finally convinced Patrick that we should invite our Greek hosts for a homemade dinner. Since we had arrived to the island we had stopped by their office twice to say hello and neither one of them had been available. I gave a note to their receptionist asking them if they would consider being our guests. I would like to make them a Portuguese dinner in their honor. They accepted.

I made Portuguese vegetable soup and *empadão*, a type of Shepherd's pie—and fruit salad for dessert. With what we were saving in accommodations, it was the least we could do for them.

The conversation was pleasant and they must have liked dinner because Lydia asked for the recipes for the soup and *empadão*. It felt good having company and socializing a little. "I'd like to invite you both to come with us tomorrow night and enjoy our local choir singing at a vineyard close by." Lydia said.

"That sounds wonderful, doesn't it Patrick?" I looked at Patrick.

He had the "gray" look.

During the fruit salad, Dio talked about the vineyards and how good the Santorini wine was. Suddenly, Patrick stood and said, "I've had enough. You both better leave, now."

Dio asked, "Did we say something wrong?" I looked at Patrick but he said nothing.

They stood. I hugged them and smiled. "Isn't my husband funny? When he gets tired, that's it. I'm in trouble too." And I put on a joker's face of total delight while putting my arm around Patrick's back.

Dio said, "Americans' humor is very different from ours. Hard for us to understand it. But that's okay, honey. We'll be here tomorrow at seven to pick you both up." They left smiling and waving back.

"Patrick, it's only nine-thirty. It's not like we have any place else to go. Why did you throw them out?"

"They were getting on my nerves with their know-it-all attitude about the vineyards. Who cares?"

"I'm going to do the dishes and clean the kitchen." I wouldn't try to understand him. The day I did would mean I was just as crazy.

He went to take a shower. I remained busy cleaning the kitchen. I knew when he was back in the room, because I could hear him recording the daily events into his tape recorder. I told him it was my turn to take a hot shower. I purposely took my time showering and then scrubbed the tiled bathroom walls and floors. I slipped into bed quietly so I wouldn't wake him up.

The next day we hiked all day under a pleasant slight drizzle, then returned to the house. We had just finished eating the leftovers from the night before when our hosts came by with their car. Patrick sat in the back seat, with his arms crossed over his chest, ignoring us. When Dio asked Patrick if he liked the island, Patrick turned his face away and stared out of his window.

As we walked into the winery Patrick said, "I'm not interested in listening to a bunch of Greeks singing." He sat by a small table in the reception area and stared into space with his arms once again across his chest. I followed Dio and Lydia to the wine bar talking to them as if the situation was perfectly normal. I figured that if I kept them away from Patrick everything would go smoothly. Dio asked me, "Would you like red or white wine?"

I hesitated because I didn't drink wine, but I also didn't want to offend him.

"White, please." Besides color I knew nothing about wine.

"Your husband doesn't want to come in, so would you like to join us inside?" Lydia asked.

They had to be kidding. I would never have heard the end of that.

"Thank you for the invitation, but I'm afraid that I must stay with him. He isn't feeling well. I'll wait in the lobby, if you don't mind. Okay?"

"We understand. Your husband has some psychological problems, yes? " said Dio while his wife nodded in agreement.

"I'm sorry. I don't know what to say."

I wanted to talk to them about what was going on, and even get their help, but they were strangers and too nice for me to get them involved in my predicament.

I brought my glass of wine to the small table where Patrick was seated.

"Look what I have. Would you like some white wine?" I smiled.

"You bought the wine?"

"No, Dio bought it for me."

"If that's true, then why didn't he buy me a glass of wine too?"

"I guess because you were not with us."

The argument escalated and soon came down to why I had asked for white wine and not red, when I knew he drank only red wine.

It was my turn to be gray. I sat across from him and blocked him out of my sight by letting the tears fill my eyes. My childhood technique for temporary blindness had come in handy once again. The glass of wine remained untouched on the table. When I heard the applause from inside the theatre I knew the show was over. I quickly picked up the glass of wine and took it to the bartender to dispose of it. He nodded his head towards Patrick still sitting. "What's the matter with your man?"

"He's not feeling well."

"He's got some serious problem." He rolled his eyes.

We were seated in the back seat of the car heading home when Dio said, "I wish you both had come in to hear the choir singing. The children were delightful."

"Yes, they were like angels singing," his wife said.

Patrick kicked the back of Lydia's seat and yelled, "I don't give a shit about your Greek choir, do you hear?"

"Young man, you better watch your language in front of my wife."

"You don't tell me to shut up. I'll say anything I want to. You and your wife can go to hell. You're a bunch of freaks that think you know everything, but you're nothing but a bunch of losers." And he kicked the seat again.

Lydia said something in Greek to her husband and the way she put her hand on his shoulder I knew that she was most likely telling him not to respond. We rode the rest of the way in deadly silence. When they dropped us off at the house, Patrick left without saying a word and went inside the house.

Before climbing out of the car, I mumbled, "Please forgive my husband. He's sick."

Dio said, "We know." Lydia added, "Please take care of yourself. In our opinion your husband is dangerous. Be careful, my friend."

Before we left the island I felt obliged to go by the medical clinic and thank our hosts. Patrick agreed, but he wouldn't go in. They were both busy with patients. I took one of their calling cards. I planned to send them a thank-you card when we returned to the US. We had spent ten days in Santorini.

On the ship to Rhodes, Patrick began acting odd by putting his face down and trying to cover it with his hands.

"Don't look now, but see those three guys seated at eleven o'clock from us?"

"Yeah. What about them?"

"I don't like the way they're staring at me."

"Are you sure they're looking at you?"

"Yes, they're staring at me."

"Don't pay attention to them then."

"They're still looking in my direction."

"Patrick, they're not looking in this direction, trust me. They're busy talking to each other."

"Don't lie to me. I have excellent peripheral vision, and I can see exactly what they're doing. I'll show them." He stood, turned his back to them, and pretended to stick his finger up his butt and scratching it, while laughing hysterically.

The three men now stared at us, along with the other passengers. They shook their heads at us in disbelief. *This is what he's going to do in Turkey. But he won't be able to get away with it there. The Turks won't stand for it.*

The sunshine was the first thing to strike me as we landed on the island of Rhodes. I put my winter jacket in my backpack. Lots of walking through ancient ruins and the delicious smell of pine trees at Rodini Park made our day as we finally found a place to stay for two nights. The hostel was like a farm and situated on top of a hill with lots of cypress and pine trees. Patrick was at his best when surrounded by nature. The next day we spent the day exploring the old town of Rhodes with its sandy colored walls through labyrinthine streets. When we visited one of the museums I played a prank on Patrick for which I was very proud.

We stood by an exquisitely carved Greek sarcophagus, admiring its historical value. I nonchalantly moved my leg to the side of it and then, looking away, kicked the stone twice.

"Did you hear that knocking?" asked Patrick.

"What knocking?"

"There was a knocking coming from inside this old coffin."

"No, I didn't hear anything. Whoever is inside has been dead for hundreds of years." Quickly I hit my foot once again and then turned around as if paying attention to a Persian carpet hanging on the wall across the room.

"Veronica, there's someone alive inside the sarcophagus. We need to get one of the guards to open it."

I couldn't hold it anymore and broke down laughing. I showed him how I had used my foot to tap on the side of the sarcophagus.

The rest of the day he kept saying, "You really got me back there. I'm impressed. You sure are amazing."

He definitely had a great sense of humor, but I never knew what would amuse him.

Traveling through the Mediterranean countries, where the average height of the population was a lot shorter than Patrick, gave him a sense of supremacy. He held a grudge towards his sister, Nancy, for being taller than him, as if it was her fault. Several times he said, "I wish Nancy was traveling with us so she could feel what it's like to be a minority."

We were the only two guests at the hostel. The owner was a young man in his mid-thirties whose wife had left him because he drank too much. Patrick took a liking to him and gave him some pep talks on how to get his wife back. At the end of each day Patrick was anxious to get back to the hostel so that he could continue to give further advice to the owner. When we left he commented, "I did good. The poor man needed a friend. I hope he'll get his wife back so he can experience the same happiness I have being married to you." We kissed. Rhodes was good to his spirit, he was happy and so was I.

~ *Chapter Twenty-Six* ~

Turkey

Patrick insisted that we take the Hydrofoil boat to Turkey because it apparently used wing-like structures to lift the boat off the water during forward motion. We spent almost two hours at the Rhodes harbor waiting for the boat to arrive. Patrick wanted to be the first one to board so he could pick a seat upfront. Supposedly, where we stood waiting was the exact place a statue of the Greek god Helios had stood astride the harbor's mouth. It was called the Colossus of Rhodes, and it was considered one of the Seven Wonders of the World because it was the tallest statue in the world until an earthquake knocked it down hundreds of years ago.

The harbor and its history were more impressive than the boat ride. It didn't feel any different than a speedboat. Patrick agreed.

The Turkish port police charged us twenty five dollars each to enter their country. Patrick called them crooks and bastards out loud. I was shocked that they didn't jump on top of him and beat him to death. Perhaps they didn't know the English language that well.

After exchanging two hundred dollars into Turkish money, he picked Pamukkale as our destination. Before entering the bus, he purposely pushed a taxi driver out of his way by turning abruptly and hitting him with his backpack. Patrick had stopped shaving since we had left Santorini. Between his rough appearance and the way he looked at anyone that dared to glance in his direction, no one was going to mess with him. If anything, they were going to avoid him and rapidly walk away.

My plan to get rid of him in Turkey would fail, and I had to accept that nothing was going to happen to him in Turkey or in any other country. I was stuck for good. I was his free ticket to the world of traveling. In exchange for that, I looked forward to being part of his life, because when he was normal I couldn't resist him. He barely took any photos. He still had the original roll of film in his camera, but he continued to tape our daily events, even mundane information such as, "Today it was cold but it didn't rain until the evening." He would go into detail about anything he thought was funny, and a day didn't go by that he didn't mention the beauty of each country we visited. His intention was to share the tape recordings with his family. I thought the idea of keeping a daily log of the trip was great. He was a mad man, but also a genius.

The emotional abuse I sustained on a daily basis was balanced by his loving attention, and those moments where he would hug me and tell me how lucky he was to have me in his life always made up for everything else. Still, as the days and weeks went by, I learned to talk to him as little as possible. I didn't want to trigger his gray side. I'd become skilled at keeping my eyes on the outside world from my window seat in the buses, trains, and ships. Nature's beauty fed my spirit and kept me strong from within. He never let me out of his sight, except for when I went to the bathroom where I would cry and take my time before coming out. Mama had taught me well, "If you keep washing your eyes with cold water as you cry, there will be no vestiges of tears."

We rode by bus to Denizli, Pamukkale where he wanted to see the famous hot mineral ponds up in the mountains. We were back to winter. Snow and ice covered the roads ahead of us, in the distance the mountains covered with snow were no different from the snowy mountains in the US. We arrived four hours later. The sun was setting when we found a hotel. Our room had nice furniture and a large bed, it looked pretty new, but it was so cold we could see steam coming out of our mouths. He complained to the hotel manager, who told us that he would take care of the problem. We decided to go and explore the town before it was too dark. With luck, the room would be warm by the time we got back.

While walking I was very cold. My goose down jacket had seriously thinned out and didn't provide much help against the icy mountain winds. As always, we carried our backpacks, since we had everything we owned inside of them. Besides the bags of sand, Patrick had put brochures, tour books and maps from the countries we had been inside my backpack. My back felt weak, but I knew complaining wouldn't do any good.

The ground was covered with thick snow that crackled with each step and I felt it appropriate to hum Korobushka, an old Russian song I used to play with my Russian guitar teacher, Mr. Zorkovich.

Everything was closed except for a small grocery store, the type one sees in small European villages. The old Turkish lady behind the counter took a fancy to me.

She couldn't speak English, but we understood each other. She offered me a cup of hot tea and gave me a gesture to sit down on a large wooden barrel. Patrick reprimanded me for buying tea.

"I didn't ask for the tea. She gave it to me." I said, shivering.

The old lady came back from the back room, with a small portable heater, and with hand signals she told me to remain seated. Patrick was upset because the woman hadn't offered him the same attention. She didn't like him and, just like he was rude to others, she was just as rude to him by ignoring him.

When he put his hand on my shoulder and said, “Let’s go.” She put her hand on my other shoulder and made the signal for me to stay seated.

“I’m leaving,” he said.

I turned to her and said, “I’m scared, cold and hungry. Thank you for the tea and the heat. You’re an angel.” I put my finger to my mouth so she would not acknowledge out loud the five-dollar bill I gave her, and I said thank you in Portuguese and in English and then waved back at her.

There was no heat in the hotel room and no water from the bathroom faucet. We couldn’t even brush our teeth. We slept with our shoes, coat, gloves, and wool hats on, under a single thin blanket.

In the morning Patrick was rightly furious. “I’m not paying for the room. The manager lied to us. Let’s get out of here.”

The manager saw us walking out and came running after us. “Hey, you can’t leave. You have not paid me for the room.”

“There was no heat and no water. I’m not giving you a cent.” Patrick kept on walking as I followed him.

“I can’t afford to turn on the heat and water because in the winter there are no tourists and I can’t afford to pay for utilities. Please, sir I have a family to feed. You must pay me for the use of the room.”

I looked at Patrick. “Just give him half the money we owe him. We did have a bed to sleep on and a roof over our heads.”

“Yes, I’ll take half the money you owe me. Please.” He put his hand out.

“No. You and your family can starve to death.” Patrick walked away as I chased after him.

“May death follow you, you cheap bastard! May you go to hell! You’re a ruthless, wicked man.” He kept cursing as we walked away.

Chills ran through my spine, and they weren’t from feeling cold.

When we arrived at the region near the mineral waters, Patrick looked up at the mountain, and said, "This is an easy climb. Let's go." I looked and all I saw was a steep icy cliff going up a huge mountain covered with snow. The mountain was bigger than the one I had climbed in California with him and his family.

"Patrick, let's not climb the mountain. How much are they charging to get in, anyway?"

"It doesn't matter. I'm not going to pay a dime to get in. C'mon let's start climbing."

"It's covered with snow and ice. I don't have hiking boots like you."

"There's nothing wrong with the shoes you're wearing. If you don't want to go with me, you'll have to wait here, until I return. It's your choice." He walked away.

The cold wind was whipping me hard, and I felt that I was better off moving than staying still in the middle of nowhere. The snowy mountain glittered in the sun. I caught up with Patrick and followed him up the precipice ridge. I focused only on where to put my feet. With my backpack pulling me backwards and the water jug on my left hand, I had to climb on my knees to pull myself up with my right hand. He never looked back to see if I was behind him.

Half way up the cliff, my right foot slipped off the rock, and no matter how hard I tried to pull myself up and put the foot down, it kept slipping.

"Patrick, I need your hand. Please help me," I screamed. "I'm going to fall."

He yelled back, "I'm not going to help you. Forget it. Just watch where you step." He kept climbing.

I cried out, "Patrick, I need your help quickly, please, just give me your hand; I have no place to put my feet securely."

I pressed my body flat against the cliff. I let go of the water jug to grip an overhang with my left hand. I stretched my right hand towards him. I closed my eyes and prayed that I would faint before falling into the rocks below. The whole thing was happening as if in slow motion I had just given up when he grabbed my wrist and pulled me up.

The rest of the climb he wouldn't let go of the fact that he was tired of my dependency on him. I asked God to punish him for having endangered my life, over a few bucks, to enter the thermal ponds.

Patrick was an adventurer, and he loved danger. He liked to live life as if it were his last day. That was fine with me as long as he didn't push me to do the same. He was domineering, abusive, selfish, and out of his mind. I was sure the only reason he pulled me up was because he realized if I tumbled down the mountain he would lose the money I had in my money belt.

Twenty minutes later we reached the top. As we walked across a flat white field I expected the crunch of snow but was surprised to meet the resistance of rock. We walked around several shallow ponds like bowls sticking out of the massive whiteness of the mountainside. A surreal feeling of overwhelming beauty took over us. Except for the blue skies everything was glittering white including the valley below stretching out as far as one could see. We stood speechless. The wind slapped us hard, besieging us to surrender and get inside the hot thermal ponds. It was a joke; a marvelous joke of Mother Nature. I took my coat off, and stripped from the waist down. He yelled at me for taking my pants off. I wasn't worried. No one else was around. I stepped carefully into one of the white pools of hot, jelly-like calcium deposits and sat like a chicken ready to lay eggs in the comfort of her coop. He took his shoes and socks off and stepped into the pool next to mine. He slipped and fell so hard on his bottom that his pants ripped.

I refrained from saying, "So, experts like you also fall, hum?" I wasn't happy he had fallen, but it was nice to know he was as imperfect as I was. Luckily he had another pair of jeans with him; the pair he was wearing was beyond sewing. I took a handful of calcium deposit and put it into a small plastic bag for our sand collection.

"If we get searched for any reason, they'll think it's cocaine." He laughed.

When it was time to leave, he wanted to go back the same way we had come up. If I showed any fear I knew he would insist on doing it. The thought of sliding down the icy cliff pushed my survivor's button by making me act calm enough to say, "I wonder what it looks like from the other side of the mountain?"

"How do you intend to find out?"

"We take the exit through the main gate and walk on the road which should be even shorter a distance to reach the valley below."

He fell for it.

Half-hour later he yelled, "This sucks, it's the long way into town."

"I've never been here before."

"It was your stupid idea to take this road back. I shouldn't have listened to you. This is the last time you tell me where to go. You're pathetic, useless, and nothing more than a burden to me."

I hummed the tune from the movie *The Bridge on the River Kwai.* It fit my mood but failed to cover the sound of his voice echoing in my head. I followed him, swearing that even if I were to break my neck on another wild hike of his, not a sound would come out of my mouth. Too bad he helped me when I was sliding off the cliff. I would have finally been at peace.

A thunderstorm rolled in and poured down on us. By the time we boarded the bus to Konya, I was drenched. Patrick had done well with his heavy-duty leather jacket and my water repellent leather pilot hat. The umbrella we'd had in Florence was long gone due to a gust of wind before we left to Rome.

He wanted to go to Konya because according to his travel guide it was supposed to be the oldest known human community, 7500 BC. I borrowed his book to read more about the town. Konya was famous for Sufism and the whirling dervishes, a group of religious people who prayed by twirl dancing. I made the mistake of sharing that information with Patrick. Once he knew it had to do with a religion that was not his own, he was no longer interested.

The bus let us out at the Konya bus station, but upon walking two blocks he decided that he hated Konya and wanted to leave at once.

"According to the pictures in this tour book Nevsehir looks a lot more exciting," he said.

We went back to the bus station to take the bus for Nevsehir, but there was a half-hour wait. Patrick left for the bathroom inside the bus station and when he returned I told him I had to do the same.

On the way into the station, my eye caught a candy counter with a large variety of freshly made Lokum. I recognized them as the same sweets the Portuguese ambassador to Turkey used to send to my Aunt Heydee every Christmas. I was the only one at home who ate them. They were made of one inch squares of delicate chewy gummy jelly scented with rosewater and dipped in powdered sugar. Oh, the small innocent memories of childhood; how much joy they could bring into the present.

I looked out of the large glass window to make sure he couldn't see me and I bought two pieces. I closed the door to my stall. There was no toilet. As a seasoned traveler, the hole in the ground was no longer a shocker. Standing against the wall I took my small water bottle and the toilet paper roll from my backpack and held them between my legs. I carefully opened the wrapping paper that held the Lokum pieces. First I licked them clean from the powder sugar so it wouldn't get over all my clothes. I felt intense pleasure as I took my time eating the Lokum, inebriated by its gummy chewy flavored rose water. I drew a slug from my water bottle and swished it inside my mouth from one side to the other, using my tongue to pull out any leftovers still stuck between my teeth. I repeated the procedure three times to make sure nothing remained. Then I took another mouth full of water and used it bit by bit to pour it over my hands and clean my lips. I dried them with the toilet paper. I used the same paper to wipe myself after peeing. I couldn't afford to run out of toilet paper before Patrick did otherwise he would be upset.

"What took you so long? I was getting ready to come and get you," he said.

"Number one and number two." I smiled. Two Lokum pieces.

It was getting dark when we arrived to Nevsehir. Its quietness reminded us of Delicias, Mexico. By the time we found the cheapest hotel with heat we were exhausted and went to bed.

The next morning we looked around the city but there was nothing interesting to see. As we started walking into the bus station, a young man sitting on the steps motioned to us. "Don't bother getting tickets there, unless you want to spend a fortune."

Patrick said, "We are interested in seeing the Cappadocia sites. Do you have any advice?"

"Nevsehir is just a transfer spot for towns such as Göreme, Uçhisar and Ürgüp. Don't take the bus, use one of the guided excursions that include lunch, you'll get a lot more for the buck." Stephen was from Australia and had been traveling in Turkey for a month with two other college students.

After some inquiries we found the best deal in town, two days of sightseeing for $20 each. A guide that could barely speak English picked us and an elderly Turkish couple at the town's square the next morning. On the first day we were taken to the fairy chimney rock formations of Ürgüp, the mountains of Göreme, and on the second day to the underground cities of Kaymakli and Derrinkuyu.

Surrounded by miles and miles of odd shaped rock formations at Ürgüp I felt like I was in another planet. I needed something tangible to look at later, so that I knew I had not dreamed it. "Patrick, you've got to take at least one picture of the scenery. No one at home is going to believe that there's a place on earth that looks like this."

"I'm not taking pictures. I don't want to spend a fortune developing film when we get home."

At noon, our guide stopped by a park close to Göreme, took an icebox from the back of the van and served us a wilted green salad, cold, greasy chicken soup and a piece of stale bread. Patrick said that the food was not fit for human consumption and eating the chicken might make us sick. The next day we would bring our lunch. Our guide gave us the freedom to explore the mountains of Göreme on our own and be back to the van by 4.

Just then an older woman approached us selling postcards from the area.

"Patrick, look, ten cards for two bucks, that's cheaper than film. What do you think?"

"I don't know..."

"For two bucks we have a great collection of twenty postcards, to remember the sights and we can also show them to the folks when we get back."

He agreed to buy two different sets of cards. Taken at the best angles by professional photographers, they were better than pictures. I put them in my backpack.

As we hiked a steep snowy hill my back felt weak. By the time we got to the top I was starting to experience radiating pain down my right leg with every step. From my past experience with a herniated disc, I knew my downfall was carrying heavy weights. The pain down the leg was a vivid reminder of my orthopedic surgeon wanting to do back surgery. I didn't want to tell Patrick what was happening. I was scared he wouldn't stand for it. I began taking small steps to help alleviate the pain and prayed we wouldn't have to hike too many steep cliffs. When we reached the top of one, he said, "Lets cross the path-like bridge connecting to the cliff on the other side. That way we don't have to backtrack."

The ice covered "bridge," created by Mother Nature, was about two feet wide by twelve feet long, but she had forgotten to put a handrail on either side. I experienced an overwhelming fainting feeling much like the first time I had to make a speech in school. My legs went weak, and my stomach became queasy.

"Patrick, I'm afraid to slip on the ice. It's straight down on both sides. I can't do it."

"What are you afraid of?"

"Falling."

"You've lived long enough." His laugh angered me. He didn't value my life. He didn't even value his own life. What he wanted to do was insane. My life was in his hands, and I had no doubt that when we ran out of my money he was going to kill me. My father had been right when he had called him a woman user.

"Let's go," he said sternly. "You get in front of me, and I'll be right behind to catch you if you slip. Look straight ahead as you walk and don't look down on either side."

I walked heroically across the bridge. Like he said, I had lived long enough. If it was meant for me to fall, then that's what it was, and there was nothing I could do about it.

"When we reached the other side, he said, "We both beat death. Wasn't it exciting?"

"Patrick, there's no such thing as 'beating' death." I felt a deep wisdom that I wasn't aware of having. "I don't find any excitement in that. We all die sooner or later, and it only happens when death wants you."

He began hiking down a steep cliff to reach the valley below. I did it too but the unconventional way. I sat on the frozen ground, facing the sheer drop, removed my pack and put it across my chest, and began sliding down with my legs straight out, so I could use my heels as breaks, while holding my back and head as far back as I could, so I wouldn't tumble forward. With my elbows slightly pointing away from my body I used them also to help control the speed of my descending. Not once did I ask for his help.

When I was about ten feet from reaching the ground below he shouted, "Stop right there. Throw me your backpack first, and then jump into my arms. I'll catch you."

I did.

At that point I could care less about myself. Besides, my lower back pain was gone.

"Veronica, I've never seen you this way. You're fearless. I'm proud of you." He hugged me.

"I'm not afraid of anything anymore." I said to him, knowing that's what he wanted to hear.

On our way to Istanbul, the passengers on the bus, mostly men, sang a festive Turkish song.

"Maybe they won a soccer game." I told Patrick, who sat with a sourpuss face.

"I'm sick and tired of listening to them and putting up with their smoking. I've had it."

He spoke loud enough for everyone to hear. It didn't matter if they didn't understood English, his demeanor matched his rude tone. He took a small red white and blue cotton cowboy scarf from his backpack and, after soaking it in water; he wrapped it around his face.

"Patrick, you look like a bank robber. Maybe you shouldn't use it that way."

"This will help me from breathing their shit into my lungs." He said aloud.

I kept quiet.

"What we need here is some good American tunes." He began singing the US national anthem.

"Are you trying to get us both killed?"

The bus driver stopped the bus. Pointing at us he yelled, "You! Get out now!"

He left us in the darkness of the night, in the middle of a road surrounded by snow-banks on both sides. No trees, no signs anywhere, just a long road leading to nowhere. I wondered if there were wolfs in Turkey. And if there were wolfs, would they be hungry. I walked as fast as Patrick did and about an hour later we saw what looked like a lit-up town ahead of us. We got out of the road by climbing a small hill that led us to an open field of white snow. To my delight, we came upon the town's main street. It looked just like any other town, except that all the stores were closed. Against Patrick's strict orders not to do it, I walked into the only store that was still open. It looked like a small travel agency, with two desks and two chairs and a few scenic posters on the walls. The two men inside greeted us as if they were expecting us. They gave us their chairs and one of them brought us two hot teas, served in small tulip-shaped glasses with two sugar cubes on the side.

"They may have put poison into it. Don't drink it."

I drank it. And then asked one of them if there was any place we could rent a room for the night. There was one hotel up the street, and that was it.

There was heat in the room, but we discovered the toilet wouldn't flush when water over-flowed into our bedroom. All that mattered was that we had a place to sleep.

The next morning we learned there was one bus to Istanbul at noon. We strolled around town, looking for something to do. It was a simple country town with not much to see. The aroma of fresh bread baking drew us into a bakery and we bought a large loaf of bread still warm from the oven. They used newspaper to wrap the bread.

"Nothing like ink for extra taste," I told him as I took a big bite. He laughed and did the same. When he was in a good mood, he was a great companion.

Afterwards we walked into a quaint little grocery store, with burlap bags by the door filled with dried fruits and nuts. It reminded me of the old-fashioned grocery stores in Portugal.

"I love dried apricots," I said to Patrick. "I wonder how much they cost for just a couple of them." I smiled at the grocery man. "Good morning, how much for a handful of apricots?"

He smiled back. "One dollar."

"You don't need apricots, let's go," said Patrick.

As I followed Patrick towards the door, the man said something in Turkish so I turned. He walked towards me, grabbed a handful of apricots, and put them in my hands. He made a curtsy with his head and said smiling, "For you only. Not him."

I thanked him and put them in my coat pocket.

"Well, you got what you wanted. Now it's my turn to find something that I like."

We had walked two blocks when Patrick saw another grocery shop. He pointed to a metal can with salty dried corn kernels. "That's my favorite snack. I'm going to get some for myself."

I took my time eating the apricots on the way to the bus station. He was popping the kernels into his mouth when one of them slid the wrong way. Tears ran down his face and he had difficulty taking a breath. He coughed all the way to the station. I didn't have an ounce of pity towards him.

Hum, hum, hum. Pop goes the weasel. Hum, hum, hum.

On the bus to Istanbul, Patrick decided to get even with the smokers in front of us. He put his hand over his mouth and made farting sounds. He picked boogers out of his nose and flicked them at the guy in front of us. I could tell they were aware of what was going on by the way they watched and spoke Turkish among themselves. I closed my eyes and pretended I was sleeping. If I didn't see what was going on, it didn't exist. I was dozing off when I felt a drop of liquid on my left hand. I figured that the guy seated across the aisle was spitting at us. I awoke Patrick and told him about it. "I have my eyes on everybody, and if that was happening I'd see it immediately."

"You're sleeping. You can't see anything."

"I was faking it. If any of them did something, I would know."

"Then how do you explain this drop on the back of my hand?" I showed him my left hand.

He looked up at the luggage rack.

"Looks like our plastic water bottle is leaking" He got the bottle and settled it on the floor between his feet. "You're having hallucinations. I'm afraid that you're getting old and starting to lose it." He laughed.

"It's your fault that I thought someone was spitting at us. How do you think I feel when you act like a spoiled child, making fart sounds and acting like you're going to vomit and throwing boogers at the passengers in front of us? What do you think my imagination is going to do when I close my eyes and there are drops of liquid falling on my hands?"

He calmed down after that and we both fell asleep.

We arrived in Istanbul at noon on January 27. Upon getting out of the bus, a man approached us asking if we needed a taxi. Patrick turned around with a smile on his face and, with the weight of his backpack, knocked the poor guy face-first into the bus parked next to us. I kept walking. He caught up with me, bragging about what he had done to the taxi driver.

I wasn't feeling well. I was coughing. My nose was running like a faucet, and it was difficult to hold my head up. I had chills. I felt my forehead and I knew I had a fever. I was determined not to complain because it wouldn't do me any good. Sooner or later I would get better.

Just like the other countries, as soon as we arrived we visited the tourism office at the main train station, which is where we usually found free maps and brochures on important sites to visit. Patrick needed only a few minutes to study a map and he was ready to go.

We spent most of the day looking for a cheap hostel but oddly enough we found a hotel that was not only more economical than any of the other places, but had many amenities. The front desk staff spoke perfect English and breakfast was included. The elevator to the third floor had all its parts. Not only did our room have heat, but it also had a working thermostat, plus a large comfortable bed, private bathroom and a television. Besides all that, it was situated in the heart of Istanbul amid all the tourist attractions.

Breakfast was a feast for the gods. Delicious hot bread, cheese, butter, olives, eggs, tomatoes, cucumbers, jam, and honey. When our server turned around, we put as much bread and cheese as we could into our backpack. Lunch was taken care of.

We spent the day exploring Istanbul, but we lingered the longest at Topkapi Palace, which was indeed a palace to the full extent of the word. We walked along a wide hallway leading to rooms (the leaflet stated 400 rooms) that had been the home to hundreds of concubines, who resided there only to please the sultan. Rich tile detail and colorful paintings adorned the fountains and fireplaces along the way. I stood at the Sultan's quarters now just a large empty room, with stained glass windows. I imagined him lying on his bed, covered in silk and precious jewels, too old and fat to get up, while some beautiful young girl, a political pawn between two countries, acted like she really enjoyed making love to her new husband. But nothing compared to what we found in the treasury section of the palace, composed of four rooms packed with exquisite Turkish jewelry, ceremonial costumes and housewares covered with gold and precious stones and works of art that had survived from the Ottoman's Empire. Each room had its own throne. Seeing a throne made of gold and then the original Topkapi Dagger in all its glory justified the reason why I shouldn't be in bed recovering from a lousy cold.

While walking to our hotel, we found a restaurant with pictures of veggie dishes in the window, each costing roughly two dollars. I said with no shame, "Sorry, but for that price, I'm having dinner."

He sat across from me with his leather coat on and wool hat pulled down to cover his face, not talking and refusing to eat anything.

Screw him. I ate a large round flatbread stuffed with spinach, potatoes, parsley, and cheese. I was happy.

Afterwards, we looked for something for him to eat and soon found a tavern that sold take-out platters of roasted chicken and fried potatoes. That did it for him. We remained in our room for the night playing Uno and Yahtzee. My cold was far from improving and I was glad when he said that sex had to wait until the next morning since he was tired.

The next day, we were crossing a square when we saw a bunch of people gathered by a tall massive stone structure with several glass semi-domes and brown wood doors under a continuous vaulted arcade. Only one door was open. It was a Mosque. Its steps were covered with shoes from those who had entered the building.

"I've always wondered what it looks like inside a Mosque. Do you want to go inside with me?" I began taking my shoes off.

"No. This place is for devil worshipping. It's evil."

"Don't worry. I'm not going to change my religion." I laughed.

"No, you're not going in there. I forbid you." A stern look crossed his face.

"Sorry, Patrick, but I've never been in a Mosque. I want to see what it looks like."

He took off, probably thinking I was going to run after him like I always did.

I stepped inside. Wow! It reminded me of a Jewish temple because there were no paintings or statues of saints to pray to, except that it was one hundred times bigger than a temple. In the center there was a gigantic super-duper round dome with four levels of stained glass windows with intricate designs below that provided natural light in contrast with the round black metal chandelier dripping with sharp white lights. There were no seats. The floors were covered with multiple layered carpets of all sizes, where some people stood while others were on their knees praying. The walls were sheathed with ceramic tiles of blue and gold with complex patterns of flowers, possibly tulips.

I had seen it, and I was content. That was until I came out.

Patrick stood by my sneakers. "What would you have done if they had stolen the only pair of shoes you have? Hum?"

"Patrick, there are hundreds of shoes out here, a lot better than mine. Why would anyone take my crummy shoes?"

"They are not Christians! They are religious fanatics. I'll never forgive you for leaving me and going in there when I specifically told you not to."

He was so angry I thought he was going to hit me. He didn't, but he cursed and yelled and made my life miserable for the rest of the day. I turned up the music station in my head and hummed, "It's my party and I'll do what I want to…."

Later that day, when we stood across the street from Taksim Square, Patrick pulled out his map to see where he wanted to go next. When he saw a man walking towards us, Patrick said, "I bet he's going to offer help because I'm holding a map. These so called good Samaritans, they really piss me off. He better not even come near me or I'll break his face."

I freaked out and put my hand flat out towards the man and yelled, "Please, stay away. My husband doesn't want any help." I couldn't control my cough and I had run out of toilet paper to blow my nose.

The guy looked at me and then Patrick for a second and kept on walking. I wiped my nose on my sleeves, shivering. My head weighed a ton. "There must be a pharmacy close by. I need to get an antibiotic to help me get rid of the fever."

We found a pharmacy, but when they told us the price of the medicine Patrick said, "That's a fortune for a drug that we don't even know if it works." I agreed with him.

That evening I skipped dinner and stayed in bed, while he left to get dinner for himself. I didn't know how much fever I had. I only knew I couldn't lift my head off the pillow and food was the furthest thing from my mind. May God forgive me, but that night I crossed my fingers that he wouldn't make it back. It would have been quite possible given how he behaved. Several times since arriving to Istanbul, drivers had stopped to let us cross the street. If Patrick thought the driver had not given him enough room to walk straight across, he would kick the side of the car, flip them his middle finger, and yell, "Freakin' Turks! Why don't you learn how to drive?"

Sometimes he would hit his fist on the hood. Usually the driver looked at him not believing his eyes, but not do anything except rollup the window as fast as he could.

It was just a question of time before someone got out of his car and let Patrick have it. With luck, tonight would be the night.

He came back an hour later, and I felt guilty for having such desperate thoughts.

I took a hot shower and went back into bed. I prayed he would get the flu, or whatever I had, so I could stay in bed for a day or two.

The next morning he woke feeling weak and had a sore throat. He still wanted to go out, but he couldn't walk as fast. I no longer had to struggle to keep up with him, and instead we walked side by side. My dog days on a leash behind were over—at least a while.

That didn't stop Patrick's obsessive behavior. Since we had arrived to Istanbul, Patrick had been collecting paperclips, rubber bands, nails, screws, and small plastics of any kind. Before getting a cold, he would walk briskly and pick up his "treasures" from the sidewalk just as fast, but now he would take a few steps, study the pavement ahead and if, anything looked important, he'd put it inside a large plastic bag he carried just for that purpose. If he saw a stupid rubber band that I had missed, he would yell at me.

That night, when I got up from bed to go to the bathroom, I walked into the wall and bumped my head. I cried out, "Patrick, I'm tired of living in hotels. When I get up from bed, I don't even know where I am. I want to go home."

"We have a lot more to see. Don't give me a hard time now."

"How much longer do you want to travel? Please, I want to go home."

"We're far from being finished traveling. We still have the northern European countries to see."

"I don't care about the northern countries. Patrick, I'm begging you, let's go home." I put my palms together as if begging.

"You feel that way because you have the flu."

"We're both sick with the flu. Let's not go out today. Let's try to recover and then go home."

"You're being selfish by denying me what you promised me in Greece."

"What?

"You said that after Turkey we would visit the northern countries. You're nothing but a liar. How do you think that makes me feel, knowing that I married a liar?"

"Okay, okay, stop it." I put my hands to my head. "If I said that then that's what it is. I'm sorry. I forgot."

While walking the next morning through a covered bazaar market, I came across a shop with a variety of Turkish brooms. I was attracted to the one without a handle. We had been traveling through so many countries, and I didn't have a single item to show for it, except for the post cards in my backpack and the sand bags. The vendor wanted three dollars for the broom, but after I did my Portuguese bargaining, he was willing to sell it for seventy-five cents.

"You can't go wrong for that price." Patrick said. "Back in the US it will be worth a lot more. But if you buy it, you'll have to carry it."

He wanted to see Istanbul's famous Basilica Cistern, Europe's largest medieval underground sewage system. Although we saw a lot of structural corrosion, we noticed no unpleasant odors and found it very clean. With its maze of water channels, it possessed the surrealistic look of an underground Venice. Presently it was being used as a water reservoir and for "plumbing" the houses above. I would have enjoyed it a lot more if it wasn't so damp and cold. My flu symptoms grew worse, and I felt chilled to the bone. Patrick wasn't doing much better than me.

On the way back to the hotel, Patrick vomited violently into the potted flowers outside our hotel. I felt weak and coughed and had a fever. He felt weak and had a fever as well, but his stomach ached and now there was vomiting.

January 30 was engraved in my memory, because for the next two weeks we both remained in bed too weak to get up, except for taking the elevator to the first floor to grab breakfast and load on enough food to take us through the day. We slept most of the time. It didn't matter if it was day or night; we were both too sick to get out of bed. I knew he was getting better when a week later he asked me to go out and bring him his favorite meal, a roasted chicken and fries. I took my time while food shopping; it was like being on vacation.

When we had been in Santorini, he had mentioned a few times that when he returned to the United States he intended to create what he called *The Red Nipple Campaign*, which I took as being part of his wackiness and it would go away soon enough. But it didn't. Now it was all he talked about. He planned to climb on every billboard he saw and draw red nipples on the female models. He was also going to buy every modeling magazine he could get his hands on and personally paint red nipples on every picture.

"What do you think? I came up with the idea from seeing your breasts. Just imagine all over the US, big huge billboards showing women with red nipples."

The fever had to be affecting his brain. He was crazier than ever and my common sense told me to be careful and go along with whatever he said.

"Oh, yeah, I see what you mean, like using lipstick, right?"

"No. As always you're not paying attention to what I'm saying. How many times do I have to say the word paint? I'm talking about paint, real paint."

"Oh yes of course, real paint so it lasts longer."

"That's right, permanent paint. And it would be mandatory for all women. I will be known for getting such movement started. I'll be famous. I can see it happening nationwide, and then worldwide. You better not tell anyone about my idea. They would steal it for sure. You hear me?"

This kind of talk made me even more scared for my life, I was sure that at that point, he had lost whatever he had left of his faculties and one night he might turn over and choke me to death.

We stayed in our room day after day. When we weren't sleeping, he would talk about nipples or we would play Uno and Yahtzee. Every time he won, he would tell me how dumb I was and that I didn't have the brains to win a simple game of cards. When my luck turned in my favor, I gave him the same talk back even though he was still feverish.

"Maybe I am smarter than you thought."

"You must stop talking to me like that. If this continues when we get back to the US, I want a divorce."

The idea that he was willing to give me a divorce over a game of cards was like music to my ears.

One night he stood by the closed bedroom window, opened the curtain, and said, "I can't stand listening to them praying to the devil over the loud speakers."

I loved the sound of the prayers over the speakers. I was sure that it was heard all over the city. It didn't matter that they were Muslims. They were people praying to God. It felt like how a lullaby must feel to a child.

"Before we leave Istanbul, I intend to blow up at least one Mosque." He said looking at me seriously.

"Patrick, please, don't even say that."

“I mean it. I’ve been thinking about it day and night, and I know I can do it.”

I knew that whatever he said he was going to do, I couldn’t stop him. I was scared for both of us. He was out of control.

“I want to confess my sins. I have not been a good man. But I believe in Jesus Christ, and he’ll forgive me.”

I sat on the bed with my legs crossed, and asked God to give me the inner strength to remain calm. I didn’t want to hear his confession. “You know I’m Jewish, right?”

“Yes, of course I know. You’re lucky because as a Jew you’re automatically accepted in heaven. You’re one of the chosen people. But these Muslims, they worship the devil and as such they’re all going to hell, including their children.”

“Not their children.”

“Yes, their children too.”

“Just because the parents are Muslims, doesn’t make their children guilty. Why would the children go to hell? It’s not their fault for being born to them.”

He opened the window and yelled out, “You are guilty! You are all guilty! When I blow up one of your mosques, I hope it’s filled with your families!”

“Patrick, the children are innocent. They didn’t choose their parents.”

“So what? They are their seeds!”

I squeezed my hands between my knees.

“Death is God’s will,” he said.

He reminded me of one of those men I had seen so many times in the street corners of New York City preaching about Jesus and the end of the world.

He went on. “A year ago, Josh, my best friend, his wife, their baby, and their three year old son were in a car accident. They all died, except Josh who after a few months in coma, survived. They all died to benefit him. It was God that chose it to be that way.”

"I'm sorry, Patrick, but I believe that God is good and doesn't kill people to benefit others, much less your friend's family."

He wasn't hearing me. He left the window and stood at the bottom of the bed and raved about Jesus being God's only son, and throwing in excerpts from the bible. He didn't seem to hold a grudge against the Jews, but that didn't make me feel any safer. I began humming, The Doors tune, "People are Strange."

He said, "If something happens to me and I need to have tubes and machines to keep me alive, like it happened to Josh, so it shall be."

"I don't want tubes and machines to keep me alive," I said. "In that case, I let God make the decision over my life."

"Not me, and remember that. I want whatever it takes to stay alive."

That night, I closed my eyes but couldn't fall asleep. In the distance I heard the Muslim prayers. I prayed to God and my mother to please take Patrick or me away. I'd be happy either way. But if Patrick died, I promised that upon my return to Portugal, and before leaving to the US, I would get the pink marble tombstone for my mother like I had promised her.

The next morning Patrick was still in bed when he said, "Let's take a plane to Germany."

"Yes, sure, but remember what we learned in school that flying isn't safe when you have a cold or congestion. The pressure on the sinus can cause extreme pain and rupture of the ear drum." I smiled. "Then we'll have something in common. You'll be deaf like me."

"I still have a cold. Let's find another way to get there."

The next morning, we walked to the American Embassy for advice on the best way to travel from Turkey to Germany. While waiting at the embassy we met a young American couple. They had been robbed of their money and passports while sleeping in a train from Bulgaria to Turkey. We decided to take the bus out of Turkey.

Patrick had not let go of his red nipples obsession. Even after I agreed with him that it was a genius idea, he kept repeating the same plans over and over. He wanted my complete attention. When he asked me a question about his plan, I'd better be ready to respond. I didn't know how much longer I could go on. I could only pray that God would keep me sane until we were back in the US. Once home, I would be getting a divorce even if he killed himself over it.

We bought two bus tickets to Munich, Germany for $50 each at The Cameron Travel Agency not far from our hotel. At Patrick's request, the friendly man behind the counter called to confirm that the bus would be leaving Istanbul at five in the afternoon. We would be crossing Bulgaria, Romania, Hungary, and Austria, and arrive in Munich at nine in the morning. The whole trip was going to take approximately forty hours.

We planned on leaving Istanbul, February 6.

~ Chapter Twenty-Seven ~

Please, Don't Take the Bus

We considered ourselves lucky to have missed the pouring rain that started just as we entered Esenler Otogar, Istanbul's main bus terminal. We looked for the #62 bus line, as we had been instructed at the Cameron Travel Agency. The people working at the bus station barely spoke English. Jug, a young traveler waiting for the same bus spoke well enough for us to understand that he came to Istanbul once a year to buy spices and grocery items unavailable in Yugoslavia. When, our bus reached Budapest, Hungary, his family would be waiting for him with their car. Buses avoided Yugoslavia for political reasons.

A man in his late thirties, and quite handsome, wearing a dark gray suit and a matching wool cap, introduced himself as our bus driver, took our tickets and told us and Jug to follow him to another part of the bus station. We followed the driver like sheep.

Before entering the bus, I told Patrick we should get rid of his Turkish change and put it to good use by buying some goodies from the small shop at the bus station.

"We have more than enough food for the two days of travel." I was not surprised by his response.

I knew I wasn't supposed to spend any money without his approval but I wanted cookies. I needed sugar.

"Patrick, honey, let's get rid of some of your heavy change. The weight is just plain hard on your back. If you can spare a few coins, I'll buy us a small box of dried cookies. It can't be much."

"Go see how much they cost first and hurry back so we don't lose our bus."

I ran as fast as I could.

"It's only a quarter for a package of Maria cookies. C'mon, Patrick, it's not going to break our bank account."

He handed me a few coins from his pocket. "That's all you get. Now hurry."

I bought two packages of cookies and put them in my backpack. I saw four men dressed in business suits seated in the waiting room, and wondered if they would be boarding too. I caught up with Patrick as he entered the bus.

I noticed there were two other passengers already on board, an elderly Turkish couple and Jug seated behind them. Patrick took a seat on the right side of the bus, three quarters of the way back. Patrick and I were impressed that our bus was like new on the inside and resembled a modern Greyhound bus.

The bus driver offered to put our stuff in the compartment under the bus but we declined. We had a large water jug filled with water, the backpacks, and two large plastic handbags. One of the bags had our food and the other had my broom, two bath towels taken from the hotel in Istanbul, two rolls of toilet paper, and his new personal effects of three empty water bottles, plastic bags, rubber bands, paper clips, rope pieces and other paraphernalia he had found on the streets.

Patrick was putting our belongings on the compartment above us when a thirtyish, heavyset, blonde-haired woman climbed into the bus. She sat on the seat closer to the front door, and got busy talking to the driver. They spoke Turkish and seemed to know each other. Two more men came aboard, dressed in the same style as our bus driver and headed toward the back of the bus, carrying three old-fashioned large leather suitcases. They stacked them flat along the back seat and covered them with a bunch of blankets.

When the driver walked by, Patrick said, "Is there a bathroom in this bus?"

"No bathrooms. We stop often."

Patrick pointed toward the back. "Who are those men back there?"

"My cousins. They help with driving." He walked to the back to talk to them, then returned to his seat and turned on the engine. The four businessmen must have taken another bus. Patrick commented on the bus company not making money with six passengers. I told him they probably would be picking up people along the way, in other towns.

"I don't believe that. We must be in the wrong bus. Ask the bus driver if we're going to Munich."

I walked up to the driver.

"Excuse me, but my husband wants to know if this bus is going to Munich."

"Yes, Munich. Everything fine, yes," he said, while waving his hand impatiently, as though to say, *move away and go sit down.*

The bus had barely left the station's parking lot when two police cars with flashing lights surrounded the bus. Two policemen raced in, grabbed the blonde woman, handcuffed her, and hauled her away, while she screamed what sounded like Turkish profanities. Then the police grabbed her large suitcase from the luggage compartment at the bottom of the bus.

Patrick said, "Probably a criminal trying to escape from Turkey." He smiled.

We finally got on our way at seven o'clock. At eight o'clock, we pulled out our dinner. Patrick ate half his chicken, the fries and some of the bread. I ate half of my salad and three Maria cookies for dessert. Each box of Maria cookies contained twelve thin butter cookies. I had no idea if they were any good, until I took a bite. They were deliciously crunchy.

A half hour later the bus stopped at a small village. The driver, his two cousins—and the old couple climbed off the bus, entered a quaint looking country house, and returned with several large black plastic bags stuffed full. They shoved some of the bags in the compartment under the bus. Once back on the bus, they lifted the aisle's rubber mats, pulled up the floorboards, and stuffed more bags into the floor spaces. Next, they filled the compartments above the seats with huge round cheeses and breads and covered them with black plastic sheets. On top of the sheets, they arranged in neat rows bags of onions and potatoes.

"This doesn't look Kosher." I whispered to Patrick.

He whispered back, "I agree. We need to know what's going on. Let's talk to Jug."

When we approached Jug, he jumped to his feet and nudged us over to our seats. "I know you want to know what's happening." He put his finger to his mouth. "Better not ask questions."

"Don't tell me to be quiet." Patrick said. "I want to know…"

Jug cut him off. "Shh. These men are carrying contraband, and a lot of other things that you don't want to know about. For your wife's and your own safety, sit down and don't ask any more questions. Just behave and you'll be fine…"

"I want to know…" Patrick said.

"Mister, if you want to stay alive, what's going on here is none of your business. Do not talk to me anymore." He returned to his seat.

Patrick sat down. "Jug is a looser. From now on only one of us sleeps while the other stays awake in case they want to cut our throats in the middle of the night."

~ *Chapter Twenty-Eight* ~

Bulgaria, Romania, Hungary

The bus moved at the speed of lightning through the icy deserted countryside road. On and off the silhouette of a tree became more visible, when a monster branch covered with snow rubbed against our window. I did my best to stay awake by staring at the whitish gray highway ahead illuminated by the headlights which made the snowflakes look like flying cotton. It was mesmerizing. The windshield wipers played a steady soft tune except for every fifth beat one of them would scrape the windshield like a fingernail on a chalkboard. I dozed off while I was supposed to be keeping watch.

At midnight, the Bulgarian border patrol stopped us at their border. Our driver and his cousins left the bus to talk to them. Ten minutes later our driver returned and apologetically asked us to give him $100 to pay the soldiers our "tourist taxes."

"I'm not paying a dime. This is your problem. We already paid enough when we bought the bus tickets."

"My friend, these are not nice people. If you don't pay the "taxes" they will get very angry and take you away." I handed the bus driver the money.

Then he went in the back of the bus and took from one of the black plastic bags, two boxes of cigarettes and a bottle of whiskey. We left without the bus being searched.

It was Patrick's turn to stay awake. He woke me up when the bus stopped in front of a small farmhouse in the woods. The only ones left in the bus were Jug, who seemed to be sleeping, and the two of us. We were parked close enough to see through the farmhouse window the two old people and the bus crew seated at a table drinking from large mugs with another couple. "How nice. They're probably visiting family," I told Patrick.

"At this rate we'll never make it to Germany."

An hour later, the people from the farmhouse helped their guests carry large plastic containers and more cheese, out to the bus which they stored inside the bus floor, laying the carpet down afterwards. Patrick and I pretended we were sleeping. We were sure those enormous cheeses were stuffed with contraband drugs, otherwise why would they hide them?

At four in the morning, the bus driver stopped for gas and announced, "Bathrooms."

Patrick went first. "Miserable bastards, none of them speak English but they know how to ask for a dollar to use their toilet. I peed behind a tree."

"I'm paying the dollar, just so you know. I ain't going into the dark woods."

There was plenty of light around the building, despite being in the middle of nowhere. It reminded me of a rest stop in the U.S.

On the way back to the bus, I took my time, enjoying the fresh air and the way the snow crunched under my feet, though I walked carefully so I didn't slip. The bus loomed in the parking lot, larger than I had realized. That's when I noticed that the name Cameron Company on the side of the bus had been switched to Ali Baba Touring Company.

I was very familiar with *Ali Baba and the Forty Thieves*. It was one of my favorite fairy tales when I was a child.

As much as I hated telling Patrick about the bus, he needed to know. He went out, making believe that he had to use the toilet again.

When he returned, he whispered, "We're in serious trouble." He had a grim look on his face as he sat down. "We've been kidnapped by the Turkish Mafia. This confirms that our lives are in danger."

"Listen, honey." I held his hands and looked straight at him. "We're in the middle of nowhere and there's no one to come and help us. If you put up a fight now or have a fit, they might kill us both. Jug already told us to keep quiet, now you know why."

"We need to make plans on how we're going to defend ourselves, when the time comes."

"Yes, but for now let's make believe we don't know anything."

We didn't sleep the rest of the night.

The bus grew unbearable cold. At one point, we asked for some heat. One of the cousins said, "Heat, broken." We wrapped the stolen hotel towels around our legs.

At seven-thirty the bus turned off the snowy highway and into a secluded area of tall trees. The panorama of heavy snow-covered trees, reminded me of a Christmas card except for the silver glitter missing. The driver saw us looking at him and said "Broken down. Bad snow storm. Be back." Then he left with his two buddies and the old couple. Jug stayed to himself and would not talk to us.

Patrick and I each ate three cookies and drank water. We played Uno until noon, when Patrick finished the leftover chicken and I finished my salad. Then we played Yahtzee. I wondered, if the driver and his buddies were going to return.

Jug began to snore, and even though it was very cold, we also dozed off. At six the sun was going down and I was glad to see that the driver, his cousins, and the old couple had returned. The bus started fine and we were on our way. Patrick and I had a slice of bread and cheese. When we passed through towns, the driver didn't stop at stop signs. Patrick couldn't get over it. I stood to stretch my legs and told him not to worry; I would talk to the driver.

"Excuse me, sir, but aren't you afraid of driving through a stop sign? What if there's a car coming the other way?"

"You very nice. I like you." He smiled. "Don't worry, we have a big bus. They can see us." Then he lowered his voice, "Stop signs for people who don't know how to drive." He laughed joyfully.

"Oh, I see what you mean." I laughed along with him. His answer was too insane for me to respond in any other way. I told Patrick the driver said he was going to drive more carefully.

"We need to ration the food we have left," Patrick said. "This is going to be a longer trip than we were told." Patrick said.

We took account of what we had. Four slices of bread, four slices of cheese, a tomato, a green pepper, and one and a half boxes of Maria's cookies.

"We don't leave the bus. As long as we stay in the bus we can fight them." He showed me a radio antenna he had hidden in his pocket. "As you can see this antenna is small enough to hide in my hand, because it is collapsible. I brought it along in case I needed a weapon."

"A collapsible antenna isn't much of a weapon."

"As long as they don't have guns, I can blind them by poking them in the eyes. Can I count on you to at least hold one of them down for me?"

I nodded my head but I knew damn well that I didn't have what it took to hold anyone down that was bigger than me.

"Here is a cigarette lighter. Put it in your coat pocket. You see trouble, start a fire," Patrick said.

He went on for hours, going over and over again on how we were going to defend ourselves if they tried to assault us.

He figured the old couple had to be the parents of one of the drivers, and being so old, he wasn't concerned about them.

We slept a lot the next morning, after staying awake through the night. Patrick believed that if we slept during the day, we could keep a better eye on them at night.

For breakfast, we each had three Maria's cookies and just enough water to wash them down. At noon the bus stopped by a large wood cottage. The bus driver came over to our seat. "You, come and eat at restaurant, good for you."

I stood ready to join them, but Patrick pulled me by my arm and said to him, "We're staying in the bus. We're not hungry."

Everybody left for lunch, except us.

We each ate a slice of bread with a slice of cheese, and a quarter of the green pepper. Patrick said we should urinate before they returned. While standing in between two seats in the back of the bus, I managed to fill up a paper cup without reaching the brim, and passed it to Patrick who put it inside one of the empty water bottles. I did that three times in the row. He opened the bus door ever so slightly and emptied the bottle out of the bus. He also managed to pee from inside the bus by keeping the bus door slightly open. Being a man had its obvious rewards.

I sat next to him. "I've a feeling that these people are harmless and they're most likely using us as decoys to help smuggle their goods into Germany. Let's join them. Jug is with them."

"You're far from smart. Can't you see that if we go out there they can easily rob us and leave us to die in the woods?"

Two hours later the crew returned with the old couple and Jug, who looked at us momentarily but showed no signs of emotion.

At the Romanian border, as we were about to leave Bulgaria, the frontier cops entered the bus and nabbed one of the cousins. Patrick couldn't have been happier. He was sure he could easily handle the two remaining drivers.

Throughout the night, we traveled back roads, avoiding the main highway. At three in the morning, the bus stopped stranded by a massive snowdrift. We watched from our windows. Several men came out of the woods, possibly nearby villagers and helped the bus driver and his cousin shovel the snow around the bus. It took about an hour before we were again on our way.

There wasn't much to see of Romania as they drove through the night, except for when the headlights hit some grey cement buildings along the road, covered with snow.

It was almost daylight when the Romanian police stopped our bus. They climbed into the bus and told us to leave all our belongings and follow them. I had never seen Patrick so quiet and obedient as we hiked up a small snow-covered hill to a large abandoned barn. Taking us into the woods like that, the so-called police could only be up to no good. My feet and hands were numb and I shivered violently. My cough had returned at full strength. Even though I wasn't coughing up blood I was sure I had Tuberculosis, because when I coughed my lungs hurt.

The barn was nothing but a decaying structure, with the icy wind blowing through the large gaps in the wood plank walls. I blessed my cousin, Meta, for the wool scarf she had given me.

The driver told us to stand in a corner of the barn next to Jug and not to say a word. The two policemen wore pistols around their belts and one of them carried a rifle over his shoulder. "This barn must be their police station," I told Patrick. He didn't answer. The policemen sat behind a wood table stacked with papers. The old couple spoke with the police. They seemed to represent the driver and his cousin. We didn't understand what they were saying but their manners and body language told us that they were bargaining some kind of deal, which seemed to work because the driver came back and told us to keep our mouths shut and follow him to the bus. Our backpacks had not been moved from under our seats. Patrick stared out of the window and remained silent. The bus driver walked past us mumbling angrily to himself as he went to the back of the bus and opened one of the large suitcases hidden in the back where his cousin sometimes slept. I was seated on the aisle seat and couldn't help looking up at him when he went by. He stopped by me, and opened his hands to show me a roll of money, as he mumbled, "They get paid well. Thieves! Robbers."

"I'm sorry." I said to him.

"Don't you dare talk to him," Patrick yelled.

A few feet from the bus, our driver and his cousin handed the money to one of the policemen. The old couple rearranged their onions and vegetables in the compartments above them and I knew that soon we would be back on the road. Patrick was sure that we weren't going to make it, but at that point I was convinced that the driver and his cousins who never drove (most likely they had come along to help load the bus along the way) were just trying to make a living and were using us as decoys.

It was only10:30 in the morning when the driver stopped at a secluded turn off. He, his cousin and the old couple left. Jug slept wrapped comfortably in a blanket. As he had told us, he did this kind of trip regularly and knew what to expect. They returned at five that evening. We stopped for gas and then, a few miles down the road, stopped again in front of a rustic wood building that looked like a tavern. The sign outside read, "Alexandru Restaurant, welcome."

The bus driver came to us and said sternly, "You two come with us. Have some food."

"We're staying."

"No. You come with us!"

"You can't make us leave the bus." Patrick crossed his arms in a defensive manner.

"What's wrong with you, man?" the driver yelled and then pointed at Patrick. "You're getting off the bus! It's my bus and I'm ordering to leave. You need to wash up. Don't you even go to the bathroom? Wash your hands, freshen up. Buy some food for your woman. She's a good woman." I liked him. He was concerned about my wellbeing.

"Let's go Patrick." I picked my backpack and slung it over my shoulders. We left the bus but to my dismay Patrick told me that we weren't eating anything and were not joining them.

Patrick chose a table against the wall so he could keep an eye on everyone. Jug sat with the others. One of the waiters brought us hot tea. Patrick forbade me from drinking it. He was sure they wanted to poison us. I was not to go to the bathroom either. He believed they were up to no good and, as long as I didn't leave his side, they would not dare murder him. He was going nuts again, and the only thing I could do was to play along. I had to stay coolheaded and keep him entertained enough so he wouldn't throw a tantrum. If that happened, our lives could be in jeopardy.

The inside of the restaurant was no different from the outside, plain dark wood walls that matched the picnic-like tables and long benches. The waiter approached us twice to see if we wanted something to eat. Patrick wouldn't look at him. I smiled and said, "Thank you, but we're really not hungry."

When we returned to the bus, I gave him my bread and cheese and ate three Maria cookies. An hour later my stomach was growling and I took another three cookies from the box.

He went off his rocket. "Those cookies are to be eaten only when we're hungry, do you hear me? You only think about yourself. How about me when I get hungry later?"

His remarks didn't even bother me. I was humming in my head, *These are my cookies, and I'll eat them when I want to. If I had listened to him he would still have a few miserable extra coins in his pocket and these cookies would still be on the shelf at the bus station in Istanbul. It's because of me, me, me, that we have enough cookies to live on for at least two or three more days.*

That night I had to pee badly. He gave me a paper cup and instructed me to sit in one of the back seats, since everyone else was busy talking and smoking up front, with the radio blasting. I sat on the second row from the back close to the window and slid down ever so slightly. Patrick sat next to me. I pulled my pants down and peed into the paper cup. He poured it carefully into one of the empty water bottles. Then peed directly into the water bottle. I had to admit, we were pretty slick about it.

We were awakened when the bus stopped at a corner of what looked like a city and Jug climbed off the bus, carrying his luggage. It was close to two in the morning. Apartment buildings and stores surrounded us, but it was too dark to see much else. The city was asleep. We had no idea of where we were, except that we were somewhere in Romania. Jug waved at us but didn't smile. We were even more on our own.

We had both fallen asleep when the bus stopped. It was the Hungarian border police. The bus driver asked for our passports. When he returned with the passports, he asked Patrick if he was okay. Patrick didn't answer and grabbed his passport abruptly from the driver's hands.

"Sorry, but my husband isn't feeling well." I said.

"There must be an error in your passport," he said while handing me my passport. "You can't possibly be fifty-one. You look a lot younger."

"Thank you. You're very kind to say that."

He winked at me, smiling, but when he saw the way Patrick looked at him, he walked away and started the bus.

"How dare you flirt with the driver."

"I was just being civil after he gave me a compliment, that's all."

"It will be on your conscience when they kill me and then rape you."

I waited until he calmed down, and told him that I was going to use the seat behind us to take a nap. That way he would also have more space to put his arms and legs.

I needed a brain escape. I sat fantasizing about the bus driver. He was very handsome, tall, dark eyes, dark hair, a unique sense of humor and he liked me. True that he was dealing in contraband, but at least he was normal. Maybe he would kill Patrick after all, and I would become his lover and run contraband with him for the rest of my life. I imagined the driver giving the wheel to his cousin and then walking down the bus aisle to bend over and kiss me softly on the lips. I responded to it. Wow, it felt so real that I opened my eyes.

It was Patrick.

"You looked so beautiful, dreaming. I had to kiss you."

I felt horrible to be daydreaming about someone else, so I sat next to Patrick the rest of the night. He removed the curtains from our window and the window behind us. We used them to cover ourselves along with the two bath towels from the hotel in Istanbul.

Between the dried ration of Maria's cookies and all that seating that's most likely what bound our intestines so that neither of us needed to have a bowel movement. We drove during the night and "broke down" during the day, usually next to a small shack where the drivers and the old folks spent a few hours.

We had crossed whole countries and all we saw were shadows in the dark, mere glimpses of buildings, trees and back roads.

~ *Chapter Twenty-Nine* ~

Salzburg, Austria

An Austrian border policeman entered the bus, checked our passports, gave us a radiant smile and wished us a good trip. "We are finally in a civilized country," Patrick said. We felt more optimistic. We were getting closer to our final destination, Germany. With the night, came sleep, and when he fell asleep I moved to the other side of the bus, trying to find a comfortable position between two empty seats. I woke shivering from the bitter cold. There was no sound of a running engine, only some clunking sounds from beneath the bus. I stood, and noticed that the bus was empty, except for us. It was dark outside except for the white snow that covered what seemed to be a large plaza. Patrick was on the other seat, but he wasn't moving. I sat wondering if they had killed him. If that's what happened, the driver must have felt sorry for me and decided not to kill me. "I'm going home now. This is truly a miracle. Thank you, dear God." Tears of joy filled my eyes. Then I heard Patrick snore softly.

I looked outside. The bus driver, his cousin and the old couple loaded the black plastic bags into a large van. I shook Patrick. "We're the only ones in the bus, and it looks like they're leaving. This is the perfect time for us to escape. We're in Austria. Someone has got to speak English. Let's get out of here, now."

Just then the bus driver and the old man entered the bus. The driver handed me two small paper stubs. "We buy these train tickets for you to go to Munich, Germany. We are in Austria and the Salzburg Central Station train station is right over there." He pointed to a long, massive building across from us.

"What are you talking about? We paid for the bus trip to Germany not Austria." Patrick was furious. "You'll take us to Germany, like you were supposed to, by bus!"

"Patrick, please let's go." I put my backpack on. He had to be kidding. What did he want, a refund?

"We aren't leaving this bus, until you take us to Germany." He remained seated.

"The bus trip is finished, you ignorant man. Get out of my bus, and consider yourself lucky that we bought these tickets for you." The old man spoke with a British accent. Until now we were convinced that he and his wife were Turkish.

I picked up the water jug, one of the bags, and my broom and walked off the bus. Patrick followed me.

We stood for a few minutes in the center of the huge, empty parking lot. The Salzburg Hauptbahnhof Station towered before us, in all its stone glory. It looked like a palace with its long rows of windows and doorways.

It was four-thirty in the morning, Saturday, February 10.

We entered the train station. Patrick took off in search of a bathroom, and I stood with my back against a large iron radiator. Feeling like a frozen steak on a grill, I kept flipping over. My clothes warmed quickly and soon I felt my skin burning. For some people that might have been a bit extreme but for me it made me feel alive.

I told Patrick several times I wanted to go home, but he disregarded my wishes. We were going to Germany whether I wanted to or not. The bus trip from Turkey had likely been only a fragment of my nightmare, one that would not end until he had run out of countries or my money, whichever came first. I felt sick, physically and mentally. I was hungry, exhausted and burning cold. No one was going to come to my rescue. I knew only that I couldn't take another step and asked God for inspiration as to what to do next.

"Why don't you answer me? What's the matter with you?" I heard Patrick's impatient voice.

"Sorry. What was that?"

"Like I was saying, the train to Germany doesn't leave until the afternoon.

"Let's stay in Salzburg for a day or so. We need to take a rest after what we went through, please." I begged with my eyes.

"Okay. It makes sense. Let's do that."

After exchanging money for Austrian currency, Patrick recalled writing down the address that Barbie and Ken, the young couple we had met in Greece, had given us about a charming and yet inexpensive bed-and-breakfast in the outskirts of Salzburg. We learned we could get there by bus. Twenty minutes later the driver gave us the signal we were in Maria Plains.

We walked and walked, but the lodging was nowhere to be found. We were in the middle of a residential area. I couldn't even imagine a hotel nearby. The snow blizzard was whipping us hard. Our backpacks grew heavier with each step. Suddenly Patrick stopped walking.

"This is it. I can't go any further. I'm not moving from here." He dropped his backpack on the ground along with his other stuff and turned his back on me, facing the stone wall on our left.

"Patrick, we can't just stop. This isn't Portugal. We'll freeze to death."

He pushed his face against the wall.

"Patrick, we need to keep moving and find refuge from this storm. We must get back to where we came from."

He began punching the wall. It was up to me to do something.

"I'll go find someone to tell us how to get back to the train station." I headed up the deserted icy road, praying I wouldn't fall. If I fell and broke my back I wouldn't be able to rescue Patrick from freezing to death, and I would freeze to death too. Then a car approached. I waved but they kept going. It wasn't any better than asking for help in New York City.

I walked back as fast as I could. Patrick stood in the same position. A woman yelled from her second floor window, "Can I help? Is he okay?"

I yelled back, "We're lost. Do you know how we can get back to the train station?"

"I'll be right down." She closed the window.

When Patrick heard her voice, he turned, and smiled like an angel, posing with his hand on his hip. My goodness, the power of a woman on a man was immense, and in Patrick's case it worked magnificently. He was back to normal, grinning and very pleasant.

We had been given the wrong directions at the train station. Maria Plains Street was different from the Maria Plains north of Salzburg on the other side of the city, and it was too far away to walk from here. We needed to return to the station and take the train. She gave us instructions on how to get the bus stop, which was right around the corner from her house.

Soon we stood in front of the train station, but before entering, Patrick noticed a McDonalds. My hamburger tasted horrible, and after two bites I wanted to throw it out. Patrick ate my burger. I thought I was hungry, but I was just exhausted. All I wanted was to sleep.

At the Maria Plains train station, we found out that the inn was on the top of a steep road. Patrick was back to his obnoxious self. I did my best to keep up with him but it was hard. My backpack and water jug felt the heaviest they had so far, as if my legs had turned into lead. I began to cry, "Please show me some compassion. I just can't carry all this weight."

He walked back to me and grabbed my backpack. "Don't get used to it. I'll do it just this one time, because we went through a lot on the bus trip, but as you can see I'm invincible and I can endure a lot more than you do." He walked up the hill without stopping.

The view of the mountains from the inn was breathtaking, and so was the price of $150 per night. It included breakfast, a warm room, a full size bed, and our own bathroom outside our room, because we were the only guests. In less than ten minutes we were both unconscious on top of the goose down duvet. We woke at seven that evening. I ran to the bathroom. My body functions were back and I thanked God for that. I took the best hot shower in my life with a rich sudsy soap and thick, clean, fluffy towels.

Rosemarie, the inn's manager, recommended a *real* Austrian restaurant. "At the bottom of the hill, go over the train tracks and a small pedestrian bridge on your right and you'll see it."

Patrick tried to be chummy but he didn't win her over. She was all business.

On the way to dinner, he said, "She's a bitch. I hate her."

Rosemarie told us she ran the inn by herself. I could understand she had more important things to do than to chat with us.

We walked briskly to our dinner destination. The restaurant felt appropriately Austrian, with dark wooden walls, a large chandelier in the center of the dining area, and a boar head surrounded by animal horns over a large stone fireplace. The seats were comfortable and the tables were covered with starched white tablecloths and matching napkins alongside with shiny silverware. Instead of sitting across from each other, we sat side by side. The waitress brought us menus.

Patrick smiled and didn't seem to mind that we were seated at a "real" restaurant with "real" prices. We took our time reading the menus. I wasn't looking at prices. I just wanted solid food.

"Everything looks so good, doesn't it?" I said.

"I'm very hungry. Let's enjoy a good dinner tonight." I rejoiced. I had his blessing to order whatever I wanted.

When the waitress came by for our orders, I pointed to the menu eagerly. "The Goulash, please."

"I'm not ready to order." He had the gray look.

The waitress said she would be back.

"How dare you order your food without discussing it with me?"

"I'm sorry. I didn't think."

"That's the problem with you, you don't think. It was understood from the very beginning of our travels that neither one of us would buy anything without talking to each other. You know very well that I like goulash and you went and ordered it for yourself without regard for what I want."

"Why don't you order goulash too? I'm just so hungry, and anything with meat sounded good. I'm sorry."

I began to cry.

"Why are you upset?" he asked, a lot calmer.

"You're right to be angry at me. There was no excuse for me to order ahead of you without asking you first. I'm so lucky to have you as my husband. You're always right about everything. You're the best husband I could wish for. I don't deserve you. Please forgive me, will you?" And I cried wholeheartedly.

He wiped my tears with a tissue from his pocket and kissed me. "I forgive you because I love you so much. More than words can say." He kissed me again. "Let's splurge tonight. We'll order a dessert after dinner and we'll share it. I'm also going to order a beer with my meal. And, what are you having for dinner?"

I looked at the prices on the menu. The least expensive was a plate of steamed vegetables. Veronica didn't exist. My spirit had been pulled out a long time ago. I watched him eat his goulash and was happy to see him so content. I understood at that moment what it meant to be indoctrinated in a religious cult and not being able to escape. He was my cult.

Walking back to the inn he stopped at the narrow wood bridge and looked down at the frozen river. "Pretty deep down there, hum?" he said. I felt like I was at his mercy. I felt like a gazelle about to be torn to pieces by a lioness. I was in danger. He had his arm around my waist. "What a night. I had a great dinner with the girl of my dreams, what more can I ask for? Would you like to dance?"

There was no one around to hear me scream when he would squeeze my neck and throw me over the bridge. The darkness of the night was on his side. I didn't trust his hands on me. *May God forgive me for feeling this way but I'm scared.* I didn't want to be held by him. I held my hand outwards and curtsied. "How about a waltz?" I sang "Shall we dance, tom, tom, tom? Shall we dance tom, tom, tom?"

He laughed and then we danced, while I maintained the space between us. He was in a great mood when we went to bed and had sex. I was glad when it was over.

Sunday, February 11

The next morning, I found his usual little love note tucked into my coat pocket. I went downstairs so he wouldn't see me. On a piece of paper, I wrote, "I love you too." Then I quickly shredded it into tiny pieces and threw it in the garbage can.

We ate our free breakfast in Rosemarie's spotless kitchen, where crumbs didn't fall and counters remained uncluttered. She served us a cup of tea and thinly sliced toasted bread with two thin slices of salami and apricot jam. When Patrick complained about breakfast being only two slices of bread each, I gave him my second piece.

I was surprised when he told me he wanted to take *The Sound of Music* tour that morning. He wouldn't buy me medicine in Istanbul when I was sick with the flu, but he was ready to spend $60 for the tour.

Hans, the tour guide, was a 24 year old, handsome blonde man, until he smiled. The preceding year he'd lost control of his paraglider and crashed face first into a tree. He was trying to save enough money to have two front teeth implanted. The mini bus tour turned out to be a rip-off and I was surprised that Patrick didn't react about it. Hans just pointed to different parts of Salzburg where Hollywood had filmed the famous movie. An hour later, he dropped us off by a metal bridge and told us to have a great day. Supposedly, the Von Trapp family had used that same bridge to escape from Austria. I took a handful of gravel from the bridge and put it into a plastic bag, knowing in my heart that once we were back in the US and I asked for a divorce he would take away from me all the sand I had managed to collect. I was sad.

Of all the places we could find for lunch in Salzburg, he chose a pizzeria. Patrick ordered two glasses of water and one slice of pizza for both of us to share, the pizzeria guy said, "One slice and two glasses of water? That's ten dollars American money." Once again Patrick didn't react to the price, and I wasn't quite sure of what to make of it. I chose not to say anything.

Afterwards, Patrick wanted to walk around the city and look for a place for dinner. I followed him quietly. He wasn't talking much, which I found wonderful. At five o'clock precisely, he stopped walking and said, "Let's go back to our room and get cleaned up. We'll have dinner in the same restaurant we had dinner last night. I really liked the food there."

It was seven o'clock when we sat at the restaurant sharing a most delicious fresh salad. Patrick was still in a quiet mood. We ate all the bread in the basket, soaking the pieces in the salad dressing. Then we shared a cup of onion soup, I had a spinach omelet. He had dumplings with two veal ribs and mushrooms, and, of course, a tall glass of beer. The last two nights had been the biggest most expensive dinners we had since we started traveling.

When the waitress approached him with a large tray of various desserts he put his hand out to her. "We've had enough food for dinner." Then he said to me, "If you even mention dessert, I'll kill you."

I could have gone for a slice of their Austrian chocolate cake, but I knew better than push my luck.

Patrick sipped from his half full glass of beer. "I took my second wife once to a restaurant like this. I'll never forget it. It cost me a hundred dollars for both our meals. We were having problems with our marriage and I was trying to impress her because she wanted to leave me." He pushed his chair back and sat very straight. "I think I ate too much. It's hard to breathe."

"Maybe it's a little indigestion."

"I need some fresh air." He pressed his hands against his stomach.

I had seen him do that before when he had eaten too much at one of the casinos at Lake Tahoe. I wasn't worried.

"I'll be back. Just stay here." He left.

I dreaded leaving those comfortable surroundings to walk back to the inn. It was freezing cold and the snow had started falling as we entered the restaurant an hour earlier. But it was so pleasant here, with the warm decor and the low conversations of the people at the other tables. It would be so nice to just have a simple chat with someone, but it wasn't worth upsetting Patrick.

Our waitress approached the table. "Your husband has asked me to tell you that he needs to talk to you." I looked over to the doorway. Patrick stood there, trying to get my attention.

I eased out of my chair and walked over.

He was now bent forward, holding his stomach. Then he shuffled over to the wall and leaned against it, trying to keep his back straight.

"I threw up a lot of blood. I believe I hurt my back from vomiting. I need you to adjust my spine."

"You vomited blood? You need a medical doctor."

"No. No doctor. I just need you to adjust my back, at T6 and T7."

"I'll be right back." I ran to the waitress for help.

"My husband needs a doctor immediately; he's been vomiting blood. Call an ambulance."

When I returned, he was on the floor in a fetal position. I kneeled next to him, crying. He put his arm around my back. "Don't let them take me to the hospital."

Fifteen minutes later, the ambulance arrived. "Good, I need to go to the hospital as soon as possible. I can't take this pain anymore."

In the emergency room they had Patrick strip off his clothes. Dr. Arkin, the ER doctor, examined him and then had him taken in a wheelchair to the radiology department. A nurse gave me a large plastic bag for Patrick's belongings.

In the hallway, Dr. Arkin told me, "I'm a new doctor. I graduated a few months ago, but I'm convinced that your husband suffers from a condition called Boerhaave's Syndrome. I could be wrong since I've never seen a patient with it, but I remember reading about the symptoms when I was still a student in medical school."

"What is Boerhaave's Syndrome?"

"It's a ruptured esophagus. I've already called a specialist. If that's what he has, he's going to need surgery immediately to stop the internal bleeding."

I followed the doctor down the hallway to the room where Patrick was seated in the wheelchair. He called out, "I need stronger pain medication."

I was asked to wait in the hallway. When I entered the room, Patrick was lying naked on his back. One nurse had just finished to put the IV into his arm the other was inserting a catheter into his urethra. I looked away. "Don't leave my side," Patrick said. "I want you to keep an eye on what they do to me during surgery. You know how I feel about medical doctors."

They began putting him under and prepped him by shaving his chest. Everything was moving very fast. Two surgeons arrived.

"Now you'll have to make all the decisions." He closed his eyes.

One of the surgeons gave me a paper to sign, stating that I allowed them to do the surgery. "Sorry, but I can't sign it. I want him to have a second opinion before having surgery."

"If we don't operate at once, he'll die."

I signed the paper and followed the team of doctors down the hallway. When they entered the surgery room behind the double doors, I followed.

"You can't come in," said one of the surgeons. "You're not allowed in here."

"My husband wants me to be near him during the surgery."

"That's absolutely out of the question. You must wait outside in the hallway. When we are finished one of us will let you know how he's doing."

A nurse named Hermine led me to a wheelchair and gave me a pillow and a heated blanket. She brought me a cup of hot tea and a small plate of cookies. I drank the tea and ate the cookies, and then I fell asleep.

It was one-thirty in the morning. One of the surgeons with a heavy German accent woke me. "A cut three centimeters long in the lower esophagus spilled stomach contents into the mediasteum and lungs. We sewed the esophagus and used part of the stomach lining to reinforce the rupture site. Our biggest fear now is complications of lung and mediasteum infection. His condition is life-threatening, and we are keeping him under observation in intensive care."

He told me to go home and not to come back until visiting hours the next day. Home meant flying back to California, not going back to the inn in Maria Plains.

I asked Hermine for directions from the hospital to the train station.

"At this hour, you're better staying at a hotel closer to the hospital. I know a short cut from the back of the hospital. The hotel is across the street. Follow me."

We crossed a large grass lot and stopped when we reached a tall black metal fence. She tried to open it, but it had a lock on it. "I didn't expect this. Look, you see that street across from us? That's where the hotel is. You can't miss it. Once you leave the hospital through the front gate stay to your right. When you get to the corner make a left and then you will see the hotel on your right."

The sidewalks were slippery enough to ice-skate. But my attitude at that point was *I will not fall.* I welcomed the cold soft breeze on my face and the hollowness of the dark, as I diligently followed Hermine's directions. But after walking around the hospital's ground two times and taking a brief walk into the side streets, I gave up looking for the hotel. There wasn't a soul in sight to ask for directions. My best bet was to find my way back to the train station. I followed a street with an array of wires above. The wires meant that buses ran there during the day. When I reached an intersection where the wires stretched into different directions, I followed the wider street, hoping it would lead me to the train station. A drunk zigzagged towards me so I crossed the street and walked in the opposite direction. When I had to pee it was no problem finding a bush to squat by. At four in the morning, I found myself at the front gate of the hospital premises. I had a runny nose, a hacking cough, and horrible back pain. Hermine helped me sit back in the wheelchair in the hallway, and wrapped me in a heated blanket.

Monday, February 12

Hermine woke me up at 6:30. She was ending her shift and offered to drive me to the hotel that was supposed to be across the street from the hospital. I could see why I had been lost trying to find it. She couldn't find it either and drove around the block twice, before she did.

The hotel wanted $250 per night, but as Hermine had pointed out, it made a lot more sense to remain close to the hospital. I needed to go back to Maria Plains and get our belongings. I bought a package of five bus tickets and then took the bus to the train station. The bus driver didn't collect my ticket, and told me to sit up front; he would let me know when we were close to the train station.

At the train station, I called California and spoke to Patrick's sister. We both cried.

"Nancy, will you come to Austria?" I begged.

"I'll have to get a passport. Call me every day, and I'll let you know when I'll be there."

Patrick had been right about Rosemarie, the innkeeper. She couldn't have cared less about him being in the hospital. When I told her it might have been from the food at the restaurant she grew offended and said those things didn't happen in Austria. It was more likely he had caught a nasty disease in Turkey.

She was heartless.

"You don't get your belongings until you pay me for the room."

"Of course. Here is $150 for Saturday."

"No, you still owe me for Sunday. The total is $300."

"I couldn't call you from the hospital to let you know what was happening, and I couldn't come back that night."

"I don't want to hear about your husband. I want my money. I kept your belongings in your room, so you must pay me for both nights."

"This is very unfair. It's not like all the rooms were taken and you couldn't rent another room."

"I'll give you a break for last night. $150 plus $100, you owe me $250."

I handed her the money, but she still wasn't happy.

"Next, you go to the restaurant and pay what you owe them for dinner. How dare you leave without paying for your food."

"My husband was bleeding. When the ambulance came, that was the furthest thing from my mind. My husband was fine until he ate at the restaurant. I've been wondering..."

Her German accent became more pronounced, "There's nothing wrong with the food we serve there."

"How do you know? It's your restaurant?"

"That's right, it's my restaurant, and they have the bill ready. I expect you to go there right now, and pay what you owe them."

"Of course," I said.

I left the inn carrying one backpack on each shoulder, the two bags with our extra belongings, my broom and the large water jug. I had no intentions of going to the restaurant to pay for the dinner that had put Patrick in the hospital. I was sure he had swallowed a sharp object in the food they had served him. Nothing else made sense.

I walked down the hill and stood on the platform, waiting for the train to Salzburg. The weight on my back from both backpacks was beyond what I could normally carry. My shoulders were burning and going into spasms. My arms felt as though they were being pulled from their sockets. My lower back felt weak. My clothes sagged and I had to keep pulling my jeans up. I felt frail and was sure that I had fever and my cough was a deadly lung disease.

"Please, dear God, don't leave me. I need help to carry on. Please give me strength." Suddenly I felt as if most of the weight had been lifted from my shoulders. I knew God was carrying me the best he could.

Two young women, carrying their own backpacks and also waiting for the train, said they had never seen anyone as small as me carry so much stuff.

"It's not heavy. I have help." The train arrived just then and I was glad I didn't have to explain what I meant.

I dropped our stuff off in my room at the hotel and then called Nancy to let her know where I was staying. When I was leaving for the hospital, the ambulance driver who had taken Patrick to the hospital was waiting for me in the hotel lobby.

He handed me a bill. "You owe us $250 for yesterday."

"Do you take Visa?"

"No mam. Cash only."

I stopped at a restaurant for lunch and had to decide between a cup of soup or a salad for ten dollars each. I had both.

Patrick was unconscious, as one of the nurses explained, *way under* the effects of pain medication. He was breathing though a respirator. Tubes drained from his stomach, from his lungs. Computerized machines pumped him with fluids, drugs, antibiotics. Everything that anyone could do to maintain life, Patrick was connected to it. It gave me the willies to think that only a few days before he had insisted on having them if he was in that type of situation. I cried and cried and couldn't breathe.

I was convinced that I had the same condition as he did, except that it was gradually taking over my body, slowly, like an alien from another world. The nurses standing by his bed told me to leave and not come back until the next day. I would get a half-hour with him each day, at two o'clock sharp.

I headed to the emergency room and told them my husband was dying upstairs and I had chest and back pain and a nasty cough, probably from TB. I was shaking from the inside out and feeling so feeble, I was sure I had a high fever.

They took my temperature. It was normal. They listened to my chest. I had a chest cold. They told me I needed food and rest. I bought a bottle of iron and another of multi-vitamins at a local pharmacy.

I knew that once Patrick recovered he was going to ask for his money belt and count every penny. I needed to save all my receipts. My goodness, he was going to be angry. *I'll worry about that when the time comes.* Meanwhile, I was determined to have three decent meals a day. One of the caregivers gave me the address to an Austrian restaurant not far from the hospital. I needed protein in my diet. I looked for steak on the menu. It came with mashed potatoes and a green salad. I didn't check the price. I didn't care. It wasn't until I finished the last morsel that I thanked God for everything. I charged the $85 meal on our Visa.

That night, when I was lying in bed, I felt Patrick enter my room. I was going to ask how he had gotten out of the hospital, but I took it as something that he would do if he felt better. He seemed tired and wasn't talking. He lay next to me the way he always did, holding on to me. I couldn't stand the thought that he was back. I cried as softly as I could so

I wouldn't hurt his feelings. When I woke in the morning I knew it had been a nightmare.

Tuesday, February 13

I called Ralph. He had never heard of Boerhaave's Syndrome, but in his opinion a three-centimeter cut in the esophagus was too big to be from something Patrick had swallowed.

I went shopping for a bottle of brown hair color. Mama always said, "A man looks distinguished in white hair, a woman looks like an old rag." I had looked at myself in the mirror that morning and had to agree with Mama.

At noon, I ate lunch at a small restaurant that advertised spaghetti with tomato sauce for seventeen dollars. Any kind of pasta sounded good. The waiter barely spoke English. He pointed toward the sign advertising the spaghetti and then sliced his finger across his throat. No more spaghetti. He pointed to the menu and smiled. I picked another item on the menu for seventeen dollars.

He brought me an extremely large plate of fries with ketchup and large twisted link-sausages, dripping with grease, three of them. I patted the sausages with the napkins, and when the napkins were soaked I used the toilet paper from my backpack. I ate two sausages. A bit of fat might do me some good. I dipped the fries in ketchup to help chase the sausages down. I left the restaurant, and within a block, I vomited lunch.

It was still too early to visit Patrick so I stopped in a coffee shop. The heat inside wrapped me like a warm coat. The delicious smell of roasted coffee impregnated the very air, and I could almost taste it. Everyone wore a wool outfit that radiated a warm fuzzy feeling. I could spend all day there, among those who had no significant problems other than make sure their coffee wasn't too hot. Then I did the unthinkable. For the first time in my life I ordered a cappuccino. It made sense that if I was going to be part of that crowd I should drink with them. I made it just in time to catch the bus to the hospital.

I ran into Hermine, in the hallway and thanked her for taking care of me. I told her I was in a financial predicament. Between the cost of buying food and paying for my hotel, I would soon run out of money. She gave me a brochure with a list of places to stay that might be less costly.

Patrick's doctor was in the ward when I arrived.

"If your husband doesn't improve by tomorrow morning we'll have to proceed with a surgical procedure to clean his lungs. No one has ever survived Boerhaave's Syndrome, but given that he's so young and in exceptionally good health, he has a good chance of making it. Was your husband sick prior to arriving in Austria?"

"We were in Turkey, when we came down with a cold, but he seemed to have a stomach virus also. I remember in Istanbul he vomited violently one night."

"Maybe vomiting damaged the lining of the esophagus, but even that's questionable." He left.

"What can I do to help?" I asked the nurse sitting by his bed.

"Just in case he can hear you, talk to him. It might help with his recovery." She left.

I told Patrick how nice it was outside. The snow had not stopped falling and since he was a great skier, he needed to get well soon so he could enjoy it. As long as I remained cool and didn't think, I believed I could control my emotions. When I touched his forehead, it felt like sand paper. My chest felt heavy and I struggled to breathe. I cried until I got outside the hospital, where the cold breeze quickly dried my tears.

When I entered the hotel lobby the manager's wife yelled, "We do not want phone calls from America. Do you understand?" Her husband added just as angry, "Use your phone in your room to call your sister."

"Are you telling me that I can call but I can't receive calls? Why can't you let me know when my sister calls me?"

She cursed at me in German. I didn't have to understand German to recognize the same angry tone my father had used when he was upset. German already sounded harsh and when you added a higher pitch, an enraged red face, tightened lips that spit words out, one didn't need translation.

I visited a library, but all I found on Boerhaave's Syndrome were two pages of research written in 1993. The abstracts didn't mention the cause but assured the reader that if a patient was lucky enough to get diagnosed before the esophageal rupture, there was a better chance of survival. I made copies and saved them.

I skipped dinner and walked until the streets were deserted before returning to my hotel for the night. Upon reaching inside my coat pocket I found the list that Hermine had given me. According to the brochure, there was a hotel a little further away from the hospital, called The Wartenberg House. It was my father's last name. I wondered if the owners were my cousins.

Wednesday, February 14

Before going out that morning, I stopped at the hotel's front desk and asked if anyone had called. The same couple was still there. Perhaps they owned the hotel. They ignored me.

"Excuse me, did my sister from America called?"

The husband growled, "We are very busy. We are not responsible to let you know when someone calls."

"I'm sorry to bother you, but your phone is the only form of communication with my family." With what they were charging, they should be happy that all I asked for was to be kept informed if Nancy called. I made up my mind to visit The Wartenberg House before going to see Patrick.

Jana, the girl at the front desk of The Wartenberg House, was very sympathetic about my situation. She was the owner's daughter, although not my cousin. She showed me a room at the end of the house with a bathroom right next to it for ninety-five dollars a night. It included buffet breakfast and they took Visa.

Jana told me that the Wartenberg owners had disappeared during World War II, and for a long time the building had stood abandoned. Her family had bought the house from the government a few years back and had decided to keep the name of the original owners. The building was a prime example of old Austrian architecture. The furnishings looked like relics, or what someone in America would call, antiques. I knew Nancy would enjoy looking at their vintage furnishings when she came to meet me in Saltzburg. The hallway's dark wooden panels gave the impression of secret doorways. A light scent of floor wax filled the air, the wood floor squeaked. I loved that.

After I left The Wartenberg House, I stopped at a restaurant that advertised a lunch special that included a hotdog, sauerkraut and dumplings for the unbeatable price of fifteen dollars. The hotdog tasted like ladybugs, and after the first bite, I couldn't force myself to eat it. I'd never eaten a ladybug but I had played with them as a child while growing up in Portugal. I enjoyed watching them crawl from one of my fingertips to the other, and sometimes they would sit very still in the palm of my hands without fluttering their wings. The myth was that before blowing them gently away you should say, *ladybug, ladybug, find my love and tell him I love him.* They would diligently look for your mate and whisper to them they'd found you. I was only 9 or 10 years old and ladybugs were the closest to fairies.

Al used to call me weird when I associated certain foods with peculiar odors and taste like soap, ink, or rotten eggs. According to my alarmed mother, when I was three years old, she found me eating crude soap. Between first and third grade I had to use a dip pen into a small inkwell inserted in my desk. Using just enough ink to write without making a mess and using the blotter to dry each word was in itself an art. I quickly learned to lick my fingers so I would stay out of trouble. The rotten eggs was a given, we didn't have a refrigerator. There's only one odor and taste that I don't know how it came about. I've never shared this with anyone, because I would be locked up as a lunatic, but the flavor is death. Yes, death. I can't explain the association all I know is that my senses tell me the information and my perception agrees with it.

Nothing was new with Patrick. The doctors hadn't performed the planned lung surgery. They were waiting to see if he would improve on his own. After fifteen minutes, the nurse encouraged me to leave because I didn't look much better than him. "This hospital is one of the best and we are doing everything to make him comfortable. Go home. You need to rest."

I intended to get to the cause of what had happened to Patrick. I read the research I carried with me several times, but they were cold medical conclusions that provided few answers. I stopped at a medical school close by to ask the staff for their opinion. I believed that a sharp pointy object in his food had cut him, but they all told me the same thing as Ralph; a three-centimeter cut couldn't possibly be from anything he had swallowed. I wasn't convinced.

Back at the hotel, I informed the cranky couple downstairs I would be leaving the next morning, and then I returned to my room and started packing. Soon the manager knocked hard on my glass door, yelling that someone from America was calling. I picked up the phone. It was Nancy. "Phone call from America, no more!" He pounded on my door so violently I thought he might smash the glass.

I cracked the door. "Excuse me, I already heard you. I'm talking to her. No need to yell."

He shoved the door open and walked in, yelling in German. I backed away and raised my arms in defense.

"Tell American sister to call you upstairs directly!"

What a moron. Why couldn't he have told me that like a human being instead of yelling like a jerk?

Nancy heard the noise and asked why he was so nasty to her every time she called. I gave her the phone number at The Wartenberg House and told her that I was moving there the next morning.

I spent the rest of the afternoon going in and out of shops. I didn't plan to buy anything; I just wanted to get a feeling for Salzburg's way of life. For dinner I stopped at a deli and bought a sandwich for fifteen dollars. It included only a thin slice of ham and one of cheese, but the slices of thick bread had seeds and grains and it was very fulfilling. I retired early looking forward to leaving in the morning.

Thursday, February 15

I couldn't wait to enjoy the peaceful surroundings of my new lodgings at The Wartenberg House. I set my belongings on the floor, closed the door and dropped onto the bed, a thick queen-sized mattress that was neither too hard nor too soft. I lay on my back and stretched my legs and arms and then rolled over from one side to the other. A side table sat next to the bed, where I could keep my glasses and toilet paper in case I needed to blow my nose. My life didn't seem too bad at that point.

I murmured, "Thank you, God," Then I sat up and hung my legs over the side of the bed. An old-fashioned cream-colored armoire towered before me, its doors hand-painted with tiny flowers of blue and gold. Even though the delicate patterns made it look like a happy piece of furniture, its age was apparent in the chipped paint and dented edges and I felt that if it could speak it would tell me many stories I would be afraid to hear. I was sure the armoire had witnessed the ins and outs of the family that had lived in that house. I could feel it breathing. I could fill its menacing look upon me. I had no clothes to put in it. What I had was what I wore. I brushed aside the fact that I was simply too scared to open the armoire.

I lay Patrick's belongings in the corner of the room, next to a small writing desk and a chair. I planned to buy a pad of paper the next day and start writing my diary once again. There wasn't much to see outside my window, except for a few snow-covered roofs and a narrow alley with two garbage cans. I closed the heavy maroon curtains. When pulled closed, they would block all sunlight and let me sleep in as late as I wanted.

I didn't see any need to carry my backpack any longer. I felt confident everything was safe in my room. All I needed with me was the money belt with the passports and airline tickets. Before leaving I slipped the bus tickets and some money in my jeans' pocket for easy access. I locked the door and headed out for my usual walk before visiting Patrick.

Patrick's condition remained the same and he was still heavily sedated. I would bring his camera the next day to take pictures of him, before he improved. Back in California, he had laughed while showing me several pictures he had taken of cadavers he had dissected in school. Given his morbid sense of humor, I knew I had better take pictures of him so he could enjoy them later on.

I didn't stay long. I felt bad for being such a weakling, but every time I visited him I became physically sick and mentally disturbed. I knew I didn't have TB, but that only meant I had some unknown disease.

I rode the bus to the train station just because I had extra bus tickets and nothing else to do and then walked the rest of the afternoon. I ate a cup of hot vegetable soup for an early dinner. Afterwards, I stopped at a mini-market and purchased laundry soap and a large pad of onion skin writing paper. I hurried back to The Wartenberg House.

When I walked in, Jana informed me that Nancy was on the line.

"How is Patrick?" she asked.

"No change. I'm sorry." I cried.

"I'll soon be there with you. I expect to get my passport in a week. I already bought the airline ticket, which is contingent on getting the passport on time. You hang in there, you hear?"

"It's so horrible, Nancy. I don't know how much longer I can stand it." I cried harder.

"Remember that we love you and the family is all rooting for you. Stay strong. I'll call you as soon as I have more details."

Nancy would faint if she saw how dirty my clothes were. It was time to do laundry. I crossed my fingers that none of the other hotel guests would come knocking on the bathroom door. First I took a hot sudsy shower and then put all my clothing into the tub. I tossed what I felt was about the right amount of detergent powder over the clothes and covered them with hot water. I stepped back into the tub and beat the clothes with my feet. But that wasn't getting out the dirt, so I kneeled in the tub and scrubbed. Soon I was covered in detergent. I turned on the shower to wash the detergent off my body and then stepped out of the tub. I had to rinse the clothes several times to get rid of the soap. The tub was deep and wide and my lower back was going into spasms from bending, but I felt a lot of satisfaction knowing that in the morning I would have clean clothes.

When I tried wringing the water off each piece, my jeans and coat resisted. I stuck my head out of the bathroom to make sure the coast was clear. I wrapped myself in a bath towel and ran to my room, carrying an armful of wet laundry. I hung everything over the hot radiator by the window and then returned to the bathroom to clean it. I took the towel I had wrapped myself with and wiped the floors and the tub. Then I sat on the toilet to consider how to get back to my room naked. Someone knocked.

"House cleaning," a sweet voice said. "How much longer before I can come in to clean the bathroom?"

"I forgot my clothes in my room. By any chance do you have a dry bath towel I can wrap myself with?"

She returned with two large heated towels.

I lay in my warm bed and stared at the ceiling. I could hear the crackling of footsteps by my door. I thought little of them, until I heard them from inside the armoire in my bedroom. I had no doubt that the house, and my bedroom in particular, was haunted. My heart was beating fast when I fell asleep.

I woke in the middle of the night after hearing them coming into my room. They were going through all my things. One of them lifted my head to look under my pillow. I opened my eyes but it was too dark to see any of them. I could feel their breath on my face, the heat emanating from their bodies. They spoke in excited voices, all at the same time. A few even laughed.

One stood on my left side and spoke with a German accent. "Let's see where she has the money belt." I heard from the one with a German accent, standing on my left side. My heart was pounding hard. I fought them with closed fists and legs kicking as hard as I could.

They pulled my blanket and bed sheet off.

"Let's turn her over. Tummy up!" said a female voice harshly. Then someone else yelled out, "Here it is. I found her money belt!" She laughed with contentment.

They must have used a scissor or knife to cut the money belt off my waist. Their efficiency told me they were professionals. Then they were gone, along with all my sand bags and my broom.

I waited for the room to grow quiet, and then yelled for help as hard as I could, but no sound came out. I was enveloped in silence, my eyelids glued shut. I felt at a complete loss and time seemed to stand still.

A sliver of sunlight protruded through the partially open curtains, allowing enough light for me to survey the room. My heartbeat echoed throughout my body. I turned on the table light and quickly realized it had all been a nightmare.

Friday, February 16

As I had hoped, my clothes were dry in the morning. Feeling brand new in my clean attire I headed downstairs for breakfast.

Next to the fireplace stood a long table, laden with an all-you-could-eat Austrian breakfast.

Three types of artisan bread, including bread rolls, butter, cheese, ham slices, soft-boiled eggs to perfection, the most delicious Muesli made with raisins and nuts—yogurt, honey, fresh fruit, four kinds of homemade jam, freshly squeezed orange juice, coffee and tea.

Adolph, the waiter, was a middle age man with a heart of gold. He brought me a cup of hot chocolate and whispered, "Jana told me about your predicament. Take all the food you need to your room, but don't let the other guests see you do that."

I waited until everyone was gone before approaching the buffet table with my backpack. I made a ham and cheese sandwich and wrapped it in one of the cloth napkins and then added a banana to my booty. I returned to my room to turn the heat off, put my food on the window ledge and opened the window ever so slightly so the cold would keep everything fresh.

Patrick looked worst. His eyes had sunken in and he had the look of death. I cried harder than ever. Just in case he could hear me, I said, "I swear, when you get better, I'm going to punch you with all my strength if you complain about stupid things that are of no importance whatsoever. Health is the only thing that's important, nothing else matters, do you hear me?"

Feeling emotionally strong again, I pulled the bed sheet up and moved it to the side so that I could take pictures. He would be impressed. Cuts and stitches covered him. Fluids pumped in and out. Blood ran through tubes. Wires stretched from the machines to the pads stuck to his chest, where the color of iodine was as prevalent as the bruises around his chest. Like mama had told me several times, may God never show us how much we can endure. He looked absolutely horrible. Then I heard him in back of my mind, "You would look horrible too if you were going through all of this crap."

The nurse walked in and yelled, "Stop. You're not allowed to take pictures."

"You don't know my husband. If I don't take pictures to show him what he looked like when he was in the hospital, he'll make my life hell."

"That's appalling."

"No, it's sad, it's pathetically sad." I walked out of the hospital, into the streets of Salzburg. My cough wasn't improving. Every time I coughed up phlegm, my lungs hurt even more. Walking in the cold was not conducive to healing, I needed to stay warm and get some sleep.

Once in my room I closed the window and turned the heat back on. I ate my sandwich and banana, and then took a hot bath. At six o'clock, I sat on my bed and stared at the armoire. I had no doubt the people who used to live in the house hadn't left. Their spirits hid inside the walls and armoire. I couldn't go through another night of terror. I would have to appeal to their human souls. I closed my eyes and put my hands together in prayer. Inside my head I spoke softly to those I couldn't see but whom I hoped could see me.

Okay guys, friends, perhaps family too, I'm not sure. You came into my room last night to hassle me, probably thinking it was funny. It wasn't funny at all. I didn't like it, okay? Look, I'm very, very sick with some kind of lung disease that's taking away all my strength. I can barely make it through the course of the day while waiting to hear if my husband is going to live or die, and I need to sleep if I'm going to make it through my own nightmare. I need your help. Please, give me a break and leave me alone. I'm asking you, from one soul to another, to let me be. Thank you for respecting my wishes.

I waited for a response. When I didn't hear anything I knew the ghosts were gone.

Saturday, February 17

After breakfast I stashed my rations for the day in my room and then sat at my desk. I first made a quick entry into my diary and then wrote letters to my family. Jana's mom gave me the address and directions to the American Embassy, where I hoped they would help me find a job. Perhaps they knew an American family looking for a babysitter. I needed an income, and something to occupy me besides walking all day.

The secretary to the ambassador was a clone of Rosemarie, the inn's manager. She was not cooperative. "Forget suing the restaurant, because there's no litigation in Austria."

"That's not the reason that I'm here. I'm hoping that you can help me find a part-time job."

"Americans are always trying to sue for everything, so if you're even thinking about it, forget it." She shook her head and asked snottily, "Does your husband have insurance?"

"We have International Student Insurance."

"Get ready to pay the bill."

"One more reason I need a job."

She said she would call if something came up, but I could tell she was just trying to get rid of me.

I had two hours left before visiting hours. I walked back to The Wartenberg House. In my room I wore my coat while eating lunch. To maintain the freshness of my foodstuff it was essential the room remained cold until dinner time.

When I arrived at the hospital the doctor told me they had tried to cut back on the drugs that morning, but he didn't open his eyes. He just began coughing.

I left the hospital. A dirty gray mush covered the streets. Everything was gray; the tunnels, the buildings, the sky, and my thoughts. I was trapped in an expensive colorless world of hopelessness and doom.

I turned on the heat when I returned to my room and then took a long hot shower. After dinner, I sat at my desk to write in my diary, but instead I tore out two pages and wrote my last will and testament. At present all I had of value were the sand bags and the broom. I gave a lot of thought to what I did own back home, and did my best to write as professionally as possible. "This is my Last Will and Testament. Saturday, February 17, 1996. Me, Veronica Esagui, being of sound mind, decrees that my Japanese doll and my grandmother's dress go to my granddaughter, Shayna Esagui. The stamp collections, including all three bags of loose stamps, go to my grandson, Jacob Esagui. All crystal, silverware and other family heirlooms should be divided equally between my sons, Ralph Esagui and Steve Esagui. The broom goes to Nancy for her fireplace, the sand collection to Paul, Patrick's son, the large wooden jewelry box from China goes to Christine, his first wife, and the smaller one goes to Lauren, his daughter. All my jewelry goes to Diane, Steve's wife."

I put the document in an envelope and addressed it to Ralph. *If I send this letter out I'm sealing my fate. It will mean that I gave up. My family will remember me as a coward.* I tore the envelope and the letter into small pieces and threw them into the wastebasket. The next day I would have chest X-rays and go from there.

Sunday, February 18

The alley I walked through every day to get to the hospital was less slippery. It rained during the night, washing away some of the mush and ice. My lungs ached every time I coughed, even with shallow breaths. When I arrived at the hospital, I headed to the ER. I told them that I wanted a chest X-ray to rule out tuberculosis or pneumonia. I didn't care what the price was; I had to find out what I was dying from.

The out-patient radiology department was in a massive brick building across from the hospital. It stood alone. The automatic glass doors opened to a large empty waiting room graced by a few black metal chairs. The empty hallways, closed doors and the lack of anyone around reminded me of the mental hospital in New Jersey where I had almost been taken for an inmate when I went to pick up a straightjacket—a prop needed for a play I was producing at the time.

I picked up one of the black phones in the hallway and said, "Is anybody home?" A young girl dressed in a nurse's uniform, with a matching cap took my voucher and asked me to follow.

The first X-ray came out blurry. She told me I had moved and needed to take another one. The second time she forgot to put the film in the cassette. I believe she was learning to take X-rays and was a bit nervous. The third X-ray worked fine. I waited in the hallway for the radiologist to look at it. He told me he couldn't see anything, but said I should stay in the hospital for further testing. He wanted to rule out a possible embolism. "Radioactive injection will show the problem more clearly." He spoke with a heavy German accent.

"I'll be back later."

I left the building talking to myself. *You better start taking care of yourself.*

Given my circumstances answering seemed just as admissible. *Yes, I better. I will continue with my daily intake of vitamins, and treat myself with three meals a day.*

Hum, what about sleep? You need to sleep more.

Okay, okay, I'll sleep as much as I can.

One of Patrick's doctors assured me his condition was stable even though his heart was severely enlarged. A specialist would be arriving from his trip to Italy on Monday morning; he would be examining Patrick and most likely insert a drainage tube deeper than the pericardium.

I returned to the hospital later in the afternoon. I wanted to know more about what was going on with Patrick's heart, and why they were waiting until Monday to do the procedure. I was told not to come to the hospital unless it was visiting hours, which was when doctors made their rounds. I left to get a present for Hermine. I bought her a small box of chocolates and returned to the hospital's floor where she worked.

She hadn't given me her last name, and no one knew who I was talking about even when I described exactly what she looked like. They told me there was no nurse who looked like what I described or by such a name. I couldn't have been that much out of my mind. I knew I had not imagined her. I would carry on with my investigation the next day.

While walking the streets and feeling sorry for myself, I wondered what the future held. I asked God to help me and apologized for bothering him when he was most surely busy with other things around the world that were a lot more important than me. I finished my prayer with one request. *Please send me an angel. I really, really need one.*

Monday, February 19th

Before going to see Patrick, I stopped in the ER to ask for information about the night Patrick was admitted to the hospital. I confirmed with them the floor where he was first operated on. It was the same floor I had been to the day before. I asked to speak to the head nurse.

"I'm looking for Nurse Hermine. I would like to give her this box of chocolates as a thank you for taking care of me."

"I don't have anyone working for me by that name."

"She was here the night my husband had surgery. She gave me hot tea and cookies and took care of me that night. She's a little taller than you, slender, very light complexion, blue eyes and light brown hair parted to the side, mid-forties and spoke English well."

"Your description doesn't ring a bell. Also there is no one by the name of Hermine working on this floor."

"What about Ermine or Jermine or Fermine. There must be a nurse on this floor with a first name that sounds like Hermine. Maybe her last name was Hermine."

"Miss, I know all my staff. You are confused."

"She had a car. The next day, she drove me to the hotel across the street."

Two nurses that had joined her looked at me as if I had lost my mind. I told them that they could keep the chocolates and went upstairs to see Patrick.

A nurse introduced me to a doctor who had worked on Patrick early that morning.

He shook my hand and said, "Good to meet you. A team of surgeons including myself performed open-heart surgery on your husband early this morning. It was a very successful procedure and he should be returning to his ward very shortly."

I dropped to my knees. "Oh my God! Do you mean you opened his chest again? I thought you were just inserting a tube for drainage."

He helped me up and pointing to a bench. "Please sit down." He sat next to me. "I couldn't drain the heart with the tube; the fluid had coagulated. The only way to save your husband was to open the chest cavity in order to make an incision into the heart. The infection of the mediasteum was quite severe. The thickness of the fluid meant it had to be taken out by hand."

"So now he's going to recover and get well?"

"Your husband is going to get better now," he said, calm and reassuring.

I didn't believe him. I left without seeing Patrick, crying without restraint. It felt good to cry and not be reprimanded. I took the elevator down into the lobby. No one was there.

I walked in circles around the empty chairs in the center of the lobby, around and around, mumbling to myself. The chairs were the only objects that I could hold on to, my only friends. When I was a little girl I used to hide and play under my Uncle Augusto's office chairs, hoping to escape from having a shot of penicillin, the miracle drug of the 40's for running noses, coughs and anything else that ailed me. Now there was no place to hide. I felt exposed to the merciless white walls. Guttural sounds rose from my throat, a sense of crying without tears. I refused to allow the walls to close in on me. As long as I kept walking, I couldn't be crushed. I *'m crazy. I know I'm crazy, I'm totally out of my mind. If I could fit, under one of these chairs I would be fine. This is not fair.* Then I said loud enough to hear my words bounce off the white walls, "This is not fair". I walked between the chairs, and then I climbed on one and jumped from one to another.

Anything to help to cope with the pain. He was dying up on the fourth floor all alone, cut-up and bleeding. I felt a sudden sense of vertigo a spinning effect that drew me to the ground, but I knew if I did I would never get up again. A man appeared at the end of the long empty hallway, wearing pajamas and a flannel plaid robe. I didn't understand German, but I could tell by his tone that he was asking me, "What is the matter with you?" or perhaps, "What in the world are you doing?"

Finally, a human being! I stretched out my arms towards him.

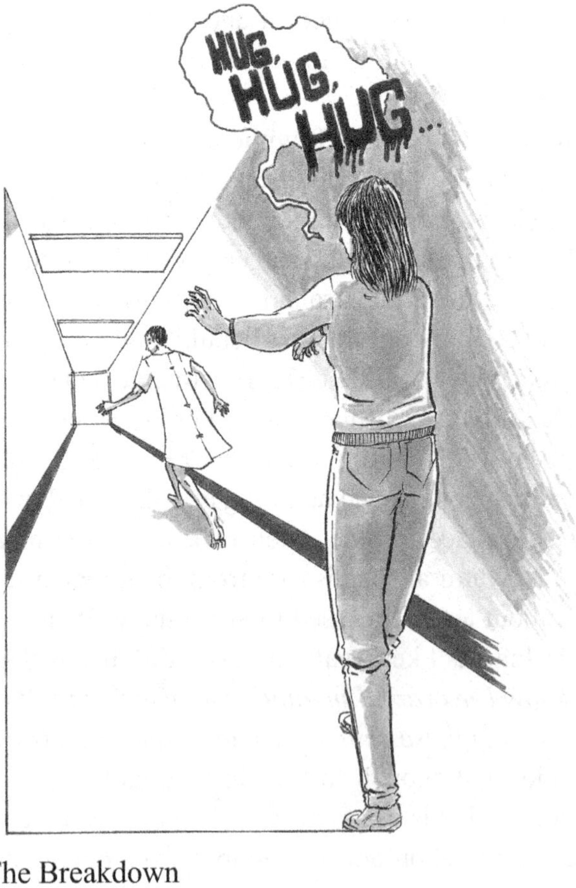

The Breakdown

"Please, I need a hug." I walked towards him, my arms stretched out and my hands opening and closing. "Hug, hug, hug!"

The poor man ran in the opposite direction, yelling at me in German, "Stay away from me you wacko!"

What are you trying to accomplish with this irrational behavior? You are out of your mind.

It's called a nervous breakdown, and I'm entitled to it.

Oh yeah? Well, you better get the heck out of here before someone takes you to the loony ward and give you electrical shocks to bring some sense into your head.

I rushed out of the hospital, and didn't slow down until I reached the warmth of The Wartenberg House.

Mrs. Vector saw me, she said, "Mrs. Veronica, you don't look right. I'll bring you some medicinal tea to your room. You need to rest."

I closed the window, sat on my bed, and stared at the curtains, wondering how many yards of material it had taken to make them and whether they'd been sewn by hand or made in a factory. Before I knew it, Mrs. Vector was knocking on my door, carrying a cup of tea and two English novels: *Dare to Dream* and *Mistral's Daughter.*

I slept the rest of the day, bundled up in blankets. I woke at eight, turned on the heat, and ate both my lunch and dinner. Then I propped myself up in bed and started *Dare to Dream.*

It was snowing again and staying in my room reading was the best thing I could do. I read half the book and at eleven o'clock I fell asleep again. I awakened to the sound of creaking. The house creaked all around me and that felt good. I was among family. Even if they were dead, they were my friends. They looked over me while I slept. Everyone at The Wartenberg House, dead and alive, took care of me.

Tuesday, February 20

A knock at my door woke me at eight. I climbed out of bed and opened the door. No one. One of my dead Wartenberg relatives must have been making sure I was up in time for breakfast. At this point in my life, I didn't dwell on anything that to others might be considered unusual. I mumbled thank you and close the door.

I took a leisurely shower and dressed. Then I waited a few more minutes until nine, thinking the breakfast room would be almost cleared of guests by then. It was easier to get my food into my backpack that way, and I didn't want to get Adolph in trouble. Even though I had his blessing and the staff looked the other way, every time I took food, I still felt like a street beggar.

I finished reading *Dare to Dream* after breakfast. The book gave me a positive feeling about myself, that *yes* I could endure being in hell every time I saw Patrick.

Adolph asked me to return for lunch because he was going to prepare his specialty, a liver dish just for me and at no charge. In his opinion I was too skinny and too pale.

I took the bus to the post office to mail my letters home, and then walked to the train station so I could call Ralph collect. I took the bus back to The Wartenberg House. I didn't want to miss my liver lunch.

It had been prepared the way my mother used to make it. Marinated in vinegar and then well-cooked with sliced onions. Adolph told me that it was a compliment to him as a cook that I had licked the plate clean.

At 1:50 p.m. I was seated in the hospital at my usual bench in the small ICU foyer of the fourth floor. I faced the elevator door. To my right an etched sliding glass door to the ICU floor remained closed unless a nurse or doctor stepped out of the elevator, walked to the glass door, pressed a button and identified themselves over the intercom. No one else was allowed until two.

I stared at the closed elevator door like a watchdog. I had my mind made up, whoever came out next I was going to make human contact. A short square-bodied older woman stepped out. She wore a thick dark green wool coat that matched her gloves, scarf, and Austrian feathered hat. Her boots were shiny black and knee high. She remained standing in the foyer and looked at me with a blank look on her face. She could have spit fire on my face and I would not have changed my mind. She was a woman, an older woman, perhaps a mother or a grandmother I felt comfortable reaching out to her.

I stood from my chair, took two steps forward and asked, "Do you speak English?"

She looked suspicious at me. "Yah, I do. Why you ask?"

"Please forgive me. But my husband is dying inside there. Would you mind if I gave you a hug?"

She stiffened for a moment and then said very nicely, "Of course, my dear."

We hugged each other, and I cried quietly, afraid to scare her away.

She asked me all kinds of questions and told me her husband was also in intensive care and she understood how I felt.

"Do you have family in Salzburg?" she asked.

"No, I'm alone. I was traveling with my husband on our honeymoon when he became sick. I'm hoping to find a job to pay for my living expenses. If you know anyone, please pass the word around."

"Where are you staying, my dear?"

"I'm staying at The Wartenberg House, not too far from here."

"I know where it is."

The sliding glass door to ICU opened.

"Will I see you tomorrow?" I gave her another hug.

"Yah, I will be here to see my husband."

We waved at each other as we parted.

I entered Patrick's ward with a more optimistic attitude. But something strange was happening to him. His body, arms, and legs had expanded with every muscle looking toned but larger than life. He looked like the Incredible Hulk. I couldn't take it anymore. My legs shook so much the nurse had to help me to stand. She led me out of intensive care and into the foyer, and then went to call Patrick's doctor to come and talk to me.

"We're sorry," he said. "Your husband's chest muscles are bleeding. The tube we inserted after the heart surgery ruptured an artery. He'll have to be in intensive care for at least two more weeks."

I was dumbfounded. I went back to ICU to Patrick's side, but couldn't look at him. I was thinking how his father had ruined Patrick's lungs by smoking next to him and how hard Patrick had worked out all his life to keep his lungs strong. I heard him telling jokes, making me laugh, and pushing me to the limit to keep up with him. The moments he had embarrassed me or made me feel worthless now seemed like wonderful times. I looked at him, but no longer recognized him.

I headed to the hospital's administration office.

A woman sat behind the wide wooden desk. She reminded me of my high school principal. Late forties, lacking any female endowments, her blonde thick hair combed back as if glued to her skull and tied in a bun. She looked very sanitary in her starched white shirt and brown pleated wool skirt. I felt humbled sitting in her presence. I placed my hands between my knees and sat on the tip of the chair. "With my husband here in the hospital and me having to live in a hotel, I need a job as soon as possible. Do you have anything available for me to do?"

"Do you speak German?"

"No, but I'll do whatever. I'll clean toilets if that's all you have available."

"If you don't speak German, how can your supervisor tell you what needs to be done?"

"They can point."

"No, my dear, that's not going to happen in our hospital. There's no work here for you." She stood and showed me the way out.

I spent the rest of that day going from store to store inquiring about a job. They were all run by family members and weren't hiring.

Nancy called. I could use the phone for only two minutes. The hotel had only one line. That probably was the case at the previous hotel with the cranky managers.

I turned on the heat in my room. I ate dinner, washed my clothes, took a hot shower, and lay in bed reading. It felt like I had just fallen asleep when Mrs. Vector knocked at my door. "The International Student Insurance Company called from the United States and left a phone number for you to call. You must use the telephone at the post office or at the train station to return the call."

I lay down and tried to put my thoughts in order, but didn't wake up until eight the next morning. Whatever disease I had made me sleepy as all hell.

Wednesday February 21

I rode the bus to the train station and called the insurance company. Mrs. Simpson, the insurance liaison as she referred to herself wanted to confirm Patrick's social security number. They would cover his hospital bill up to $100 per day for sixty days and provide his transportation back to the US. He was covered up to twenty-five thousand dollars. I was in shock with the good news. Mrs. Simpson promised me she would stay in contact with the doctors and every few days call me to find out how I was doing.

It wasn't until I hung up that it clicked what she had said. They would be paying for his transportation to the US? That didn't make any sense. The next time Mrs. Simpson called I would have to tell her that Patrick already had a return plane ticket.

I got to the hospital at 1:45 and was very disappointed the lady I had met the day before didn't show up. I walked into ICU determined not to fall apart and did my best to remain calm and detached as I stood by his bed. If I were in his shoes, I would definitely feel better if someone held my hand and told me I was going to get well, rather than having someone spilling tears all over me as if I were dying. Suddenly, I had a feeling that someone was staring at me and looked up. An older woman with a bright smile and a purple fuzzy hat stood by the doorway. She smiled as if she knew me. I threw her a kiss, and she threw one back. She was gone as fast as she had appeared.

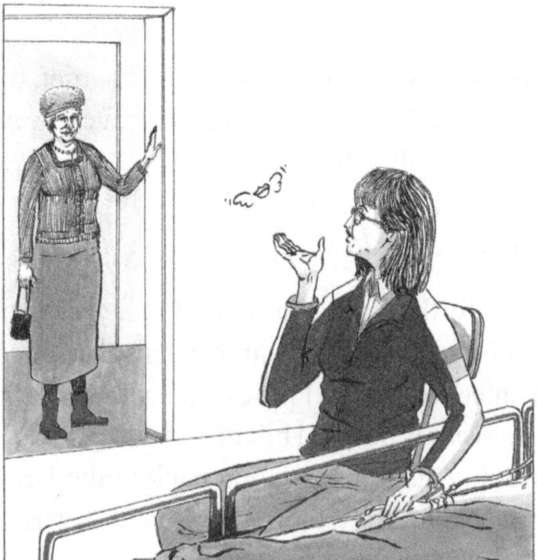

Brunhilde

I didn't think much about it and returned my attention to Patrick. I took a deep breath and, even though he looked the worst ever, I smiled. I kept that smile going the whole time as I spoke to him about the weather outside and told him not to be afraid because I was right next to him. I sang a few of his favorite tunes, mostly from the Rolling Stones, his favorite group.

"I know you like country music, but I don't think you want to hear me botch up some of what you call good music." If he was listening, he was no doubt laughing at my wit. As always, a doctor stopped by the room to see if I had any questions.

"It's very nice that there's always a doctor available when family members are here during visiting hours. How is my husband doing today?"

"Your husband isn't any worse. In two or three days we are going to try to wake him up again. His internal bleeding has stopped."

"That's great news." I lifted his bed sheet. "What about these red circles on his chest. Is that from shock pads to make his heart work?"

"Oh, that's nothing. This morning his heart was going too slow and we speed it up just a little. Nothing to worry about, my dear."

Smile Veronica. Smile.

"Thank you Doctor, for taking such good care of my husband. Now I know he's going to get well soon." I spoke loudly enough for Patrick to hear.

"Just a little fever," the nurse told me after taking his temperature.

"That's right, just a little fever to get rid of the infection and those little white cells. Hey Patrick, we survived the bus trip from Turkey and you'll make it through this one too."

I took my time walking to The Wartenberg House and used the occasion to have a heart-to-heart talk with God, who I felt was always there for me.

Dear God, I do not wish for Patrick to die. I ask you, God, to save him, if you believe that's a good idea, of course. He told me several times that he couldn't take drugs because they affected his brain. I can't even think of what he will be like if he lives. I've asked you for an angel and I know how hard it must be to send someone from heaven. So please send me an earth angel who will offer me a place to stay. The longer I stay in Austria, the less I'll have left to buy my mother's stone, as I promised her in Turkey. Please, dear God, send me an angel as soon as possible.

When I entered the hotel, Mrs. Vector told me that a lady named Mrs. Hilpold had been waiting for me for over an hour and had finally left to go home. Mrs. Hilpold had left her phone number and wanted me to call her as soon as I came in.

"I don't know anyone in Salzburg. Who could it be?"

"I'm supposed to tell you she's the one you blew a kiss to in the hospital. She wants to take you home with her."

"Did she have a round fuzzy purple hat on?"

"Come to think of it, she did."

"Did she have wings?"

"Just the fuzzy purple hat. No wings." Mrs. Vector smiled.

Of course, my protecting angel had to have wings, but they were hidden under her coat. I had better not make a fuss.

Mrs. Vector made the call for me.

I picked up the receiver and turned away from her so she wouldn't hear me.

"Hello? Are you Hilpold, my angel?" I asked.

"Yes, I am," answered a sweet voice. "Call me Brunhilde."

"Brunhilde, that's a very nice name."

"I speak English not good. Would you like to see me? Will you come to my house tonight?"

"Yes, Brunhilde, my angel. I want to be with you."

"I'll be there immediately." She hung up.

Adolph saw me waiting in the lobby and signaled me to follow him to the kitchen.

"I told my wife about your situation. You can come live with us until your husband gets out of the hospital. We will take care of you until then."

"You and your wife are wonderful, and I thank you from the bottom of my heart, but I can't accept your kind offer. Adolph, I know it's hard to believe what I'm going to say, but God has sent me an earth angel and she's coming to take me with her."

"An angel? Did you say an angel?"

"Yes. You're the only one who knows about it."

His eyes narrowed and he stepped back. "There's no such thing as angels, Ms. Veronica. You better be careful."

Brunhilde ran into the room, still wearing the purple fuzzy hat. Adolph shook his head and walked away. Brunhilde and I hugged each other as if we had known each other since childhood, I held on extra-long, afraid to let go. She grabbed my arm and led me to her warm car left running outside by the front door. I couldn't help smiling at her small figure, and high-spirited character. *So that's what earth angels look like.*

Her driving convinced me someone was definitely looking out for her. An angel would never drive so haphazardly. She was too short to see above her car hood, or perhaps her eyesight was not good enough to measure distances, like the cars in front of her. Not once did she slow down at crossings, intersections, or red lights. I blessed myself when she drove at the same fast speed through a filled-to-capacity, semi-lit parking lot and into her compact parking space underneath her luxury apartment complex. "Me, get license to drive, three months ago. Me very proud, pass test."

"Congratulations. It's never too late to do anything in life if you really want to."

"Yes. Correct, and why you in Wartenberg House? Not good for American girl. Not good place to stay. You must stay here in my house. I take care of you. Please, I like to do that. Say yes to Brunhilde, me, my first name."

She showed me "my" bedroom and her bedroom, the living room and kitchen. She was very proud of being a good housekeeper. There was a certain German flair of neatness, old dark furniture without a speck of dust, everything equally spaced, the chairs, the bookcases, the bed covers with the decorative pillows, right down to the smallest details of the small side tables covered by dainty lace doilies. After being a theatre producer and designing most of the set designs, for almost ten years, anytime I was at someone's home I couldn't help but to take an overall inventory of its contents thus providing me a clear image of the residents' personality. She planned to pick me up from The Wartenberg House the next morning at eight.

I thanked her whole heartedly and she drove me back to the hotel. We both hugged and cried and then said goodnight.

~ Chapter Thirty ~

My Austrian Angel

Thursday February 22

Brunhilde picked me up at precisely eight. I hugged everyone at the Wartenberg House and thanked them for taking such good care of me. I went to the kitchen to say goodbye to Adolph. "I saw who is taking you home. Are you sure you want to go with her?"

"Of course."

"Be careful, my friend."

Brunhilde zigzagged through traffic easily, her driving not nearly as scary in the daylight. She made me laugh. She was a fearless racer and I admired her superhero personality.

The rest of the morning we sat at her kitchen table and cried and laughed and shared stories. Brunhilde must have been a blonde in her younger days, her short curly hair was a mixture of white and dirty blonde now and her white complexion except for a few age marks and deep lines around her eyes and lips made me think that she was in her mid-seventies. It's a fact that most people about her age start to lose muscle mass and since Brunhilde was not overweight, she looked elegant. Her English was not very good but decent enough to understand. Hans, her husband had died the previous month, after suffering for five years with a heart condition. The days before he died, he lay in his bed and stared at the bedroom door, hoping to see his daughter one last time. Brunhilde felt that he had died from a broken heart, when their daughter refused to see him.

Brunhilde's brother was in the same hospital as Patrick, in the room next to him. He had suffered a stroke, and she wasn't sure if he would live. Ana, the woman I had hugged coming out of the elevator, was Brunhilde's sister-in-law. That evening, Ana had called Brunhilde and told her about our encounter by the elevator at the hospital and my situation. Brunhilde woke that night from a dream in which her husband had told her to take me home and to do everything she could to help me. That's what she had done.

Her first husband had died during World War II, just six months after they were married, and Hans, her second husband who just died, had been a prisoner of war in the US. I didn't quite get the complete story, but didn't want to pry.

Brunhilde was a great cook. For lunch she served a delicious beef and vegetable stew she had made the night before. I ate all the bread she gave me by soaking it first in the sauce. From her kitchen window on the third floor, I could see the Austrian mountains covered with snow.

We walked to the hospital, holding on to each other's arm. She left to see her brother and I stayed with Patrick. His condition remained critical.

On the way home, Brunhilde saw an older couple walking towards us. They had a very distinct stern look. Their dark green hats matched the heavy wool material of their coats. She squeezed my hand as if alarmed by their presence and whispered, "I must say hello to them. Please don't follow. Stand here and don't move."

She was visibly disturbed about what they said to her, and when the couple was out of sight, she grabbed my arm, shaking.

"They are bad, stupid people. They not hurt you. I protect you."

"Thank you, Brunhilde."

I wondered who the couple was and why they had frightened her. If she was an angel, they must have been two devils.

On the way home she bought a beautiful bouquet of fresh flowers to put in my bedroom. Once home, she put them in a vase and then we sat at the kitchen table, talking while we held hands and cried together. She had lost her husband and her only daughter would not speak to her. Her grandson was a student in Berlin and she saw him only during Christmas. She had no one in her life to comfort her. I was lucky. I had family in the U.S. I hugged her, and tried to console her every time she cried. She needed a lot of affection and someone to talk to. I wondered if Patrick would consider us taking Brunhilde with us to the U.S.

For dinner she served radishes, soup broth, toast, and cheese. I saw her take a pill and asked her what it was for.

"Blood pressure very high. Me needs medicine."

Before bedtime, we ate vanilla pudding. I noticed that if I didn't cry, Brunhilde didn't cry either. Crying seemed to be contagious for both of us.

"Brunhilde, you have cried a lot since your husband died. If you don't cry any more I won't either. How about we protect each other from crying? Do you want to be happy together?"

She was like a child, and her spirits grew. We agreed that we would talk only about happy things, even if we had to make them up. "Deal, Veronica, American girl! I glad you here. I love America and Americans." She shook my hand as if we were sealing a contract.

She was so sweet. Her daughter had to be a nut case not to love Brunhilde.

After taking a very difficult shower—there was no shower curtain to keep the water from splashing all over—I put on the blue flannel pajamas she lent me. She tucked me into bed and covered me like a mother would her child.

"And now I tell story before you sleep." She described her life as a girl on the farm her parents used to have on the outskirts of Salzburg. She promised that the next day she would show me pictures of the farm and her family before the war.

When I closed my eyes, she kissed me on the forehead and tiptoed out of my room. When she left, I thought about how kind God had been to me and began to cry. I was in a warm bed, wearing fresh, clean, flannel pajamas. Brunhilde was not a celestial angel, but she was definitely an earth angel, and God had put her in my path. I couldn't have been more thankful than I was that night.

Friday, February 23

For breakfast, Brunhilde served toast, cheese, and jam, and then offered me tea or coffee.

"Just hot water please. No tea bag. Any chance, do you have a slice of lemon to put in it?"

"Interesting. Americans drink tea with no tea bag?"

"That's right. Healthy Americans don't drink anything with caffeine."

I was hoping to influence her enough that she would follow my example and give up caffeine all together.

"Caffeine bad?" She asked in a childlike tone.

"Yes, it increases blood pressure. That's why I drink hot water with lemon, so I'm healthy. No tea and no coffee."

"I want to be like you. No more sick. No more pills."

She poured her coffee into the sink and prepared a cup of hot water with a lemon peel. Then she sat next to me with a big, bright smile. "I want to be American. No more blood pressure high."

"Salt isn't good for blood pressure either."

"I like very much salt."

"Me too. I like salt, but if you don't use salt in your food, I promise to eat without salt too. How about it?"

"You are my true friend. You like salt, but you eat no salt, for me?" She hugged me and did not let go. She started crying. I pushed her away gently. "If you cry I have to cry too."

"Oh, sorry. I stop. I never have friend like you."

"If you don't eat salt, I won't either," I said. "That's what good friends do for each other and I want you to live and be healthy."

"Okay, no more salt in food." She smiled.

We spent the morning seated at the kitchen table, sharing funny stories and laughed a lot. We cried only once.

After lunch I headed to the hospital. Brunhilde stayed home to nap.

When I arrived, I discovered that Patrick had been taken for esophagus surgery. A fistula had to be stitched without delay. The floor nurse told me that Patrick's doctor had suspected the fistula for a while and the surgery was critical to his recovery.

I climbed into the elevator. I was alone. I kicked the wall. I punched it. I yelled, "This hell can't go on. They keep cutting him open like a bag of potatoes. How many times are they going to cut open his chest?" I hit my head once on the wall but I was afraid my skull was too soft and I would get brain damage. I kicked and punched until I was exhausted. Patrick would have been proud. He would have done the same thing—except he would have made a hole in the wall.

I had been expecting a long letter from Papa in response to the one I had sent him about Patrick being in the hospital. But I received only a telegram. "My blessings. Love, your father."

I called Bonnie to let her know that things were about the same with her son.

"Take care of yourself, Veronica. Just in case Patrick doesn't come home, I already withdrew the money in your joint account and hid it someplace safe."

"Thank you, Bonnie. You're very kind."

"I knew that money wasn't his to begin with. It's yours fair and square."

I could never repay Bonnie for her kindheartedness. What an incredible human being. I began crying, not because Patrick might die, but because Bonnie didn't deserve to lose her son.

On the way back I stopped at a bakery and bought a loaf of bread and some cottage cheese to take home. I wanted to help Brunhilde with some of the groceries.

She was very happy with the bread and showed me on the bottom of the loaf a stamp with the baker's name. Making bread in Austria was a bona fide craft passed down from generation to generation.

Brunhilde's English was a lot like my father's. They had learned it while youngsters in high school, and I admired how they could recall a language they barely used. There was no serious language barrier between us. We understood each other's pain.

"My daughter, perfect daughter, yah; good girl, busy, very busy, no time for me. My daughter, hard and not want to forgive. She no understand me. She ashamed of me, say me bad person. Veronica, my husband dead, I live all day here in front kitchen window, look at mountains and cry every day, here alone. My daughter no visit me, say good I am alone. My brother, now very sick in hospital, maybe die. My daughter says good, my brother die soon. My friend in Canada wants me to visit. My heart is in Canada. My daughter say me crazy; I must not go Canada. Wants me stay home, in kitchen, alone crying." She removed the handkerchief from her apron's pocket and wiped her tears.

"Would you do me a big, big favor?" I asked her.

"Anything you want I do. My husband tells me to help you. I told you dream, right?"

"Yes, you told me. You husband will be very happy if you go to see your friend in Canada, this spring. I will also be very happy. Do you promise to do that?"

"You be my daughter, better than my daughter. You love me. I promise to go to Canada."

That afternoon, Brunhilde and I took a long walk around the city. We were both in a great mood and everything looked funny to us. We stopped at a hotdog stand and she bought us a hotdog each.

"When you come to America someday, you must go to New York City. They have the best hotdogs in the world. They sell them in the streets like here, but the hotdogs are served in a bun and covered with mustard and sauerkraut and you eat it with your hands."

She said, "With the hands, hum? Americans smart. No dishes to wash." We laughed.

There was a phone message when we came home. I was to be at the hospital at six. Brunhilde stayed home.

Patrick's new surgeon came out to the lobby. He spoke with a heavy German accent. "Complete re-done of esophagus, heart re-done, left lung abscess found and removed. This triple surgery very complicated by damaged lungs. Chances? Don't know. Situation is critical. Now we wait. This is his last chance." He looked apprehensive when he added, "We have done everything we can to save your husband."

Saturday February 24

I woke at five in the morning and couldn't go back to sleep. Being careful not to wake up Brunhilde, I sat down in the kitchen and stared out the window. A pigeon landed on the outside windowsill and looked at me. I took that as a message from Patrick. He loved pigeons.

"Is that you, Patrick? If it's you, tell me what you want me to do. Should I ask the doctors to pull the plug? I know how you feel about being connected to machines, but I still think it's horrible what you're going through. They tell me you don't feel anything. I hope it's true."

I don't remember going back to bed, but I woke in it at seven. Brunhilde was still sleeping.

I showered, and dressed. When she came into the kitchen she found me at the kitchen table staring out the window.

"Beautiful mountains, ya?" We hugged followed by the customary kiss on each cheek.

The phone rang. It was Nancy.

"I'll be arriving by train from Munich, on Monday."

"Hold on, let me share the good news with my friend Brunhilde."

Brunhilde was ecstatic. "Tell American sister stay with me. I change bed sheets and clean bedroom." She marched into my room while singing an upbeat German marching song.

"Do I hear someone singing in the background?" Nancy asked.

"It's my friend Brunhilde. She's the lady I told you about. She wants you to come live with her also."

Brunhilde came with me to the hospital. Her brother was on the same floor.

Patrick looked like a corpse. I tried to keep my crying quiet so I wouldn't annoy the other patients. I felt the panic rise when I struggled for air, as though an elephant had sat on my chest. I ran out of intensive care. Brunhilde was in the hallway waiting for me.

"Good news. My brother better. Transported morning early to nice hospital. Stays until strong enough to go home. No more danger, going to live."

Patrick's doctor saw us and came over. I asked him to give the details in German to Brunhilde. I couldn't listen any more to what they were putting him through. It was plain inhumane to continue with one surgery after another. When he was finished talking to Brunhilde, she grabbed my arm and said, "Let's go. We need pray together."

I didn't want to know what the doctor said. One doesn't go praying if it's good news.

She took me to two churches, and I did everything she did. I dipped my hand in holy water and made the cross on my chest.

"Now, we go see my brother, Ja? Together, ja?

"Ja, we go together."

Brunhilde asked me to sit in the waiting room while she visited her brother. I wondered why the waiting room had no one waiting, much like the hospital where Patrick was staying. It felt creepy.

Ten minutes later, I heard several people yelling down the hallway. An old, emaciated man in a hospital gown, probably in his mid-eighties, raced toward me in a wheelchair, using both hands to push himself forward. When he reached the elevator door to my left, he rammed the wheelchair into the elevator door screaming like a maniac. Even though I couldn't understand his words, it was clear he was desperate to get away. I had not seen Ana, Brunhilde's sister-in-law, since I had hugged her at the hospital. She was now running towards us, with Brunhilde right behind. They tried to stop him, but he maneuvered his wheelchair away from their grasp. For a second I wished I had a video camera. Ana finally blocked the wheelchair with her body, and Brunhilde grabbed the back of the wheelchair and hugged him from behind. Ana yelled at him but Brunhilde held up her hand and spoke calmly to the old man. He stopped screaming and twirled his chair around. Brunhilde walked to the payphone and dialed. She spoke in German, loud enough for the old man to hear. Then she walked back to him and patted him on his back. Ana wheeled him out of the waiting room.

Brunhilde sat next to me and said, "My brother sick." And she moved her finger in a circle to the side of her head. "Believes Nazi hunters after him. My brother SS officer, for our Hitler. Gets scared, very scared. Goes crazy. I make believe I call SS for help. I must do this all the time. Works good. Very, very good. He calms down." She wore a proud smile.

I smiled back awkwardly and slipped my hands into my pockets.

Ana returned, and stood before us and crossed her arms. Brunhilde stood, and they argued in German. Ana glanced in my direction every so often. Something told me that she wasn't happy about me having witnessed her husband act the way he did. Brunhilde said something back at her and then grabbed my arm. "Let's go Veronica."

Ana pushed me back into the seat and Brunhilde away from me. She bent forward and glared at me with eyes that felt like carving knives and asked in a tone that made my skin crawl, "Are you Jewish?"

I stared at her.

"She Catholic," Brunhilde said. "Stupid woman. I told you many times, she Catholic."

"I'm not sure." Ana's look was defiant. "Answer me! Are you Catholic?"

"Yes, I am."

"I'm not sure you are." She continued to argue in German with Brunhilde. At some point, Brunhilde pointed toward her brother's room.

Ana left us grumbling. Brunhilde grabbed my arm forcefully and led me down the white marble staircase, rather than the elevator.

"Don't pay attention to Ana. I tell her to go care for husband. Veronica, you, me leave hospital now. Ana cuckoo like my brother."

Once we were home, Brunhilde made two cups of hot water with lemon and we sat at the kitchen table.

She said, "I miss my farm. I miss the farm I grew up with my family. I want to show picture of farm to you." She stood and brought me a small black-and-white picture. I couldn't differentiate the tiny farmhouse from the land that she described as the most beautiful farm in Austria. The colors of her memories were still present in that faded photograph as she pointed to it and said, "See, here? My brother and me swim in this river."

I nodded.

"My brother, I love. Sad, only nineteen died airplane fighter for Germany. Good cause, but too young to die. Too young. I still cry today." She wiped away the tears. "I was fourteen, Hitler came to power. Hitler bring hope for people. My family work very hard in farm, but happy in Germany, in Nazi party for our Hitler. My family leave farm in Austria and we live in Germany. I marry good German man, happy married, six months. War no good, guns boom, boom make plane crash after six months."

I nodded again. *Holy Christ, this can't be happening. It's her English, I'm misunderstanding everything she's saying.*

"My brother, my husband, dies for my Hitler. Later I marry again. He very lucky. Prisoner in United States, American camp after plane crash. Americans good to everyone. I have daughter. She hate father and me. Father died. She don't come to see him to say goodbye. She says we bad people, ashamed. Don't let me see mine granddaughter. Me not welcome in her house."

Brunhilde cried. My tears poured out.

"Veronica, my American girl. War no good to German and Austrian people. War make suffer. Need to pray. Need to pray for your husband."

She didn't mention the Jews, the gypsies, or all the other people tortured and killed. She left the room and then returned with a tall glass prayer candle filled with red wax and a picture of Jesus with a halo and a bleeding heart in the middle of his chest. She asked me Patrick's last name.

"Is that Catholic name?" She lit the candle.

"No, it's a Christian name. He's Christian, and he definitely believes in Jesus Christ whole heartily. He loves Jesus." I answered joyfully since I knew it was true. Then I put my hands together in a prayer position and prayed that she would not ask me any more personal questions.

"Good. That's very good, Veronica. Let's pray to Jesus." She put her hands together and closed her eyes.

I did the same and I thanked God for giving me the wisdom to keep my mouth shut and for not informing her that, like Jesus, I was also Jewish.

Sunday, February 25

When I entered Patrick's hospital room the nurse told me he'd been in surgery an hour that morning and they had removed two of the tubes to his lungs. I decided that he had suffered enough. I planned to pull the rest of the plugs. Then I recalled what he had said in Turkey. I didn't stay long.

I needed Brunhilde's hugs as soon as possible. What I had witnessed the day before and what she had told me made as much sense as to what Patrick was going through. Brunhilde was the only thing in my life that kept me from going mad.

She was waiting for me in the lobby. "Him better?"

"The same as yesterday."

We spent the rest of the afternoon visiting the Fortress on the hill and then Salzburg's Old Town, which had lots of shops and restaurants. "Me take you to fine, expensive Austrian restaurant for dinner."

"Oh, please you don't have to do that."

"There are no pockets in heaven. Delicious food here. My favorite with my husband."

We entered what looked like a restaurant for Austrian royalty. Crystal chandeliers hung all around me, surrounded by golden cherubs painted on the ceiling. Then there was the golden silverware and gold trimmed dishes and glasses, cups and saucers. Real orchids adorned the center of the table covered with a white-laced tablecloth matching the starched napkins, trimmed in delicate lace. I picked up the salt-and-pepper shakers made for kings and queens and I held them in my hand appreciating its elegance. If Tracey, my kleptomaniac friend from New Jersey had been there, the shakers would have disappeared.

"Nice, ya?" asked Brunhilde.

"Ya," I said to her. "Very beautiful."

Our waiter wore a black tuxedo. He said something in German and dropped the menus on the table. He didn't smile. He said something else and stood erect like a soldier waiting for orders from a general.

Brunhilde said, "My friend American. Speak English when addressing us, please."

"Very well. Drinks?"

"We want two cups of hot water with lemon, please." She smiled at me.

"It will have to be coffee or tea. We do not serve hot water here."

"We want hot water with small piece of lemon. We drink like Americans." She laughed.

"I'll have to charge you the price of tea."

"Very well, charge fine."

I looked at the menu with padded black leather cover and a gold insignia in the center and then turned to Brunhilde for help. "Every time I eat out I order the wrong food. Whatever you're having you can order for me. I'm sure I'll love it too."

"You like pork?"

"My favorite. I love it more than chicken."

Our waiter approached us, carrying a silver tray with two porcelain teacups. "Ladies, here is your hot water with a slice of lemon each. The tea bags are on the side, in case you change your mind. Have you decided what to have for dinner?"

"Yes," said Brunhilde. "But can the chef prepare food without salt?"

He threw his head back, and sighed. "I'll be back."

I laughed so hard my cheeks hurt, Brunhilde had tears rolling down her face. "He pompous comedian."

"How much do they charge for tea?"

"Nine dollars each."

"That's a highway robbery."

"Highway? No. Tea robbery. I keep tea bags." She laughed and so did I. She slipped the tea bags in her purse. "I keep expensive tea bags and put inside my jewelry box at home."

The waiter returned and said, "The chef will make your food without salt, but he says he's not responsible if you don't like it."

Brunhilde ordered. "Liver dumpling soup, Styria pork pot roast and Salzburger Nockerl for dessert. Make everything double and no salt. You can take the shakers."

"Do not expect your food for at least an hour."

"No hurry. My American friend and me talk."

After he left, we reminisced over our wonderful husbands. We even cried a little. Brunhilde couldn't say enough good things about her husband, and I was obliged to do the same. I couldn't tell Brunhilde how I really felt about Patrick and that my tears were out of pity for myself. She wouldn't understand.

During much of our chat and our meal, an American couple sat at the table behind us. I barely noticed them leaving, but then the wife returned and stood before us. "I'm so sorry about your husbands. We heard your conversation. It's horrifying what you've gone through. I admire your inner strength and find it inspiring to see such wonderful friendship between you two. Please allow my husband and me to pay for your dinners."

She told us her name was Marilyn. I stood and hugged her. Brunhilde started to cry. Then I cried. Then Marilyn cried. Brunhilde gave Marylyn her home address and invited her to come over for a slice of her homemade apple strudel. Marilyn paid for our dinner and left.

When we got home, we sat at the kitchen table and, as always, she held my hands when she talked. She smiled. "American soldiers like me. They nice to me and give me food. I dream one day I go to America, to visit."

"When I go to America, I will send you my address and you come to stay with me."

Monday, February 26

I finally remembered to ask Brunhilde if she had a flashlight I could use during the night when using the bathroom. If I turned the light on in the hallway I was afraid I would wake her since she kept her bedroom door open. She retrieved an English-German dictionary from the bookcase in her living room and looked up the word flashlight. She said "You need a torch?"

"No, I don't need a torch." I laughed. "A torch is used for Olympic runners." She was so sweet so vulnerable, so kind. She was my Austrian Angel.

After breakfast we remained seated at the table like we usually did. She talked and I listened. "My daughter not love me. My grandson say he love me, but busy in Vienna, going to University." She cried and held my hands. "I call my daughter. She say sick with cold, not talk. I make chicken soup take to her house. She open door and say, 'Soup with poison.' And close door. I call husband of her. He say me not welcome, me bad. My daughter say, no forgive. I must pay, go to hell not heaven. But… I am good now, see I help you." She cried.

"You have helped me a lot and I appreciate it. If you had not come into my life, I would have been living in the streets by now. You're an angel of kindness and have showed me that there's hope for humankind."

She kissed my hands and I kissed her hands and we hugged. Where she fit during Hitler's time was something I didn't want to think about and felt it was better left buried in the past.

"When you back from hospital, I take you to visit my old friend, not seen for ten years. My friend daughter-in-law is Helena. You like meet Helena and talk Portuguese?"

"I like that a lot." I smiled. "Thank you, Brunhilde." I kissed her on the cheek and left.

Patrick's doctor saw me in the hospital hallway and said he would be right back to talk to me. I waited an hour and when he didn't return I tried to get in to see Patrick but visiting hours were over.

Brunhilde and I were about to leave her apartment when the phone rang. Nancy had just arrived in Munich. She was by herself and found the people in Munich to be very unfriendly. She was exhausted and decided to get a hotel for the night. She would call back the next day before taking the train to Austria.

Helena was in her late fifties and had been a well-known opera singer in her younger days, back in Portugal. Her curly shoulder length jet-black hair didn't compliment her white skin complexion even though she had no wrinkles. According to my Aunt Heydee, the secret to maintaining youthful skin as we get older is to gain 5 pounds each year and the skin will keep stretching. Helena was obese. Brunhilde introduced me to Helena, her husband, the mother-in-law, their cousins and aunts, all seated in a circle in the living room. Helena and I sat next to each other. She told me about her life as a singer and we spoke Portuguese while eating butter cookies and mini chocolates. Everybody had tea or coffee except Brunhilde and me.

Brunhilde stood up from her chair, tapped her spoon on her tea cup and announced like a news broadcaster, "Attention, attention. Veronica, my American friend, and me, only drink hot water with lemon. Tea, coffee and salt no good for blood pressure. My friend, Veronica is my doctor. Veronica is a chiropractor. I need no more medicine." She went on to explain in full detail how her health had improved since we had met.

After that announcement, Helena told me that she wasn't sleeping well due to back pain and in the last six months it had gotten worse, especially when she lay down. I told her I would love to treat her but needed to examine her before adjusting her spine. Brunhilde wanted to go home early to bake her famous apple strudel for Nancy. Helena's husband offered to take me home.

After the physical exam I asked to see Helena's bed. The mattress was over twenty-five years old and looked as though it had been hit by mines. I told Martin, her husband, a stocky, tall man, with the shiniest bald head I had ever seen, that they needed a new mattress. He said, "I do not agree. Our mattress is fine the way it is." The sad part was that he owned a mattress factory.

After I adjusted her lower back, she gave me a small bottle of French perfume and an autographed picture of herself when she was thirty years younger and at the peak of her singing career.

On the way to Brunhilde's apartment, Martin put his hand on my leg and said, "You need to get away from Salzburg. Come with me this weekend, yah, you and me. I have a house in the Alps. We ski and rest and enjoy each other's company."

"Don't touch me." I removed his hand and scooted toward the door. I was ready to jump out of the car even while moving.

When we arrived, I jumped out of the car and slammed the door. How I hated men. I considered telling Brunhilde about him, but wasn't sure she'd believe me, or worse, she would tell Helena. The whole thing could blow up. Helena was better off not knowing what kind of man her husband was. But then, maybe she did.

After our typical light dinner at home, Brunhilde said, "My husband and me very busy with good old friends. We play cards every Wednesday evening, and vacations with friends for many years. My husband died, no more friends. They ignore me. I call telephone, they don't call me. I do not exist to them. I am sad." She pounds her chest with her fists. "I am heartbroken. I am very sad. Very lonely. I cry every day. My friends not my friends. You my only friend. True friend. Today I don't cry anymore."

I hugged her and said, "I will always be your friend."

She grabbed my arm and took me to her living room. "I want to show my photography album with pictures of my old, good friends. You like pictures?" She removed an album from the bookcase. "Come sit in couch. See here. Me, fourteen years old."

The picture showed her wearing a school uniform with a swastika on her sleeve.

"These my good memories." Her eyes and smile were bright with contentment.

She turned the pages slowly, pointing out pictures of family and friends. Some wore uniforms that proudly displayed their swastikas. When she mentioned their names her eyes lit up and her voice grew excited, "Friends, important people."

I was astonished to see so many pictures of Hitler. She put her index finger to her lips and kissed one of his pictures. I couldn't look at her after that. I was afraid she would read from my face how confounded I felt by her behavior and the kind of people she'd been associated with.

"Handsome, ja?"

In my opinion, he was far from handsome. Perhaps he just wasn't my type.

"Yes, I see what you mean." I could barely speak.

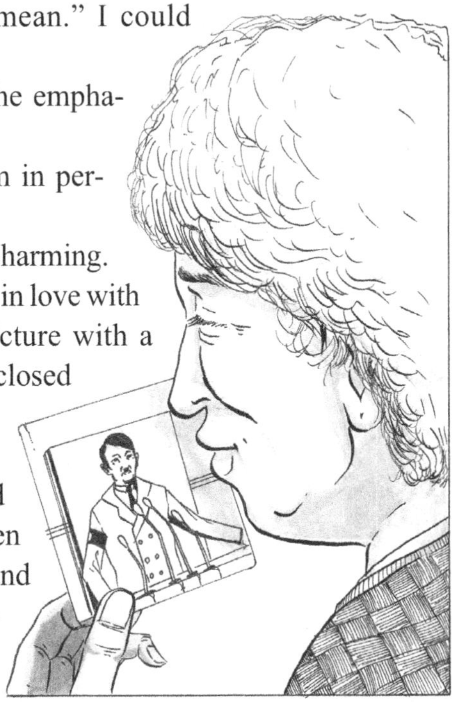

"My love. My man." She emphasized each word.

"Did you ever meet him in person?"

"Yes, many times. Very charming. Every girl my age and older in love with him." She stared at his picture with a look of adulation, and then closed the album and held it to her chest for several minutes. I clenched my hands and held them to my chest. Then I squeezed them together and covered my face. An overwhelming feeling of grief took over me. I didn't know if I could ever smile or act normal again in front of her.

"I'm tired. You too?" she asked.

"Yes, very tired."

"You are my American daughter. I love you." She hugged me. I hugged her back.

“I love you too.” I was being sincere but still felt very confused. She had been fourteen years old when her parents had joined the Nazi party. What else could she do at that age? She couldn’t go against her family. She had been a victim of circumstances.

~ Chapter Thirty-One ~

Nancy

Tuesday, February 27

After breakfast, Brunhilde drove us to the train station to pick up Nancy. I wondered how she had passed the driving test. Brunhilde pulled her car to the curb and I went into the station to look for Nancy. She was walking towards me. I couldn't stop hugging her. I cried. Her eyes were teary.

"It was a horrible feeling when I got to Munich after such a long flight and not knowing where to go. The people were so unfriendly. I'm so glad to be here. I'm absolutely exhausted."

"Before you meet Brunhilde, I must tell you about her. She lost her husband two months ago. If we cry, she'll cry too. I made a pact with her that we would not cry any more and that we would talk only about happy things. Brunhilde tells me about all the wonderful years she had with her husband. And I only tell her how wonderful Patrick was. We both laugh a lot over silly things. That's how we've survive. Nancy, we can't cry near Brunhilde."

"Sounds good to me." Nancy smiled.

Her prompt response meant to me that this was the wrong time to tell her about Brunhilde's background.

Brunhilde came out of her car and hugged and kissed Nancy like long lost friends. "Me love you. Me very happy to meet you. Veronica and you, my girls, my family." Before we could stop her, she picked up Nancy's luggage and put it inside the trunk and just as quickly she opened the back door. "Nancy please sit with Veronica in my car, talk, be happy together."

She drove out the parking lot with both hands on the wheel but her eyes were not on the road. She sang joyfully.

Nancy whispered, "Scary the way she drives." She held on tight to my arm and laughed. "My goodness, she's so wonderful, so full of life."

Brunhilde laughed. "I drop American girls at hospital. I need time to cook special dinner tonight. Be to my apartment by 5pm, okay?"

Before entering the hospital, I warned her about Patrick's condition and how horrible he looked. I expected that she was anxious to see him and was surprised when she said, "I thought I could do it but I can't bring myself to see him all cut up. How can you stand it?"

"It's not easy but I have to." I cried.

"Veronica you don't have to go in. I don't expect you to." She hugged me crying. "You're going to get sick. How can you stand it?"

"I have to. He's my husband."

I stood by his bed and stopped crying. I could stand it because I was empty of emotion. I had Nancy's blessing, I didn't have to visit him any longer. I was in and out in less than five minutes. I was done torturing myself. I grabbed her and cried.

On the way to Brunhilde's apartment, she told me that everyone at home was praying for Patrick and me. When I told her that I was ready to give up on life until Brunhilde came along, she put her arm around my shoulders and told me that she was there to take me home.

Brunhilde opened her door joyfully. "My Western Girls are here." After much hugging and kissing, she asked us to follow her to the kitchen. We stayed home the rest of the day, having a great time sharing stories with each other. Nancy fell in love with Brunhilde just like I had.

For dinner, Brunhilde served a variety of Austrian sausages with a side of mashed potatoes. Nancy didn't eat sausages. She sneaked hers on my plate and dined on mashed potatoes and a piece of Brunhilde's homemade apple strudel. After dinner, Brunhilde insisted on doing the dishes herself. Nancy tried to take over washing the dishes, but had to pull her hands away from the scalding water. "My goodness," Nancy yelled out. "The water is boiling doesn't that burn your hands?"

"Boiling water, best clean dishes good. I like pain, means clean dishes." She laughed. "Veronica always help me dry dishes. You can take shower if like. Long trip for you. Tired?"

"I'm exhausted. A hot shower would be great right now."

When Nancy returned to the kitchen Brunhilde was delighted with the fun pattern of Nancy's flannel pajamas, which featured bright little Christmas moose.

Brunhilde acted like a young girl having a pajama party. After I took two melatonin tablets that Nancy gave me to help me with sleep, we both laid down. Brunhilde tucked us into bed like twins, and then sat next to us and told us stories from her past.

"American soldiers very good to me. Americans kind. They give me food, stockings, clothes to be warm." The way she expressed herself and the funny stories she told us had us all laughing and it was late when she kissed us on the forehead and said, "Goodnight my Western Girls."

"She's unreal. How did you find her?" Nancy asked me, while still laughing.

"She found me, after her husband appeared in a dream and asked her to help me. If she hadn't taken me in, I would probably have died insane."

"The way she came into our lives is a true miracle. I tell you, she is truly our Austrian Angel." I lacked the courage to tell Nancy about Brunhilde's past. She would never believe me. The melatonin helped but I woke up three hours later. I stared at the ceiling until it was time to get up.

Wednesday, February 28

Nancy came with me to the hospital. I didn't go in to see Patrick. I told the nurse that we would wait to see his doctor. Nancy and I sat silently on the only bench in the hallway entrance, and held hands. His doctor told us, "I'm sorry to inform you, but your husband's heart is severely damaged and his kidneys and lungs are not able to function on their own." I remained seated crying. Nancy stood. "Are you telling me that there's nothing that can be done to save my brother?"

The doctor shook her hand. "You are the sister from America. I'm very sorry. In my opinion, it can't get any worse, and hope for recovery is almost gone. But we're not giving up. We will keep you posted of any changes." He left.

"Cold bastard," said Nancy.

Until that moment I only knew Nancy, as Patrick's sister, from the casual family gatherings back in California. Now I looked up to her. She was my lifesaver amidst the storm. She didn't cry in front of me, most likely for my sake just like I did my best not to cry in front of Brunhilde.

Outside the hospital, I said, "My mother died a year ago today." I held her arm as we walked. I cried.

"I'm sorry Veronica. But don't worry. You're going to be fine. I'm not leaving you. That reminds me, I need to call home and let the family know I arrived safely."

"To call long distance, we'll need to go to the post office or the train station. Look, over there." I pointed to the Wartenberg House. "That's where I stayed before going to live with Brunhilde. You have to take a look. You're going to love their antique furniture."

We climbed the sixteen steps stairway to the floor where I had stayed. Half way through one of the hallways, she stopped and said, "This place gives me the heebie-jeebies. Let's get out of here."

We left immediately.

The post office was nearby. Nancy was instructed by an impatient operator to keep putting more change into the phone and then dial the number directly. After several attempts Nancy gave up. She approached a young woman sitting behind the counter, and asked for assistance.

"We're closing soon. I don't have the time to help you."

"Excuse me? You're still open. I just need some help to use the phone."

"Too bad, but you'll have to come back tomorrow." She turned her back on us.

"You pimple-faced, fat lazy broad." Nancy yelled. "I'm going to squeeze your ugly neck."

"C'mon, Nancy. We'll come back tomorrow." I doubted that she was going to do what she said, but I grabbed her arm and led her outside, both of us laughing.

After we had walked two blocks, she said, "Look, Veronica, a bakery, my favorite place to shop."

"Mine too."

Nancy and I goggled over a small glass counter with an array of pastries. The smell of freshly baked goods was exhilarating and I decided that I had better enjoy the moment, because I was most likely dreaming.

She bought a huge apple strudel and we sat on a park bench and shared it. We agreed that apple strudel was the best we had ever eaten. The one Brunhilde had made was dry, though we didn't plan to share that finding with her. We did tell her about the pimpled-face rude girl at the post office.

Her response was delightful. "Not pimple-face, pickled-face."

That became the joke for the day, the pickled-face girl at the post office.

After dinner, Brunhilde said, "Follow me to parlor to see my photographic albums. You like?"

I panicked. “Nancy, just go along with it.” I whispered.

“What do you mean?”

“You’ll see. Please, don’t say anything.”

Brunhilde sat between the two of us holding the photo album on her lap. Just like before, she took her time turning the pages, pointing out pictures of family and friends some wearing uniforms that proudly displayed their swastikas. She had a story to tell about all of them. They were the pride of the German people. Nancy looked at me in shock when Brunhilde, upon showing Hitler’s picture, became transfixed. Then she caressed Hitler’s picture and said to her, “Isn’t he handsome?” And she kissed his picture before closing the album.

Nancy looked at me in disbelief. I covered my mouth with both hands and stared back at her. Silence was our best friend and we remained quiet until Brunhilde came to tuck us in bed and sat next to us telling us more stories of her youth. She had us laughing again.

When she left the room, Nancy said, “Holy crap. I can’t believe that this sweet old lady was a Nazi. I refuse to accept it.”

“I do too. That’s another reason I didn’t tell you about it, I didn’t think you would believe me.”

“I refuse to believe that our ‘Austrian Angel’ was a bad person.”

We talked for a long time and came to the agreement that poor Brunhilde had been an innocent victim of her parents’ decision to move to Germany and join the Nazi party.

The medicine Nancy had brought to help me sleep worked like a narcotic, even though it was only melatonin. I was marching with Brunhilde towards a tall gray building. Gray smoke from all five chimneys covered the skies. A storm of smoke particles was falling upon us. She smiled. “Gas chamber very pleasant. Everybody that goes in, don’t want to come out. You go in.” She smiled and pushed me forward. “You go in.”

"No, I don't want to go in. I want to go home with you."

"No, you must go in." She stopped smiling. "I need to go home and clean my kitchen."

"Please don't leave me here."

Suddenly her brother appeared in his wheelchair, next to her. She kissed him on the cheek and said, "Veronica doesn't want to join the others inside."

"Don't worry. Watch me throw her in." He stood and began taking giant steps towards me, I ran as fast as I could, but his arm stretched out in my direction and he grabbed me by the hair. I woke up crying.

I didn't want to wake up Nancy. I was afraid to close my eyes. I stared at the ceiling trying not to think but it didn't help this time. Even with my eyes open I could see Patrick lying in the hospital bed, as his bed twirled above us. I could see every one of Brunhilde's friends and family members, staring down at me. One by one, their faces became grotesque masks of hate, mocking my presence. I began humming, another brick on the wall, yes I need another brick on the wall. Stack them up one by one all around. Build a brick wall, girl. Build a brick wall, girl. Make it tight, make it high and they will remain outside. I was still awake, but all I saw was the bricks.

Thursday, February 29

The three of us sat at the kitchen table drinking hot water with lemon, and eating toasted bread with cheese and jam for breakfast. We could barely see outside the kitchen window through the thick fog. Even the snowy mountains in the distance were hidden. Nancy and Brunhilde talked all morning, I pretended to listen. Even breathing made me tired. Nancy commented that I should take a nap before going to the hospital. After an hour nap and Brunhilde's chicken soup, I felt recharged.

Nancy and I sat in the hospital lobby during visiting hours, waiting for Patrick's doctor to come speak with us. The floor nurse told us that his doctor was not available to see us but she was to tell us that there was a slight flicker of hope. His lungs seemed to be working better, where before they were shutting down. Even though Nancy asked me not to see Patrick because I came out of his room an emotional wreck, I felt obliged to show some form of concern for him. Knowing that Nancy was waiting for me in the hallway and was anxious to leave the hospital as soon as possible made it easy for me to go in, and look briefly at Patrick. He didn't look any different from the last time I had seen him. By now I had mastered two distinct personalities. I chose the one most suitable for the occasion. I took in a deep breath and allowed an overwhelming pain to enter my body believing with all my heart that if I cried hard enough I would be lucky to die instantly.

Nancy made me promise her that I would not visit Patrick again.

We rode the bus to the train station so Nancy could call her family and then spent the rest of the day at home with Brunhilde.

Friday, March 1

After breakfast, we remained at the kitchen table talking. Brunhilde's English had improved considerably since we had first met. She was a smart cookie.

After lunch, the phone rang. Brunhilde answered and spoke in German for several minutes. After she hung up, she said to me, "You must be strong. Need to go to hospital. Not good. Not good news. Important, we talk first." She grabbed my arm hard and pushed me into the living room. Nancy tried to follow me but Brunhilde put her hand out to Nancy. "You, wait outside." Nancy shrugged her shoulders wondering what was going on. Brunhilde closed the glass doors behind us. She cried and kneeled before me. She grabbed my hands, kissed them, and said, "Please forgive me! I didn't mean to kill your husband."

"Of course you didn't kill him. Brunhilde, what's wrong?" At this point I was sure Brunhilde had gone over the edge. I reached for the doorknob to get Nancy, but Brunhilde pulled my hand away and wouldn't let go. She was very strong.

"I am bad. My daughter knows truth. I am a very bad person." She continued to cry.

"No, Brunhilde, you're a very good person. You're my friend. You helped me. Please get up."

"I help you because I want to help me, myself, me. I don't want to go to hell. I want to go to heaven when I die."

"Brunhilde, you're an angel, our Austrian Angel. You offered us your home."

She would not let go of my knees and cried out louder. She pulled down on my hands.

"No, you don't understand. I didn't use to be good. Stop! Listen! I have done bad things, ashamed of me. Many died, I killed them. Please, forgive me. Please forgive me. I don't want to go to hell when I die. Please forgive me. I need you to say you forgive me."

"Okay, I forgive you."

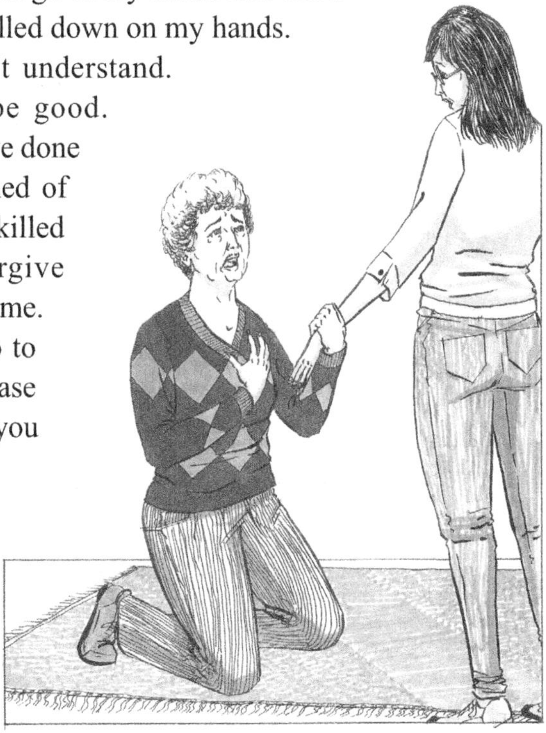

"You forgive me?" She let go of my hands and put her palms together as if praying.

"Yes, I forgive you."

She stood, smiled and kissed me on both cheeks. "Thank you to forgiving me. Now I can die and go to heaven. Thank you, Veronica. Now we go to hospital." She opened the glass doors.

Nancy had not moved from her spot. When I passed, she flashed me a look that said, *what in the world,* but she didn't say anything. Brunhilde hugged her. "Sorry, very sorry Nancy, your brother dead very soon, we need to go to hospital immediately. I drive." My legs went weak and I fell on my knees crying, both Nancy and Brunhilde had to help me to get into the elevator, into the parking lot and then into her car. When we got to the hospital Brunhilde waited in her car.

It wasn't visiting hours, but they let us into the intensive care hallway. We sat on the only bench against the wall and held hands. Two young doctors with solemn looks approached us. We held on tighter to each other. Only one spoke English.

"When your husband first arrived we thought he might survive because he was young and healthy. We did everything we could to help him, but his destiny was already set. We disconnected him an hour ago and he has since died. We are very sorry."

Nancy and I hugged each other and cried. I held her arm as we left the hospital.

It had started to snow. When we saw Brunhilde, we stopped crying. On the way home no one spoke. I focused on the snowflakes brushing my window and then melting away while Nancy just gazed forward. Before getting out of the car Nancy whispered, "Let's get out of Austria as soon as possible and go home."

The phone rang when we entered the apartment. Brunhilde answered the phone and then handed me the receiver. "American person for you."

It was Mrs. Simpson, the insurance liaison. The hospital had called her and she was very sympathetic about Patrick's death. She gave me the name and address of a funeral home in Salzburg to go to, where I should choose a coffin. They would take care of all the finances.

Brunhilde said, "Not far to walk. Good place. Very nice choice." That same afternoon Brunhilde walked with us to the funeral home. On the way, Nancy whispered, "Once we finish making the arrangements for my brother we should leave. Let's take the train to Munich tomorrow morning and then fly home. We need to tell Brunhilde."

As much as I wanted to go home I wasn't looking forward to tell Brunhilde we would be leaving so soon.

I didn't know what to expect when we entered the small vestibule of the funeral home, but as long as Nancy stood by my side, I wasn't afraid. Brunhilde introduced us to Mr. Schmidt, the funeral director and also an old friend. He was a pale, extremely thin, bald man appropriately dressed in a black suit. "I'm so very, very sorry about the loss of your loved one, please accept my condolences. Please follow me."

Brunhilde remained in the vestibule and Nancy and I followed Mr. Schmidt to another room with a desk and some chairs and were asked to wait. He came back a few minutes later. "I will take you now to a room where you will be able to pick any coffin you like for your loved one."

We were surrounded by coffins, all colors, shapes and sizes. I was hoping Nancy would decide on which one to get. Mr. Schmidt must have been reading my mind. He pointed to some. "What you see here are caskets, they have four sides, those over there are coffins and they have six sides. I recommend you pick a casket; they are a lot more reliable and last longer than a coffin. For example, this beautiful ornate casket made of mahogany is resistant to termites and rot. It's my favorite. Very elegant, agree?"

Nancy pointed to another with a more simple design. "I like that one."

"That's made of cherry wood, a nice choice, even though not as hard as walnut wood."

"My brother would pick something simple. Veronica, do you like the cherry one?"

"Yes, it's very nice."

Mr. Schmidt said, "How about this one? It's made of oak, highly resistant to water."

"My brother is being cremated; we don't care about the quality of the wood."

He took us back to the room with the desk. After I signed some papers pertaining to the purchase of the casket by the insurance company, and Nancy entered the information regarding the address to where the casket with Patrick's body would be delivered in California, he gave me a small envelope and some paper. "Would you like to write something loving to your husband and I'll put it inside the casket?"

I wrote, "Dear Patrick, I'm sorry that you died. Love, Veronica."

I enclosed the note in the envelope sealed it and gave it to Mr. Schmidt.

Back at the apartment, Nancy reminded me to tell Brunhilde our plans.

"No. You don't leave. You can't leave me." She cried. "Please stay another week."

"I'm sorry, but Nancy and I have to go home. We love you very dearly but we have to go. Our family is waiting for us."

"I understand. Family important to have."

"Yes, that's right," said Nancy. "But we love you and we'll miss you, and very soon you're going to get a letter from us inviting you to come to America to visit us. Okay?"

"Yes, I promise to come and visit you in America."

That night I didn't sleep. The brick wall I had built the night before, crumbled. I looked for all the positive things that had happened in the three months that Patrick and I had dated and the next three months traveling as a married couple. I had learned to ride a bicycle. I had learned to climb over walls and fences of all heights. He had taught me to play golf, run, climb steep cliffs, fish, play football, baseball, toss a Frisbee and play cards. He had taught me to think ahead, ask the right questions, and drive a stick shift properly because he was afraid I would mess up his ZX. Our marriage of three months had been the worst time of my life as well as one of the most adventurous and exciting. Together we had been to sixteen countries and had shared the beauty of the world with good and bad times all rolled into one. He loved living, and that he had done well.

Saturday, March 2

Brunhilde called the station to confirm the train schedule. We had time to have breakfast with her. I gave her Patrick's clothes, including his heavy leather jacket, hiking boots and extra pair of shoes. She assured me she knew some poor farmers who could use them.

I emptied his backpack of all the stuff that I didn't want to carry. I kept his camera and a few other small items. In Patrick's backpack, I found the two train tickets to Munich the Turks had given us. Nancy and I would be using them.

Before leaving, Brunhilde gave me a pair of heavy-duty wool socks. "They belonged to my husband. I want you to have them. Keep you warm."

I thanked her and put them on.

When we entered the train station, Brunhilde asked to see our tickets.

"These tickets are not first class. I buy first class tickets for my Western Girls." She ran off before we could stop her.

She stayed with us until we boarded the train and then remained on the platform smiling.

"I'm gonna miss her." I threw her a kiss.

"Me too, I wish we could take her with us."

The train whistle blew and the train moved ever so slowly. Nancy and I waved and threw her more kisses through our compartment's window.

Brunhilde looked straight at us, clicked her heels together and, with a serious look on her face, she gave us the Hitler salute.

We looked at each other stunned. I said, "Oh my God! She's reverting back to Hitler's time." I pulled up the window and yelled out, "No, Brunhilde, please don't do that. Don't revert back!"

She stared at us and gave us the Hitler salute again as the train pulled away.

My throat closed tight and a cold shiver ran down my spine. I sat silently next to Nancy. I imagined that train full of Jewish families being taken to concentration camps on a cold winter day just like that day, and under that same salute that Brunhilde had given us. Nancy watched me as I took the green wool socks off and threw them into the small wastebasket by the window. I was repelled by the mere thought of who had used those socks. Our Austrian Angel was a Nazi. I was faced with the reality of why she had begged for my forgiveness. We sat silently for a long time. Then I began talking about my two sons and how wonderful they were, and Nancy talked about how wonderful her children were.

~Chapter Thirty-Two ~

Germany

I agreed with Nancy that Munich was not a welcoming city. She was glad I had noticed, because that's what she had experienced before going to Salzburg.

Our first encounter was with a rude bank teller who wouldn't exchange the large amount of foreign change that Patrick had collected. When we tried to change Nancy's airplane ticket at the airport so we could travel together back to the US, the agent said he couldn't do anything but direct us to a travel agency that might be able to help. It was closed until Monday.

We stayed at the same hotel where Nancy had stayed before. I threw away Patrick's books and notes and gave her his tape recorder and tapes. I kept the camera and last page of a calendar where he had written the names of the countries we had visited.

We were in our beds by eight o'clock. Before dozing off, I told myself that whatever was in my future had to be something important enough to make me forget the nightmare I had been through.

Sunday, March 3

I woke crying. I finally understood that Patrick wasn't coming home. It didn't matter that I had planned to ask for a divorce. All that mattered was that he wasn't there.

During breakfast, I cried uncontrollably. While walking the streets I cried. Each time I cried, Nancy hugged and comforted me like a sister. I felt bad because I was afraid to annoy her but knowing that she loved me, I was thankful for having the freedom to cry relentlessly. I didn't have to explain why I cried so much, she knew.

We spent the day walking around Munich. The buildings were grey, tall, monotonous, and uninviting, but Nancy's company and cheering mood kept me going. The streets were covered with snow but it wasn't that cold. The way Brunhilde held my arm everywhere we went, I did now with Nancy. We ate sandwiches for lunch at a delicatessen, and for dinner we stopped at McDonald's. We retired early to our room and were again in bed by eight o'clock.

Monday, March 4

It took us most of the morning to find the travel agency. The two women at the agency could have cared less about our problem. My airline ticket was a student special, and as such I would have to fly to Portugal, and then use my original ticket to fly from Portugal to Amsterdam, Holland, and then to San Francisco. Nancy's ticket was from Munich to California only.

"My husband died two days ago and this is his sister. We don't want to be separated. Please can't you arrange the tickets so that we can travel together?" I couldn't hold my tears.

"We have to follow the rules," said one of the women, who Nancy later called a "cold bitch."

I would have to leave that afternoon for Portugal, and Nancy would be stranded in Munich until Thursday. She came to the airport with me. We both cried as we said goodbye. I promised to call her as soon as I arrived in San Francisco, and then she and Sean would pick me up.

Aunt Heydee used to say I was her best student when it came to learning to deal with the ups and downs that life throws at our faces. Being married to Patrick had taught me to never trust another man. Being in love made one weak. I had learned my lesson. I was the product of an insane man who had succeeded in killing me from inside out.

I wanted only two things more than anything in life: to go home and to go back to school.

~ Chapter Thirty-Three ~

Farewell to Papa

I arrived at Lisbon, at seven-thirty in the evening and took the local bus to the pensão where Patrick and I had stayed. The managers at the pensão were horrified when I told them that Patrick had died. They remembered him. They took me under their wing and moved me to their best room, on the same floor as their apartment. They told me that if I needed anything during the night I should knock on their door.

I took a look inside my money belt. I would be able to take care of my mother's stone, after all. I put the three thousand dollars in a separate portion of my money belt. That money was sacred. I left my belongings at the hotel and went to visit my father, keeping my fingers crossed I would find him at Luisa's apartment. He was there, seated on the couch in her living room. He wore his usual attire of suit and tie but had a large bruise on the left side of his forehead and a black-and-blue eye.

"What happened to you, Papa?"

"Your father fell in the street, when he went for a walk." Luisa answered.

"Luisa, may I have a glass of water?" I asked.

She left the room and I asked Papa, "What really happened to your head?"

He whispered, "What do you think? Luisa wanted more money from me, but I didn't have any more to give her. We argued. I was lying in bed and she picked up my cane and beat me over the head with it."

"That's it. I'm taking you out of here." I stood.

"No, I can't leave her. She needs me. Veronica, she doesn't know what she's doing, I already forgave her."

Shit! Papa had turned into a martyr. He was no different from me. He was willing to stay in an abusive relationship even if it killed him, just because he loved Luisa.

When she returned to the room I bit my lip and acted friendly, since Papa insisted on continuing to live with her. Just like my brother Max-Leão, I gave up reasoning with Papa. Our parents never took our advice. Things had to be their way or no way at all.

Luisa wanted to know more about what had happened to Patrick.

"I'm sorry, but I can't talk about it yet. Papa did you get my postcard from Italy?"

"Yes, Veronica. And as soon as I saw the picture of a damsel in distress, I knew it was a message that you were in trouble. I wasn't worried. I knew you would be coming back to see me one more time."

"How did you know that?"

"Once I received your letter that he was dying, I knew the reason for you to be married to him. Veronica, stop crying. You have no reason to cry. Your mission was to carry him until the end. It was because of you that he was able to travel to all the places he wanted to see before dying. God chose you to be the facilitator of his last wishes. You were his angel of mercy. I kept you in my prayers every day. My telegram to you in Salzburg was my way of letting you know that you had my blessings." He took a deep breath. "Veronica, my daughter, will you give me a haircut?"

While I cut his hair I told him about Brunhilde. I wasn't sure how he would react since he had lost so many family members in concentration camps.

"I don't care if she was a Nazi during Hitler's time," he said with tears in his eyes. "She took care of my daughter, and I must thank her for doing that. Please, let me have her address before you leave. I must write to her and thank her for being there for you." He added what I had always heard him say since I was a child. "There are good and bad Germans. We cannot blame a race for the actions of a few ruthless individuals. There were many Germans that helped save lives at the cost of their own. Those are the Germans we must honor. The others are just criminals, and as long as men exist there will always be good and evil. It has nothing to do with being German."

Luisa offered me dinner.

"Thank you, Luisa, but I'm not hungry.

"Please don't go yet. Here, this is good for you," Papa handed me a tangerine from a bowl on top of the dining table.

"It's late, Papa. I'm very tired. I need to go back to the pensão and get some sleep."

"Save your money on lodgings. You can sleep in my bed."

"Sorry, Papa, but I can't do that."

"I would consider it a blessing to have my daughter sleeping next to me."

"I understand, but I already have a room reserved at the pensão. I promise to be back before leaving for America."

I wasn't comfortable sleeping with my father. I hugged him and left proud of myself for standing for what I believed in.

The pleasant fresh air outside was familiar to me. These were the same streets I had walked on when I was a young naïve girl, before going to America to be married to my cousin Al. Like before I walked alone but this time I appreciated being on my own. No more Patrick. I was free. Now that Patrick was gone, I would never cry again.

I entered the hotel lobby and Maria Souza, the manager wife, hugged me crying. "I heard about your husband's death. I can't even imagine the pain you must be in. If my husband died I would ask God to take me away too. I couldn't live without him."

I wondered if her husband would give up his life for her. Love is so demanding, so pathetic. Such a nasty four letter word. Romeo and Juliet gave up their lives for love. Love sucks.

My room was cold, but it wasn't as cold as in Turkey. The bed had one thin blanket. I slept with my clothes and coat on.

Tuesday, March 5

I woke early. I climbed out of bed and washed my eyelids with icy water from the bedroom faucet, and then brushed my hair. I was ready to take on the new day.

I called my cousin Max in England and told him about Patrick. He was horrified about the news. I shared my concerns about Papa's safety in Luisa's house. He said that we couldn't force my father to do anything he didn't want to. He told me not to worry about Papa's finances. He would continue to send his monthly check, and any time Papa changed his mind he was welcome to come to England to live with him and his wife.

I went to the airport to see if I could use my airline ticket to go directly to the US instead of via Holland, but the agents couldn't help me. Just like in Munich, they referred me to a travel agency. When I finally found the address in downtown Lisbon, their computers were down. The manager said, "Why don't you return on Thursday, and we'll see what we can do to help you."

I called Dr. Grentz, an American chiropractor who Patrick and I had briefly met while we were in Lisbon. I told him my situation and explained that it was difficult for me to carry around my adjusting table after I picked it up at my brother's place in the south of Portugal. I offered to sell it to him for

$150. He said I had a deal if I brought the adjusting table to his office by ten-thirty Thursday morning.

Everything in my life seemed to be dependent on Thursday.

I took the bus to the Jewish Community Center to talk to Mrs. Beckman. We had met just a few months ago to inquire about purchasing my mother's tombstone. She was shocked to find out about Patrick.

I confirmed my agreement to honor my mother's request. The pink marble gravestone would be fifteen centimeters tall and would be carved with her name, followed by wife, mother, author, music composer, and artist.

Mrs. Beckman guaranteed that my mother's wish would be granted. She would make sure of that. I gave her three thousand dollars. I had exactly $600 left in my money belt, but my first mission in Lisbon had been accomplished.

I headed to the bus station, where I would catch the bus to the town of Ourique to pick up the adjusting table as well as everything else Patrick and I had left with my brother and his wife, Patricia. I made it to the bus station just five minutes before the bus was leaving. I arrived in Ourique at six in the afternoon.

The owners of the tavern by the bus station couldn't reach my brother by phone. I waited until seven. Then I gave up and walked up the hill towards the only pensão in town. Mrs. Lucas, the owner, also knew my brother, and kept calling his cell phone until she finally reached him.

My letters from Salzburg had terrorized my poor brother and his wife. Their son, Leo, had developed a problem with his neck, and they immediately thought Leo also had a ruptured esophagus. They sent Leo to London to see a specialist and were waiting for a call to find out if he was going to be all right. They were down to one car and asked me to stay at the pensão for the night. In the morning they would send a taxi to pick me up.

I sat on one of the chairs in my room shivering and pondered how the Portuguese could live without heat in the winter. How I had survived these living conditions while growing up was beyond me. I called Mrs. Lucas and asked if I could get some heat in the room. She brought me a tray with a hot teakettle and a mug with a tea bag. "This is the best I can do for you."

I put the teakettle under my bed covers where my feet would be, drank the hot tea, and, left my wool hat and coat on. I slept until the kettle went cold.

Wednesday, March 6

I remained in bed until seven and then climbed into the shower. There was hot water! I stayed in there until it ran cold. I dressed quickly and pulled on my coat, then jumped up and down in the middle of my room to stay warm. At eight o'clock a car horn blasted on the street below. I knew it was for me. The taxi driver was overjoyed to finally meet my brother's sister from America. He also wanted to know if President Bill Clinton and Vice-president Al Gore were my friends.

Max-Leão and Patricia were very happy to see me. They had good news from London. Leo was fine and would be home by the end of the week. But they were still stressed out. They wanted to know exactly what had happened to Patrick.

Once they were assured that what Patrick had, was something rare and had nothing to do with what Leo had been experiencing, they brought out the large suitcases that Patrick and I had left behind. They contained twenty hefty chiropractic books along with his clothes, coats, shoes, vitamin bottles and toiletries. It would be ludicrous to take Patrick's stuff to the U.S. I told my brother to do whatever he wanted with the suitcases and his things. I packed the chiropractic books into two sturdy boxes that Patricia provided. The adjusting table was still in its original box. When Max-Leão saw my stethoscope and blood pressure cuff, he asked me to check his blood pressure, which turned out to be quite elevated. I gave him a light back massage and adjusted his back and neck. I wanted to spend at least a day with them, but I needed to get back to Lisbon before Thursday morning. I had lunch with Max-Leão and Patricia at the bus station, but barely had time to finish eating because the bus arrived early.

My brother gave an extra tip to the bus driver to put my adjusting table and books, in the cargo space under the bus. I kept my backpack and broom with me, along with my water jug.

I waved goodbye to my brother and his wife, wondering if I would ever see them again.

Three hours later, I arrived at Lisbon's central bus station. Not sure how to proceed, I stood in the middle of the parking garage. Buses honked, and drove around me. People pushed me out of their way as they rushed in and out of the garage I didn't have enough arms to carry everything. After standing there for a few minutes, I decided that the best method was to move my belongings in stages: move what I could as far as I could within sight and then go back and get the rest. If I did that several times, sooner or later I would make my way out of the bus depot.

I carried one box ten feet, set it on the ground, and then brought over the other box. Next, I retrieved my broom and water jug and put everything in a neat pile. After that, I dragged the adjusting table over, moving it in short spurts. Throughout all this, I wore my backpack. I wasn't concerned about the books and adjusting table. Only Superman could have run off with them.

It took several trips, but I finally made it to the baggage counter. For five dollars, they could keep the adjusting table until Thursday morning. I also had the option to store the two boxes, but it would cost five dollars each. I couldn't afford such luxury. I had to pay for food and lodging in the days to follow.

I threw away the water jug. I could always go into a coffee shop and ask for a glass of water. I pushed my broom half way into my backpack, but the wood stub hit the back of my head when I walked. The broom worked better under my arm.

Once out on the street, I used the same technique to move the boxes. I carried one to the street corner and then returned for the second one. At one point, I passed by a store with collapsible luggage carts in their display window. A Visa sign hung on their door. I asked the saleslady if she had anything strong enough to hold my two boxes. She said, "All our carts are of superior quality."

"If the cart breaks from the weight of the boxes will you exchange it for another one?" I knew it was a dumb question. No Portuguese store accepts returns, but I had to make sure.

"No one is twisting your arm to buy it. If you buy it and it breaks it's your problem." She turned her back on me.

The books were too expensive to throw away, and I would need them when I returned to school. I bought a cart and loaded the boxes one stacked on top of the other. I tied them with a stretch cable she had included in the purchase. I pulled the cart lovingly across the uneven cobblestones, patiently easing forward each time a wheel became caught between the cobbles.

I was never more grateful for the pensão's old elevator. It beat dragging everything up to the third floor. I stashed my belongings in my room and headed to the corner tavern, where I was guaranteed to have an honest-to-goodness Portuguese meal at prices geared towards the working class. I ate a thick piece of broiled cod fish, rice pilaf and steamed vegetables.

When I returned to my room I found it warm. Maria Souza, bless her soul, had turned on the heat. It had been my fault that the last time I slept there I had almost frozen to death. I didn't know that the room had a thermostat. I slept like a baby.

Thursday, March 7

I arrived at the travel agency ten minutes before it opened. The computer was working, but no one knew how to transfer my ticket to fly from Portugal to America. "Your best bet is to fly to Amsterdam like you're supposed to and take the next flight to the United States. Would you like the three-thirty flight?"

You better believe it!

I had until ten-thirty to take my adjusting table to the chiropractor's office. I took the local bus to the bus terminal. Once again I pushed and pulled the box with the table until I was out on the sidewalk. I flagged a taxi.

Upon seeing the size of the box, the driver said, "It's too big. You need a bus."

I stared at him with my eyes full of tears and murmured, "Nothing is impossible, please don't give up on me."

He tried pushing it into the back seat but the box would not go through the door, nor did it fit into the trunk. Huffing and puffing, he tied it with a rope to the top of the cab. Minutes later, he dropped me off in the middle of a large deserted plaza and told me the address I was looking for was across the plaza facing the avenue. The box didn't budge when I tried lifting it, so I had to push it across the street through the non-stop roundabout traffic. My vision clouded with tears and I prayed, *Dear God, please help me.*

A tall woman, dressed in black, appeared in front of me. She said, "Where are you going?" I showed her the paper with the chiropractor's address. She said, "Follow me." She picked up the table with one hand and I followed her. We entered the lobby of the old building. Several steps stood between me and the elevator that would be taking me up to the fourth-floor's

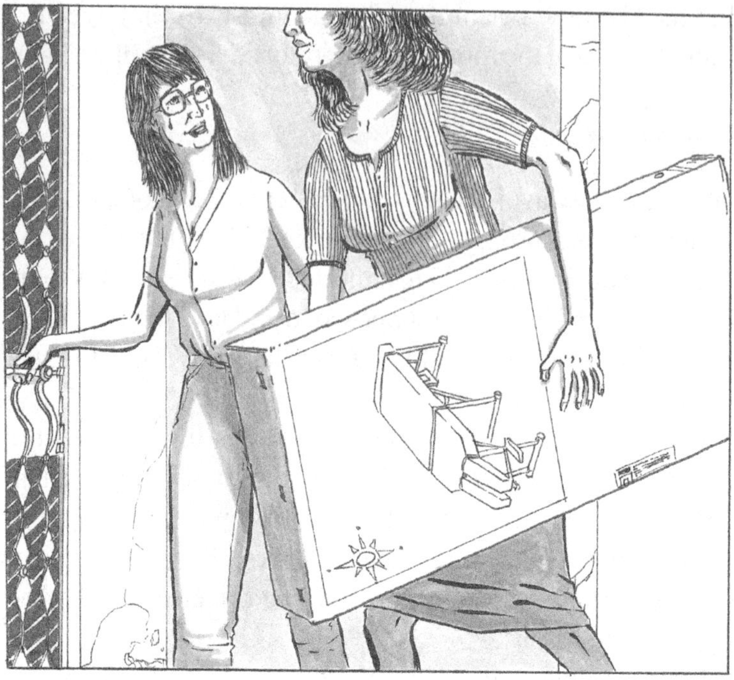

Divine Mover

office. I looked at her but couldn't see her features through my tears. She carried the table up the marble steps, opened the sliding door to the elevator and put the box inside. She was gone when I turned around to thank her.

Dr. Grenz handed me an envelope and said, "I'm sorry about your husband. The money is inside." He didn't even look into the box. He gave me a quick hug and said he was busy with a patient.

I took a taxi to the cemetery. I needed to say goodbye to my mother.

I sat on the ground where she was buried, and took from my money belt, the last poem she had written before she died. I read her goodbye poem aloud.

For you only
The day I held you for the first time
I knew you were God's gift to me.
I knew your journey ahead would take you away
to do what I could only dream of becoming,
I had no choice but to let you go.
Veronica, someday you will need my help.
Call me.
I will be there, I promise.

Your Mama, on earth and in heaven

I wrote on the dirt, "I love you too," and then said softly, "Thank you, Mama, for protecting me. I know you were my guardian angel. If it wasn't for you I would have never made it. As promised, I took care of your pink marble stone and soon it will be here." I didn't feel her presence, so I knew she was gone and at peace.

On the way out, I placed a small stone on Aunt Heydee's tomb and smiled.

I was lucky to catch a trolley car back to my father's place. It was the slowest form of transportation in the area but there were no buses or taxis available where I was.

Papa greeted me with a smile, and when we hugged goodbye he wouldn't let go.

"Papa, I have to leave. I just came to say goodbye."

"Please, my daughter, just a few seconds longer. Let me take in your image into my mind, like a picture, to keep forever in my heart." He pushed me away slightly, then held my face between his hands. He stared into my eyes, as if absorbing me into his soul. He had a glow of insightfulness about him that communicated I should not be afraid of the future, his look, one of contentment, as if he knew the meaning of life.

We said nothing. We both knew it was the last time we would see each other.

I ran down the apartment steps and crossed the street. I distinctly heard someone call my name, but I didn't turn around. I couldn't help him. I couldn't save him. I kept walking away from what I couldn't change.

On the way to the hotel I stopped to eat a slice of pizza and then went to pick up my belongings and to thank my friends, the pensão managers. Upon opening the envelope from Dr. Grenz to help pay for my lodging, I found four-hundred American dollars.

~ *Chapter Thirty-Four* ~

The Sound of Madness

When the airplane landed in Amsterdam, I felt a surge of energy. *I'm going home. I'm going home.* I kept repeating this inside my head as I looked for the KLM counter. I was shocked when the woman behind the counter told me I couldn't fly out for at least two weeks.

I wept so pathetically that even I felt sorry for myself. I felt I was having a nervous breakdown. I grabbed her hands. My tears dripped onto her fingers. I told her how I wanted to go home because my husband had just died a few days ago.

"I need to be there when his body arrives from Austria."

"Oh my. Under the circumstances, I'm putting you on a flight, even though it's booked." She winked at me.

"How can you do that?"

"We have ways." She left and quickly returned with a ticket. "March tenth at three-fifteen, arriving San Francisco at five-fifteen, same day. You can take the train into Amsterdam to find lodging. Just for three nights. The information center can provide you with places to stay."

At the information desk, two young girls stood in line in front of me. One asked for directions to Bob's Hostel.

I touched her forearm. "Excuse me, but you're Americans, like me."

"What you want?"

"I'm by myself and don't know where to go from here. Would you mind if I follow you to the hostel?"

"You have a lot of nerve. Go get your own place." She turned her back on me. Her friend threw me a contemptible look when they left.

I felt ashamed for even asking their help. The lady at the information center said, "Spoiled American tourists. They think the world owes them a living."

"Not all Americans are that way. I'm an American."

She smiled and gave me a map of the city and circled Bob's Hostel and a few other hostels and told me where to purchase the ticket for the train to Amsterdam. She encouraged me to get a round-trip ticket so I wouldn't have to worry about it on the way back.

"Beware," she said, "there's a lot of crime in Amsterdam. Keep an eye on your things."

Great. That was all I needed. But I wasn't worried; nobody was going to run off with any of my overweight belongings.

Getting them onto the train was another story. I had to lift the cart up two steps, while the people rushed impatiently in around me. I pulled and pulled and finally hauled the cart into the train, but the broom fell between the first step and the platform.

"My broom! My broom! Somebody help me!"

A woman asked her husband to get the broom as the train was about to leave.

I held the broom against my chest like a mother holding her child. I saw the look on everybody's face and felt compelled to explain.

"I'm sorry. Except for the sand bags in my backpack, this is the only thing I have left from my travels after my husband died last week in Austria." More tears flowed. "He died during our honeymoon."

The woman who had asked her husband to get my broom said she was sorry to hear about my loss and gave me a hug. Everyone standing next to us knew enough English, to understand what I said, and took turns hugging me. The couple promised to let me know when we reached the Amsterdam station. When we arrived, her husband, Mr. Smith, helped me to take my stuff off the train.

I put on the backpack, held the broom in one hand, and pulled the luggage carrier with the two boxes. I walked towards the station exit with a determined attitude. I would not be defeated.

I stood at the exit door, and faced the city of Amsterdam. It was lit up like a Christmas tree.

Then reality hit me. *It's eleven-thirty. Now what?* The little hand-held map with cute childlike drawings meant nothing to me.

Several policemen hung out by the exit.

"Excuse me officer."

He turned slowly towards me and said briskly, "What's the problem?"

"Where do I go from here to find this hostel circled in red?" I pointed to the spot on the map.

"Go straight up the avenue. You'll find the hostel you're looking for." He turned his back on me and continued chatting with his colleagues.

The little wheels in the luggage cart kept getting stuck between the dark cobblestones, but it was holding up well for such a flimsy piece of junk. I changed hands often when pulling the cart, but after a while my forearms felt as though they would come apart at the elbows. When I came to a split in the road, I headed left because the street was wider and better lit. I went from one hotel to another and from one hostel to another. They were either booked or overpriced, or I couldn't go up the steps to check them out because of my books. I had been warned about crime being high. Now that the books were on wheels, someone could easily roll them away.

The hotels ran between $150 and $350 per night. One hostel was $50 per night, but only that night was available.

Finally I found Bob's Hostel. I inserted the broom between the two boxes, and was able to slide the cart down the steps all in one clean sweep.

They charged $25 only for each night, but I would have to share the room with six others. The thought of being stuck in the same room with those rude American girls from the airport was more than I could bear. I pulled the cart up the steps to the street and continued walking. I saw the lit sign for a hotel. It had no steps either up or down. It had to do, no matter the cost.

"We have one room available for thirty dollars," said the young desk clerk with a thick dark mustache.

"Perfect. I'll take it."

"Don't you want to look at it first? It's on the fourth floor."

"Does it have a bed?"

"Of course it has a bed." He looked at the other man behind the desk as if I was a nitwit.

"That's all I need."

"Then come along. I'll take you to your room." The one with a thick mustache jumped diligently over the counter.

In front of me was the steepest, narrowest staircase I had ever seen.

"Do you have an elevator?"

He smiled. "The only elevator we have is me, Emre. I'll carry the boxes for you." But when he tried to pick them up, he yelled something other than Dutch to the other guy and then said, "My cousin Latafat will carry the other box for you."

It wasn't just their names, but their accent had a familiar ring.

I took a stab at it. "By any chance, are you Turkish?"

It was a Turkish hotel and restaurant, run by Turks! *Irony* was all I could think, so I just smiled. I couldn't have found better lodgings.

My room was the size of a large closet, with just enough space for a single bed and a chair by the window, but there was plenty of heat. I had to share the bathroom with the other guests on that floor. I used the toilet and brushed my teeth over the sink and then noticed that there was no tub, only a shower head sticking out of one of the walls. I would figure that one out in the morning.

As I dozed off I noticed a pungent sweet smell like burning rope. I woke in the middle of the night with a sinus headache. I opened the door to find that there was a smoking party in the room across from mine. Evidently I was allergic to whatever they were burning. I shoved my coat along the floor to cover the wide gap under my door, opened my window and went back to bed. The voices and music next door kept me awake. I got up, and wrote for a while. When it became quiet I went back to bed.

Friday, March 8

I was up at seven to take a hot shower and wash my hair. The showerhead sprayed water all over everything in the bathroom, except the bathroom door, which was smartly covered with a shower curtain.

It was too early to go anywhere. I headed downstairs and ate a leisurely Turkish breakfast. Afterwards, I remained seated and wrote in my diary. While in Austria I had bought a large pad of onion paper just for this purpose. Emre sat with me asking me questions about America and his cousin Latafat joined us. He wanted to know why I was traveling by myself. I told them my story and they apologized for having asked so many questions.

I returned to my room and opened the bedroom window, hoping it would clear the odor of smoke. Then I left to explore Amsterdam.

I walked with no specific place in mind. A song played loudly inside my head, and some of the words repeated over and over again. I walked with the beat, thinking how interesting it felt to have my own radio station implanted in my brain. But there was only one station and only one tune.

"I'm never going to dance again, lalalalalalalalala, I should have known better, lalalalalala. I'm never gonna dance again the way I danced with you, lalalalalalalalalala." I was sure Patrick was sending me a message. It made sense, since our dance on the bridge in Maria Plains had been the last romantic thing we had done.

I found myself in front of Anne Frank's house, where she and her family had hid from the Nazis. I stayed cool throughout the tour, until I recalled Brunhilde asking me to forgive her for her past. I cried so hard I had to leave the house. Did Brunhilde have something to do with Anne's murder as well as with so many other children? I comforted myself by recalling my father's belief that Brunhilde had been my guardian angel, and should be forgiven for whatever she had done in the past.

I found a large music store in a mall. I wanted to find the name of the song playing in my head so I could understand Patrick's message. It continued to play, and what had been fun at first was now driving me nuts. I sang the tune to several of the employees, but none of them recognized it. I left the mall and walked. I came across several churches converted into shopping malls. Even though I'm not catholic, it made me sad to think that a shopping mall had taken on more meaning than having a place to pray.

I found a pharmacy and asked the pharmacist if she had anything natural to help me sleep through the night. I also told her about the music in my head. She asked if I had suffered any head trauma. I told her the only trauma I was suffering from, was losing my husband and consequently I wasn't sleeping much. She said, "It sounds like you have a sleep disorder which many times can cause auditory hallucinations." She sold me a small bottle of melatonin, thirty milligrams per tablet, and guaranteed that two tablets would make me sleep all night.

I headed to a deli across the street and went inside. I could do nothing but stare at the splendid assortment of expensive cheeses and cured meats. A British couple standing in front of me commented on the weather, and I said, "It's a lot warmer here than in Germany." We struck up a conversation. They had to leave early the next morning and wouldn't be able to use their tickets for one of the canal tours. I was overjoyed with the gift. I didn't buy anything at the deli but sat at a pizzeria and had a slice of pizza and a cup of hot chocolate.

It was eight o'clock when I sat on my bed and took two melatonin tablets, with a glass of water.

Saturday, March 9

When I opened my eyes at ten-thirty in the morning, my head felt as though it were filled with lead. I could barely lift it off the pillow. Being that doped up went against everything I believed in as a future chiropractor. I shoved the melatonin into my backpack as an Amsterdam souvenir.

I ate a late Turkish breakfast at my hotel, and then headed to the canal for my boat trip, humming along with the music in my head. I was the first one to board. The glass roof and large side windows seemed to have a magnifying effect that caused the inside of the boat to be mercilessly hot. I took my jacket off. Not feeling like communicating with the couple next to me, I put on my sunglasses and drew into my seat next to the window. I felt awkward among the boisterous tourists that began filling the boat. I considered leaving, when I was handed a pair of headphones. Once I realized that the recording could be turned on as loud as I wanted and, my auditory hallucination could be blasted out of my head, including the voices of the sightseers around me, I smiled.

Gently down the canal we went, under beautiful bridges, and equally elegant but aging narrow houses with big narrow windows and decorative gable tops. They reminded me of the simple wood block houses I used to play with as a child. Throughout the tour the recording kept me up to par. "They were built during the 17th century, Amsterdam's golden age. The houses are about 30ft wide with very narrow stairs inside. You will notice most of them have a pulley outside. It's used to transport larger items to upper floors." That would explain the narrow staircase in my hotel. The recording continued to provide me with a good glimpse of the history behind the canals and Amsterdam. "The canals are flushed three times a week when the locks are open and water flows in from the North Sea. They are also used as sewage dumps for the many houseboats that line the city's waterways. For that reason, it's never a good idea to go swimming in the canal."

When the cruise was finished, I used my second ticket to go take another hour trip on the same boat.

After the second tour I spent the next hour sitting at a sidewalk café, enjoying a large plate of Pumpkin basil soup and a chicken sandwich, while watching the people walking by.

I finished my lunch and started to walk. The tune again played in my head, over and over, the same lines as before. I was convinced that the rest of the lyrics were a message from Patrick, saying he was sorry and wished he were still alive to dance with me again. Once home, I would sing the tune to everyone I knew until I found its name and learned what the message was.

It was only six-thirty when I climbed the steep steps to my room. Between the tune playing in my head and the cough that had started again that afternoon with a vengeance I found myself in a vacuum where time stood still. I was empty of any thoughts. The peaceful emptiness of emotion, gave me comfort. I was alone but I knew that it was only temporary.

I had been writing a little each day, but the idea of sleep meant a lot more at that point. I wrote, "Goodnight dear diary," and then curled up under the covers and fell asleep.

Sunday, March 10

Emre and Latafat insisted that I share breakfast with them. They knew my story, and both felt sorry for me. We had olives, cheese, bread, and tea. They carried my belongings down from my room. They were my big brothers. Before I left, I ran upstairs and put all my small change from the countries Patrick and I had visited on top of the bed, along with a little note. *Thank you for being my friends. Veronica.*

I arrived to the airport three hours ahead of time. I couldn't chance missing my flight.

I took my note pad out and wrote, "Dear diary, now that I have time to reflect, I promise never to be judgmental against a woman who allows herself to be pushed around either emotionally or physically and doesn't have the will power to stand for her rights as a human being. I will never say that such person is a fool or deserves what's coming to her for staying in an abusive relationship. All I can say is that such a person needs a friend. I'm still confused as to why I put up with Patrick. Maybe my father was right when he said I was Patrick's angel of death, not in a derogatory way but more like fulfilling his last wishes, to travel and see the world he loved so much. Without me he wouldn't have done it. In all fairness to him, it was because of him being a miser and dying when he did that I had enough money left to pay for Mama's tombstone. My double mission has been accomplished after all. Mama, thank you for hearing my prayer in Turkey and coming to my rescue."

When we were about to board the plane, we received an announcement saying our flight was delayed because our plane was being inspected. The airline had received a bomb threat, and all passengers had to move to the next gate until it was safe to board.

When we returned, everyone gathered at one corner of the large waiting room. I looked around and told an American woman next to me, "We're better off standing in the middle of the waiting area where there's no trash cans or seats where a bomb might still be hidden."

She followed me to the center of the room and a few others did the same. Two hours later we all boarded the plane.

I was going home. Patrick's family, now my family, would take care of me. Nancy would help me be strong when Patrick's body arrived. I had to get ready to go back to school. I had to learn to be on my own again. I had a lot to do.

Then I heard the most profound announcement I had heard in my life. "Please make sure you have your seatbelts fastened because we are ready to take off."

I bowed my head and thanked God. Then I stuck a piece of gum into my mouth to keep the change in pressure from hurting my ears.

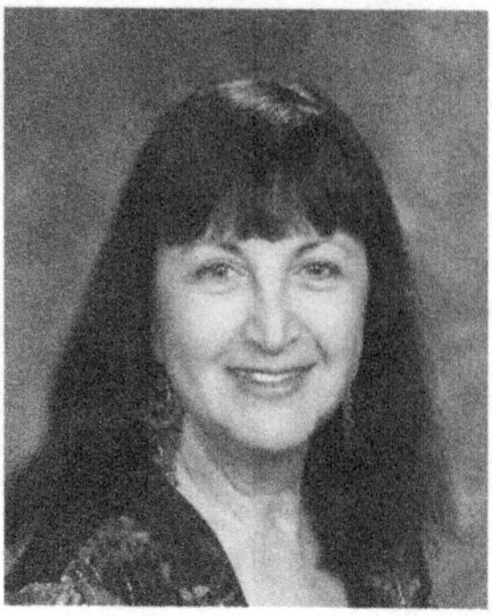

Dr. Veronica Esagui is a chiropractic physician and the internationally and critically acclaimed author of The Scoliosis Self-Help Resource Book. In addition to maintaining a successful practice in West Linn, Oregon, she hosts The Author's Forum, a television talk show featuring authors, publishers, editors, and others involved in the production of books. Dr. Veronica Esagui was the theatre producer of the Simy Theatre Company, longest running dinner-theatre in N.J. and the playwright of the musical series: *Broadville I, II, III, The Time Machine* and the musical drama, *The Black Panther Cried.* Her memoir series are: *The Journey of Innocence, Braving a New World, Awakening the Woman Within,* and *Angels Among Us.* Besides being a member of the Pacific Northwest Literacy Alliance and the recipient of the NABP Member of the Year Award, she is also the founder and Chief Executive Officer of the Northwest Annual Book Festival, and The Northwest Writers and Publishers Association. (NWPA)

Aged to Perfection a comedy in two acts she wrote in collaboration with Linda Kuhlmann, was sponsored by Fertile Ground and the Lakewood Arts Center in Lake Oswego, OR .

Aged to Perfection is scheduled for its world full stage production at the Dolores Winningstad Theatre in Portland OR, autumn of 2015. Dr. Veronica Esagui is presently working on her fifth diary book series *The Gift* and adapting to a play *She Overheard Murder,* by Jean Sheldon.

For information on upcoming events, interview requests, and comments about *Veronica's Diary IV—Angels Among Us,* or to find out more about the availability of other published works, please visit the author at: www.veronicaesagui.com.

www.veronicesagui.com
www.nwbookfestival.com

Dr. Veronica Esagui, books' synopsis:

The Scoliosis Self-Help Resource Book (Also available in Japanese) Includes the illustrated step-by-step approach to TESP (The Esagui Scoliosis Protocol), a very specific group of exercises for the spine. Through this book, a person with scoliosis will discover that they may have options other than drugs or surgery. As Dr. Esagui says, "If by writing this book, I can shed some light onto scoliosis management that is more proactive than waiting under observation, then people will understand their options and I will have done my best as a chiropractor and educator."

*Verónica's Diary—The Journey of Innocence (*1944-1962)
Describes in the most candid manner the first eighteen years of Veronica's life growing up in Portugal, until a pre-arranged marriage with her cousin brings her to the USA in 1962.

Veronica's Diary II—Braving the New World (1962-1988)
Follows her trailblazing accomplishments as a music teacher, performer, news reporter, theater director, playwright, owner of three music centers, theater producer and owner of the only American dinner theater in the world in a Japanese Restaurant.

Veronica's Diary III—Awakening the Women Within (1988-1994)
Her children are now grown up; her ex-husband is still her friend but her lovers don't fit the role model of the romance novels she used to read as a young girl.

Coming soon…
Veronica's Diary V—The Gift (1996-2003)
A stranger follows Veronica into a supermarket and hands her a small pottery, insisting that the gift is meant only for her. She accepts it. Veronica's rich life experiences as a time traveler have finally taught her to recognize that her quest for happiness has finally been granted.

About the Artists

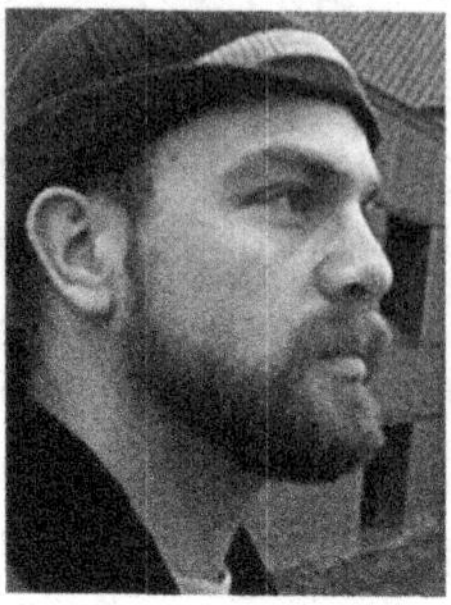

Derrick Freeland – when not engaged in the fine and subtle art of Tom Foolery, Derrick can be found illustrating the lives of others, and those who never existed in the first place. His work can be found here in this volume and with Common Ties Publishing.
Derrickfreeland.blogpspot.com

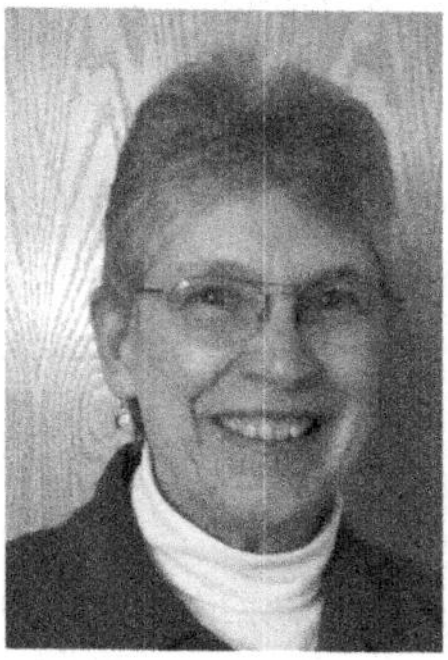

Jean Sheldon is a graphic artist and the owner of Wellworth Publishing and the fiction imprint, Bast Press that has published her mysteries *The Woman in the Wing, Seven Cities of Greed, Flowers for Her Grave, An Uncluttered Palette,* and books 1 and 2 from the Nic & Nora series: *She Overheard Murder,* and *Puzzled by the Clues.* www.jeansheldonwriter.com

Made in the USA
Monee, IL
04 November 2026

67377060R00266